tween life and death. Learn how to answer all the questions your doctor will put to you—how to comprehend what those answers mean to him and to you. Enter your doctor's examination room—a world of "percussion," "auscultation," "palpation"— where you are pushed, pounded and poked. See why the checkup is such a vital procedure; learn what to expect from your physician: how your personal habits, family and medical history can help him help you; how such clinical tests as electrocardiograms, stress tests, Holter monitors, echocardiograms, barium enemas and other routine and special examinations can send out early warning signals of trouble. Throughout, Dr. Rosenfeld offers advice on how to participate in your checkup— arming you with the understanding of what it's all about.

The anecdotes and true-life experiences sprinkled throughout illuminate the many dilemmas that face the doctor, and will make you realize how shy, intimidated and terrified we, as patients, have been— and why each one of us must take a new approach to our own health. What your doctor knows about you is critical—but what you know is crucial. The new knowledge available in The Complete Medical Exam may very well save your life.

Dr. Rosenfeld, a cardiologist, is Associate Clinical Professor of Medicine at The New York Hospital-Cornell Medical Center. In addition to his private practice and his teaching and research activities, he also serves as consultant to the National Institutes of Health in the areas of arteriosclerosis, high blood pressure and sudden death. He is the co-author of a textbook on cardiology, as well as author of several scientific publications. Dr. Rosenfeld lives in New York City with his wife and four children.

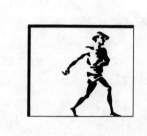

THE COMPLETE MEDICAL EXAM

What Your Doctor Knows Is Critical;
What You Know Is Crucial

by ISADORE ROSENFELD, M.D.

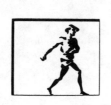

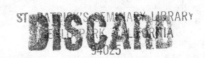
Simon and Schuster / New York

DESIGNED BY IRVING PERKINS
MANUFACTURED IN THE UNITED STATES OF AMERICA

1 2 3 4 5 6 7 8 9 10

LIBRARY OF CONGRESS CATALOGING IN PUBLICATION DATA

ROSENFELD, ISADORE.
THE COMPLETE MEDICAL EXAM.

INCLUDES INDEX.
1. PERIODIC HEALTH EXAMINATIONS. I. TITLE.
RC71.4.R67   616.07'54   78-4837

ISBN 0-671-22844-7

Acknowledgments

I wish to thank my associate, Dr. Michael Wolk, and my friend Mary Lasker for reviewing the manuscript and for their helpful suggestions. Aaron Sussman and Joseph L. Mankiewicz provided invaluable editorial comments. Several of my colleagues read sections dealing with their special areas of interest and expertise and offered important advice:

Dr. William Arnold (Orthopedic Surgery)
Dr. David Becker (Nuclear Medicine)
Dr. Myron Buchman (Gynecology)
Dr. William Cahan (Surgery)
Dr. Eugene Cohen (Endocrinology)
Dr. Lester Coleman and Dr. Wilbur J. Gould (Ear, Nose and Throat)
Dr. Murray Dworetzky (Allergy)
Dr. Mary Allen Engle (Pediatrics)
Dr. Richard Gibbs (Dermatology)
Dr. Richard Imber and Dr. James W. Smith (Plastic Surgery)
Dr. Harvey Klein (Gastroenterology)
Dr. Gerald Klingon (Neurology)
Dr. Russell Lavengood (Urology)
Dr. George Reader (Social Medicine)
Dr. James P. Smith (Pulmonary Diseases)
Dr. Norton Spritz (Internal Medicine)

My friend Jules Bass convinced me I could find the time to write this book despite my other commitments. And finally, special thanks to Alice Ross, who typed and retyped this manuscript countless times, always with skill and patience.

*To my patients—who continue to teach me
everything I know about medicine—
and to Camilla and the children,
Arthur, Stephen, Hildi, and Herbert,
for their love, patience and help.*

CONTENTS

CHAPTER 8   EXAMINING THE UPPER PART OF YOUR BODY   155
*Eyes: what they reveal; seeing spots; testing eye muscles; pupils—
constricted, dilated, irregular; inside-the-eye examination . . . Bad
breath . . . Ears: kinds of deafness . . . Nose . . . Mouth and
tongue: cancer warning . . . Gums . . . Teeth . . . Throat: gag
reflex; vocal cords . . . Cosmetic facial surgery: when it's helpful,
when it's not; face lifts; nose and ear repair; choosing a plastic surgeon
. . . Lymph glands: enlargement . . . Thyroid gland: enlargement
. . . Arteries: pulses; aneurysms; arterial disease in legs . . .
Treatment of vascular problems . . . Varicose veins . . . Phlebitis
. . . Shoulder pain: arthritis; bursitis; tendonitis; as symptom of heart
trouble; frozen shoulder; treatment . . . Elbows . . . Hands: as
diagnostic clues; color of palms; deformities . . . Nails . . . Hand
tremors*

CHAPTER 9   YOUR CHEST   188
*Structure . . . Shape: pigeon breast, barrel chest . . . Breathing
patterns . . . Lung examination: palpation; percussion; use of
stethoscope; bronchitis; asthma; pneumonia . . . Breast examination:
assessing cancer risk; looking for cancer—lumps; drugs that cause
breast enlargement; mammography—benefits and risks; self-
examination . . . Treating breast cancer: surgical procedures; use of
drugs . . . Causes of breast cancer: suspected drugs . . . Cosmetic
breast surgery . . . Heart: structure; function; replacement of heart
valves; how blood circulates; scarred lungs and swollen feet; angina
pectoris and heart attack; development of collaterals; pericarditis . . .
Heart examination: murmurs and other sounds; use of stethoscope;
looking at neck veins*

CHAPTER 10   EXAMINING YOUR ABDOMEN   217
*Location, function of organs . . . Disorders and diseases: hiatus
hernia; gastritis; ulcers—new treatment; diseases of small bowel; of
large bowel—bowel cancers; liver disease—hepatitis; cirrhosis;
gallbladder—stones; cancer of pancreas; spleen—when to remove;
aneurysm of aorta . . . Examination of abdomen: pushing,
percussing, listening . . . Abdominal angina . . . Rectal
examination*

CHAPTER 11   EXAMINATION OF YOUR GENITAL ORGANS   233
*Penis: size, shape; disorders and treatment—venereal diseases; blood in
ejaculate . . . Scrotum, testicles . . . Vasectomy . . . "Morning
erection" . . . Disorders, diseases of scrotum and testes . . . Pelvic*

"THE HEALTH of the people is really the foundation upon which all their happiness and all their powers as a state depend." So spoke Benjamin Disraeli more than a hundred years ago. Unfortunately, few of us appreciate good health, our most important human asset, until we are threatened by disease or restricted by disability.

Dr. Isadore Rosenfeld, a distinguished heart specialist, has written this book to help the average layman learn how to remain healthy and to know what to do when he becomes ill. Much can be done by each of us to prevent illness and to maintain good health. But this requires education and knowledge about how the body functions, what disturbances may occur, how they may be detected, what preventive measures can be taken, and how the physician functions in the prevention and treatment of illnesses.

Dr. Rosenfeld's book meets this need. It is comprehensive in providing practical information about common diseases as well as symptoms. Ranging widely across a panorama of medical and health problems, from a checkup examination to a heart murmur and from a swollen toe to a lump in the breast, it tells the layman simply and clearly what these conditions may mean and what he should do about them. It is a most readable and human account, which provides a better understanding of ways to select, and communicate effectively with, one's doctor, and of the reasons behind and meaning of the diagnostic and therapeutic procedures that the physician uses.

In writing this book, Dr. Rosenfeld has made a valuable contribution to the medical education of the layman and consequently to the improvement of his health.

Michael E. DeBakey, M.D.
Baylor College of Medicine
Houston, Texas

GOOD MEDICAL CARE depends on a partnership. It requires the free flow of information between you and your doctor—in both directions. The purpose of this book is to enhance this relationship. It contains much of the information you need in order to understand what the doctor does to you during an examination—and why. It also examines the reasons and rationale behind the advice he gives you, both when you're healthy and when you're sick.

What your doctor knows is very important to you. How much *you* know is crucial. An accurate medical diagnosis depends to a great extent on how *you* assess your symptoms and describe them to the physician. Successful treatment often requires that you follow instructions carefully, patiently, sometimes for long periods of time, and not without expense or inconvenience. That requires motivation. The best-informed patient is the one most likely to do what is good for him.

Here you will find the description, explanation, and significance of the most common complaints that bring people to the doctor—as well as a list of those that don't—but should. You will also have a chance to ask yourself the same questions your doctor does—and learn *why* he poses them and what your answers mean.

If you're well and seeing your doctor only for a checkup, as you read these pages you will participate in a step-by-step account of the actual physical exam he performs, and will understand what he is looking for. You will find a description of and reasons for the different tests he may want to do before he can give you a "clean bill of health."

I have concentrated on the common and important medical problems you may encounter in your lifetime—not the rare or esoteric ones that afflict the few. Reading this book will not make a doctor out of you—just a better patient. It is not meant to substitute for a visit to your own physician, but rather to help you determine if and when you need to see him. When you do, the knowledge you bring with you will help you both.

CHAPTER 1

ASK, ESPECIALLY IF YOU
DON'T UNDERSTAND

I HAVE ASSUMED you know nothing about medicine—like the young woman whose neck I was examining for enlarged glands, a routine procedure to detect leukemia, infection, cancer or the common cold. As I felt both sides of her jaw I asked her, out of curiosity, "Do you know why I'm doing this?" "Yes," she replied with a sweet smile. "Because you like me." But even if you are medically sophisticated, I hope you will find much that is new and important to you in these pages.

Most of us are anxious and worried when we visit the doctor. We don't understand what he is doing to us and why—and we're afraid of what he may discover. But we go again and again (six hundred and fifty million times a year in the U. S. alone)—to our own doctor, to hospital clinics or to various medical meccas like the Mayo or Lahey clinics. Even when we're feeling well, we're sent for a "checkup" by our wife or husband, our boss, our union, a friend. And what happens when we get there? We're asked all kinds of personal questions. We're pushed, pounded and pricked. We even obligingly bend for a stranger poking around some perfectly private part of our body. We're x-rayed. Then we're hooked up to a stationary bicycle or treadmill and forced to pedal or run—going nowhere—until we're exhausted. Finally, after they ask us to fill a bottle for them (usually when we've just finished doing it elsewhere), when they have removed what seems like altogether too much blood (not always on the first attempt either) and made us promise to bring an unspecified amount of stool, they're just about through with us—except, of course, for the insurance forms and the bill, which amounts to a small fortune.

A Welcome Invasion

Why do you and I (yes, doctors go too) submit to this uncomfortable, humiliating and expensive invasion of our physical and emotional privacy? Because even though we may feel perfectly well, we want to be sure and need to be told we really are healthy. And if we're not, we hope it's early enough so that whatever is wrong can still be treated or cured.

One would think, since the stakes are so high and involve your health and perhaps even your life, that you'd query the rationale of all the things being done to you. Is it enough? Is it too much? Is it being done right? Why all the questions? Why all the tests?

We rarely ask. We react to the medical exam much as we do to flying. When we board an airliner, we glance into the cockpit, are overwhelmed by the complicated controls and wonder for a moment. Then we shrug our shoulders, sit down, fasten the seat belt, and hope for the best.

Just think. How many times, as you stuck out your tongue, drank barium for the stomach x-ray, or ran up and down steps for your exercise electrocardiogram, did you ask what it was all about? Don't you quiz the mechanic more about your car than you do your doctor about yourself?

"I went for a checkup yesterday." "Anything wrong?" "Yes, I

have a 'condition.' " "That's too bad. What are you doing for it?" "Oh, I was given a pill to take three times a day." "What's it called?" "I don't really know. It's blue and white."

Maybe it's because you're shy or intimidated by the whole medical atmosphere—the cold, gleaming, forbidding equipment and the promise of its impending involvement with you, the antiseptic smell, the white coats. Perhaps you grew up in awe of doctors, believing everything they did was necessary and right—and no questions asked. It may also be because you're afraid to ask— "What I don't know won't hurt me." Whatever the reason, you convince yourself it's none of your business, that asking might offend the doctor, that you wouldn't understand his answer anyway, and besides which, he is much too busy to be bothered by your naïve questions.

CHAPTER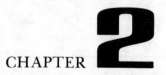

BEFORE READING ANY FURTHER

QUESTIONS YOU SHOULD ASK YOURSELF

Most of us see the doctor either when we're obviously sick or when we're frankly well—for a checkup. (More about that later.) But there are also those symptoms you may not think are important and so you tolerate them and do nothing about them. You may have rationalized them away as the kind of thing that probably happens to everyone "at a certain age." Yet these are often warning signs which, if heeded in time, may make the difference to you between life and death.

How can you recognize these early danger signals? Don't depend on self-examination (except for the breasts). That's your doctor's job. But you should ask yourself the same questions that he will during a checkup; these are the questions on which most medical diagnoses are based.

Following are some of the most important ones. *Why they're asked and what they mean are described in detail in the pages that follow.* As you will see later, your doctor will pose many more—about your personal habits, family history and past medical illnesses. But a "yes" answer to any of the following *key* questions below means you should see your doctor *now* There is a greater urgency about some than others; but each of these symptoms demands an explanation.

1. Do you usually feel very cold (or hot) when everyone else is quite comfortable?
2. Have you recently developed a persistent and unexplained ache or pain in some part of your body?
3. Has your hat, glove or shoe size been increasing gradually?
4. Have you noticed a persistent rash or itching anywhere?
5. Has the pitch of your voice dropped noticeably?
6. Have you become persistently hoarse?
7. Has your hair begun to fall out?
8. Have you recently begun to feel "old" and tired for no apparent reason?
9. Has sexual appetite or performance become so poor that your relationships are threatened?
10. Have your monthly menstrual periods suddenly changed in character?
11. Has someone in your household recently come down with TB, hepatitis or some other contagious disease?
12. Have you noticed a hard "cold sore," which cleared up all by itself, after a casual sexual encounter?
13. Have you recently returned from a trip with "travelers' diarrhea" that has lasted for weeks?
14. Do you get a "Charley horse" or cramp in the calf of your leg(s) when you walk or run?
15. Do you drink "moderately," or only when you "have to," but noticed that your breasts (you're a man) are getting bigger?
16. Have you noticed that instead of shaving once or twice a

day, as you used to, you can now get away with a shave every second or third day?

17. Have you been following some weight reduction program and noted that even after going back to your usual eating habits you're still losing weight?

18. Are you over 45 and have just started a vigorous jogging or exercise program without first seeing your doctor?

19. Have you been getting hormone shots for your potency somewhere "downtown" because your own doctor won't give them to you?

20. Have you been taking female hormones for more than six months because of "hot flushes" and not been examined?

21. Are you recently always very tired, especially in the morning, even after a good night's sleep?

22. Has your stool become jet black?

23. Are you a heavy cigarette smoker and have you developed a chronic "smoker's cough"?

24. Have you noticed blood in your sputum?

25. Do you have some heart condition that required digitalis and do you find your appetite has become very poor and that you're losing weight?

26. Have you noticed mucus and/or red blood on your stool or on the toilet tissue?

27. Are you gaining weight and feeling sluggish despite the fact that you're actually cutting down on your food intake?

28. Have you been taking blood thinners (anticoagulants) for many months without a blood test?

29. Have you been taking "water pills" (diuretics) on a regular basis to help you reduce or get rid of excess fluid in your system?

30. Are you taking your chances with an unwanted pregnancy because you've heard about the dangers and side effects of the "pill"?

31. Are you over 40 years of age and still taking the "pill"?

32. Have you noticed that your stool has become very light (the color of clay) and that your appetite is off?

33. Do you have vaginal bleeding after intercourse?

34. Do you stain between periods?
35. Have you developed a persistent headache in the past few weeks?
36. Has your nose begun to bleed frequently for no apparent reason?
37. Have you begun to faint or suffer from severe dizzy spells?
38. Do you get palpitations or rapid heartbeats?
39. Have you recently developed noises or buzzing in your head?
40. Do you see double from time to time?
41. Does chewing your food make you tired?
42. Do you have trouble swallowing solid food?
43. Are you short of breath when climbing one or two flights of stairs?
44. Do you have difficulty breathing when you lie flat?
45. Do you get a heaviness or pressure in the chest when you rush, walk uphill in windy weather, or become excited?
46. Do you have discomfort in the chest when you exert yourself, which is relieved by belching?
47. Do you almost always have pain in your stomach after eating?
48. Are you always uncomfortable and bloated one to two hours after eating?
49. Does food ever get stuck when you swallow?
50. Are you losing weight for no apparent reason?
51. Have you felt any lumps in your breasts?
52. Do you have to get up more than twice at night to empty your bladder even when you've not had alcohol at dinner?
53. Does it burn or feel hot when you urinate?
54. If you're a man, have you noticed that your urinary stream is frequently split?
55. Do you have vaginal itching that won't go away?
56. Have you become very thirsty recently?
57. Is there blood in your urine?
58. Do your feet and ankles swell?
59. Does your temperature during the day regularly exceed 99.5F (37.5C) by mouth?

60. Is your pulse rate always below 50 per minute?
61. Is your pulse irregular? (Do you often experience some skipped beats?)
62. Has your skin changed in quality or color?
63. Have you noticed any blue-black warts or moles?
64. Have your eyes begun to bulge?
65. Does your tongue have hard white plaques on it?
66. Do you have swollen glands anywhere that don't go away?
67. Are your palms discolored?
68. Is your urine the color of tea or mahogany?
69. Have your hands begun to shake or tremble?
70. Do you wheeze at night?
71. Do you have a discharge from your nipples?
72. Has your stool become narrow or ribbonlike?
73. Have you noticed blood in your ejaculate?
74. Do you lose some urine when you cough or sneeze?
75. Have you tried to have a child without success?
76. Have you suddenly developed a bad back?
77. Do you have pain going down the back of your leg?
78. Do you have numbness or tingling of your fingers?
79. Do your joints swell and hurt?
80. Have you recently begun to bruise easily?

QUESTIONS YOU WOULD LIKE TO ASK THE DOCTOR BUT OFTEN DON'T

In addition to the questions listed above, I have found the following subjects perplexing to many of my patients and have also answered them throughout this book.

Is it a good idea for me to go somewhere like the Mayo Clinic for a *real* checkup?

My "clean bill of health" is good news. But how come Uncle Jack passed his complete checkup last month, was told he was "in perfect shape," stepped outside his doctor's office and dropped dead?

C'mon, Doc, what's my sex life got to do with this checkup?

I have a good bowel movement every morning. Is it really necessary to have a rectal examination today?

Doctor, do you mean to tell me you actually plan to get all of that ten-inch sigmoidoscope in—me?

What kind of medical clearance do I need before I start a jogging program?

What's the best way for me to examine my breasts? Why do I need a mammogram if you found them O.K.? How often should I have it done? Can too many mammograms cause cancer?

You're a vampire. Why are you taking so much blood?

Is my cholesterol high? Should I have a triglyceride test too? Can a high cholesterol actually protect me against heart disease?

If my blood-sugar test is normal, why do I need to sit here four hours more for a sugar-tolerance test?

Are you suggesting I have a positive test for syphilis? That's impossible. I'm a virgin.

How can my blood pressure be high? I feel so well. Do I need medicines? Do they make me impotent?

You tell me my electrocardiogram is normal, even though I have heart disease. How is that possible?

My prostate is too big and has to be removed. Will I be impotent after the operation?

CHAPTER **3**

LET'S SUPPOSE YOU'RE HEALTHY—
WHY YOU NEED A CHECKUP

THE CLOSER A DOCTOR IS to his medical-school and internship days the more he prefers treating the sick to examining the "healthy." Medical students, interns and residents consider the routine checkup a chore, not an intellectual challenge—the same old thing over and over again. They would much rather deal with uncommon, exotic or exciting problems than with people who are apparently well. "I had a great day today—two strangulated hernias, one mysterious fever and three hemorrhages." But as the doctor matures and his experience increases, his priorities change. The attraction of and preference for emergency "last resort" medicine dwindles, and he comes to realize that it is at least as rewarding to maintain health—or to find and treat disease as early as possible. It's better to give the polio vaccine than to use the iron lung.

There are three main reasons why you should have a checkup even if you're feeling well.

(1) *To detect unrecognized disease.* Each year, in the course of routine examinations, millions of persons are found to have previously unsuspected illness. The more important disorders detected and subsequently treated include 600,000 new cases of diabetes mellitus (sugar trouble), gout (not necessarily a rich man's affliction), silent heart disease (masquerading as "indigestion"), cancer (more and more of it found early enough to be controlled or cured), tuberculosis (by no means wiped out), and high blood pressure (where early therapy will prolong and save life).

(2) *To establish an ongoing doctor-patient relationship* in which you can be advised about a healthy life-style. If you begin to drift toward trouble, the trend can be detected and reversed. Even if no disease is found, your normal baseline is established. No two persons are exactly alike in any respect and no given patient, as he grows older, stays the same. Appearance, weight, bodily function, the electrocardiogram, blood tests, all change over the years. The objective differences between "health" and "disease" are sometimes very subtle. For example, certain minor variations in your electrocardiogram are usually of no significance. But if not present in previous tracings, they may indicate early trouble. Or, suppose that year after year your blood pressure has been running around 110/76, a nice, low-normal value. Suddenly it's 148/86, still really normal, but higher—a warning that it has to be watched carefully, and at more frequent intervals. And so it is for your weight, the size of your heart, cholesterol level and many other indices. Recording these values over the years establishes a trend in your health status—permitting intervention at the earliest time.

(3) *Reassurance*—the peace of mind which cannot be measured in dollars or cost effectiveness. You may have lingering anxiety about your health because your father and uncles died of heart attacks in their 40's, or your mother and most of her sisters had cancer. It's very comforting to be told every now and then that you're all right.

What the Checkup Involves

The kind of checkup you get is not normally up to you. What tests are performed (and how reliably) will depend on where they're done, as well as on the philosophy, experience, facilities and training of your doctor. For example, at the Lahey Clinic in Boston, a 45-year-old woman in apparently good health, coming for a complete evaluation, would routinely have the following done:

1. a detailed history
2. thorough physical examination
3. analysis of the urine and stool
4. Pap test (for cancer of the cervix)
5. chest x-ray
6. sigmoidoscopy (looking up the lower bowel with an illuminated instrument)
7. tests for visual acuity and eyeball pressure (to rule out glaucoma, an important cause of blindness)
8. an electrocardiogram taken while you lie quietly (stress testing is not routine)
9. several blood tests

How Long and How Much?

All this takes approximately three days, and in 1978 costs between $300 and $400, excluding expenses for travel and lodging. You would not usually be hospitalized. Many other clinics perform checkups of similar scope. Various corporations and unions also provide basic diagnostic health packages at the industrial facility.

These centers do not usually treat the diseases they discover unless you want them to. They pride themselves on not interfering with the traditional "doctor-patient" relationship. The results are forwarded to your physician. He is either equipped to perform virtually all of these tests or has the necessary facilities available to him. He also has the advantage, because he has known you over the years, of being able to appreciate subtle changes and trends better than any machine or laboratory test.

So going to a big center is not necessary unless you have some problem or symptom that cannot be managed closer to home.

Checkups for Whom?

Who should have a regular health maintenance examination, and at what intervals? Opinions differ sharply. Some doctors believe you can't have them often enough. Others think that as long as you're feeling well, don't look for trouble. The National Institutes of Health and the Mayo Clinic suggest two checkups between ages 18 and 30, three between 41 and 50, five from 51 to 60 and an annual exam after age 60. Here are my recommendations for these age groups.

Early in Life

Parents routinely take their children to the pediatrician primarily for advice on infant feeding, immunizations, growth measurements, and to have the doctor fill out school or summer camp forms. These visits are sometimes brief, squirming and noisy affairs where subtle disease may not be detected. So I recommend a thorough physical exam once in adolescence—to detect malignancies (especially if other children in the family have died of cancer), chronic low-grade infections (many youngsters have worms, anemia and lingering diseases of which the parents may not be aware), heart murmurs (which may have been missed at birth), high blood pressure (as many as 5 percent of "normal" children have hypertension), hernias, visual and hearing defects, and other unrecognized handicapping conditions. Most of these can be treated. Many children who do poorly in school or are thought to be emotionally disturbed are in reality sick or disabled.

Some youngsters should be more frequently examined for specific abnormalities. For example, if a parent, grandparent, brother, sister or even aunt or uncle has *diabetes mellitus,* a disease which runs in families, analyses of blood and urine for sugar content should be done at regular intervals. A normal test is no guarantee for the future, since this disorder may appear at any time.

Preventing Sudden Death

If there is a history of *sudden death* in the family, especially among the younger members, an inherited heart disorder may be responsible. Fatal collapse in children is not rare. It may be due to an abnormality in the cardiac electrical system or to certain deformities in the structure of the heart that were present at birth. Some of these life-threatening conditions can be treated— with medication, pacemakers or surgery. I know of one case, a boy of 19 who died suddenly during a tennis match. Autopsy examination showed he had a certain abnormality of the heart muscle, which runs in families. It can be detected by new x-ray and sonar techniques (echocardiography) and cardiac catheterization (threading a thin tube up the blood vessels and into the heart). We therefore examined this boy's four siblings, all of whom seemed to be in good health. Three did, indeed, prove to be normal, but one brother was found to have the same potentially fatal disease. He had no complaints whatsoever, never felt better in his life—but so had the youngster who died during the tennis game. As a result of our findings, we advised the boy to avoid strenuous exertion. In addition, and more important, we gave him a medication which we expect will greatly reduce the risk of his dying suddenly. This particular medication is more effective than open-heart surgery. Other inherited disorders that render one vulnerable to sudden death can be diagnosed just from the electrocardiogram, and protection is virtually complete with currently available medicine. So if there is a history of sudden death in the family, a thorough examination can be lifesaving.

Tuberculosis (TB) is very contagious and is transmitted easily from one member of a household to another. Sometimes the infection is not suspected because the symptoms are very mild and resemble a cold. Any child living in an environment with old or recent TB infection must be examined and skin-tested. The TB skin test involves injecting a tiny amount of a derivative of the killed organism. Anyone who has had the infection, even if it was mild and unrecognized, will have a positive reaction to the test—

the injected area will become red. It is necessary to follow up a positive reaction with a chest x-ray.

Adult Life

If you were a healthy child and adolescent, and have a good family history, a routine examination should ideally be performed every five years between the *ages of 21 to 35*. However, women in this age group must continue to see the gynecologist every year to make sure they don't have cancer of the breast and cervix.

Between the *ages of 35 and 42*, I suggest an exam every three years to detect the onset of heart disease, hypertension and cancer. In women who do not have high blood pressure or diabetes, such examinations need not include a special search for arteriosclerosis, which generally becomes apparent after the menopause.

Between *ages 42 and 50*, I advise a routine physical every two years for everyone.

At *50 years, and through age 60*, the checkup for both men and women should become an annual affair. After that, a shorter, more targeted evaluation should be performed six months after the annual one. Its purpose is the early detection of those diseases which begin to take their toll in this age group. These include high blood pressure, arteriosclerosis, cancer, diabetes mellitus, gout, emphysema and chronic bronchitis, arthritis, and behavioral changes, especially depression.

Where Should You Get Your Checkup?

This depends on your geographic locality, the facilities and motivation of your own doctor and what you can afford. If your doctor has a busy general practice devoted to treating the sick, sees fifty or more patients a day and spends only five or ten minutes with each, he probably does not have the time to give you a thorough checkup. A cursory "non-examination" masquerading as the real thing is worse than none, because it gives a false sense of security.

A Half Hour Is Not Enough

Plan your checkup with your own doctor. Ask him where you should have it done, what it will consist of, and how much it will cost. Most physicians have the training and the facilities to perform the majority of the tests themselves and can arrange for the rest to be done by a colleague, a clinic or a hospital nearby. Find out how much time it will take. If you're told you'll be through in less than half an hour, that's not enough to get the examination you need. It requires at least one half to one hour exclusive of any special x-rays or ECG stress testing. Try to avoid an appointment very late in the afternoon. That's when your doctor is at his lowest peak of efficiency after a long, hard day. Monday mornings may also be bad, because he is apt to be distracted by the calls and messages that have accumulated over the weekend.

Beware the Superspecialist

Be careful about going to a superspecialist for your general checkup unless he is interested and routinely does them. If your doctor is primarily a gastroenterologist (stomach), a cardiologist (heart), an endocrinologist (glands), or a rheumatologist (joints) he may so emphasize his own specialty because of his interest and expertise in it that some other areas of your body are neglected. Make certain that he will send you wherever necessary to complete what he can't do adequately himself.

If your own doctor can and will perform this kind of examination, then it is not necessary for you to go to a famous diagnostic clinic. If, however, he cannot arrange it, don't compromise. Go wherever you must to get a complete study. But remember, there is no virtue in distance. So many patients live in a community with excellent medical facilities, yet travel hundreds and even thousands of miles because they believe that "somewhere else" must be better.

Like Choosing a Wife or Husband

I feel very strongly about the importance of the doctor-patient relationship. You should be almost as careful about selecting your personal physician as you are about choosing your spouse. You will turn to him in sickness and in health, in crises and in terminal illness. Imagine spending your last days on earth looking at the face of someone you dislike, or fear, or in whom you have no confidence. And how awful to have to confide your embarrassing personal problems to some cold, disinterested fish. By the same token, whether or not your doctor likes you will have a bearing on the kind of medical care you get. It's often said that most doctors do not become emotionally involved with their patients' problems. That's not true. It's unavoidable. What's more, unless they are involved, you won't get the best care. Treating the sick is not only a matter of drugs and machines, but of warmth, concern and compassion.

Always Ask First How Much It Will Cost

If your doctor charges more than you can afford, ask him where it can be done within your budget. Such facilities are to be found. Always ask whether your insurance policies will pay for any part of the cost; remember, however, that most individual contracts cover treatment of illness but not medical checkups. If, after a complete workup, your doctor finds you fit and answers the question "Diagnosis" on the insurance form with "No disease," you will probably not be reimbursed by the carrier. So if any abnormality is found in the course of the examination, no matter how trivial, remind your doctor to indicate it on the claim form. You may then be at least partially reimbursed.

CHAPTER **4**

WHAT NOT TO DO BEFORE
SEEING THE DOCTOR

AFTER YOU'VE MADE the appointment for your checkup, don't try to whip yourself into shape during the next few days to help you "pass the test." That defeats the purpose. It may present a false picture of your health habits and status. I have asked patients, "How much do you exercise?" only to be told "I walk four miles a day, swim 10 lengths and do 15 push-ups every morning." "Very good. How long have you been doing it?" "For the past week."

Hazards of a Crash Diet

Don't embark on a crash diet seven or eight days before your visit because you're ashamed of being fat. Sudden changes in biological life-style are usually undesirable anyway, and may also confuse the results. For example, if you go on a "starvation diet," avoiding all sugar and carbohydrates for several days, you may

34

so distort your tests as to make you appear diabetic. You will see later how that can happen.

From a Dead Stop to Sudden Death

If you are middle-aged and have been living a chair-bound, sedentary life (no walking, no exercise, elevators even to the mezzanine), and then, without having been previously examined to see whether your heart can take it, you suddenly decide to jog to become physically fit, you may have a heart attack or even die suddenly. It happens this way: Supposing your coronaries (the arteries that supply the heart muscle with blood and keep it pumping) are only modestly narrowed by arteriosclerosis ("hardening of the arteries"). They can still deliver enough oxygen to your heart so that you can carry on normally—work, walk, make love—all without any symptoms. Since you're not very "physical," your circulation is rarely called upon to handle a sudden, excessive energy demand. Then one day, instead of getting to your desk job by bus, you decide to jog—too fast and for too long. Your narrowed arteries are not able to deliver the greater volume of blood suddenly required, and the heart muscle is deprived of oxygen. This "insufficiency," as you will read later, may give you transient chest pain, a heart attack—or even kill you. And that's the reason no reputable gym or physical rehabilitation center will enroll you in an exercise program if you're over 40 years of age, until you have clearance from your doctor. What such clearance consists of is discussed in a later chapter.

"Don't Stop Smoking"

Don't kid yourself into believing that a few days before the examination you can break the cigarette habit. The chances are you're not going to be able to do it that quickly, and your resolve will probably last only until you "pass" the checkup. Then you'll make the same old excuses: "After all, how bad can my smoking be if the doctor found me in good shape?" So it's back to a pack a day until next year, and the next checkup—unless, of course, in the meantime, you get your lung cancer or heart attack. Continue to smoke your cigarettes right up to the day of the examination, so you can be shown the effect they have on your electrocardiogram, your lung function, and your exercise capacity. Ask the doctor to take your ECG before and during inhalation of some cigarette smoke, and then look at both tracings. You may see changes whose significance he can explain to you. Also ask him to put up side by side your chest x-ray and that of a nonsmoker. A picture is worth a thousand words. It may have a much greater impact on you than a thousand slogans. Finally, ask for "pulmonary function tests" to see how well your lungs are working, and compare your results with those of a nonsmoker. If that doesn't get you to stop, nothing will.

These are just some of the preparations you should *not* make before seeing the doctor. There are others. For example, don't douche before leaving home on your way to the gynecologist. This will just wash away the discharge he needs to analyze. Don't see your hairdresser just a few days before your medical exam. Hair color and texture are important clues in medical diagnosis. In short, don't do anything that distorts the actual you.

CHAPTER **5**

FIRST IMPRESSIONS

THE MEDICAL EVALUATION may start even before the doctor sees you, since his nurse or receptionist will report any peculiar mannerisms or behavior while you're still in the waiting room. One day, my secretary buzzed to tell me that a new patient had arrived early, taken off her coat, stretched out on the couch, and fallen asleep in the reception area. The other patients, some of whom now had to stand, were surprised and amused. A few minutes later the woman was gently nudged awake and shown to my consulting room where I awaited her with several possible diagnoses: (a) she was working too hard and was simply overtired; (b) she was an alcoholic and had been on a binge the night before; (c) she had chronic pulmonary trouble (the diseased lung does not blow out all the "used" air, whose chemicals then accumulate in the blood and cause drowsiness); (d) she was on drugs or sedatives; (e) she was an epileptic or had some other kind of brain disorder; (f) her thyroid function was low; (g) she had some emotional problems; or (h) she simply had one hell of a nerve. This particular lady turned out to have a sluggish thyroid. But I was prepared with at least seven other possible diagnoses even before seeing her.

Occasionally, you may form an impression of the doctor before seeing him. A local comedian, who thinks he is better known than he is, was leaving my office one rainy day. There was one other patient in the waiting room, and she didn't recognize him. He just couldn't believe it. He stared at her, ogled her—to no avail. He was determined she would never forget him. He put one of his rain boots on his head, slipped into his coat wrong way round so that the buttons were down the back, and hung his umbrella around his neck. As he opened the door to leave, he turned to the startled lady and said, "Madam, you are about to see a great doctor. I'm sure he will help you too," and with that he left.

Time Is Money

Very few patients sleep in the waiting room. They usually sit quietly, glancing at their watches, leafing through an old *National Geographic* magazine, or trying to diagnose what's wrong with the other people in the reception room. If you're kept waiting too long, your anxiety and irritability rise together. One of my friends, an eye specialist, tells the story of how he "unavoidably" kept a young woman waiting some two and a half hours beyond her scheduled appointment time. The eye examination, when he finally got around to it, took only ten minutes. A few days later, she received his bill, which she returned with a letter saying in effect, "Your time is worth $50.00 an hour. You spent ten minutes examining me. My time is worth only $8.00 an hour, but you wasted 2½ hours of it in your reception room. Please remit $10.00." And then she added a P.S.: "But I am grateful. After you kept me waiting for so long, you did rush me through the examination."

What You Reveal at First Glance

When I greet you in my consulting room, certain aspects of your personality and health status may become apparent. Take the handshake, for example. There is a certain type of patient who wants to let me know at the very outset that he is seeing me under protest. Someone has made him go for the checkup. In fact, he's sure he enjoys better health than do I. He makes his point in the handshake, squeezing mine so hard as to leave it aching for the rest of the afternoon.

Ordinarily, I note whether your handshake is firm and you look me directly in the eye. If your palms are hot, tremulous, and moist, I will be alerted to the possibility of an overactive thyroid. If they are dry and cold, and the skin is rough, I will suspect an underfunctioning thyroid gland. I also note whether your hand trembles, as in certain brain diseases or chronic alcoholism. Finally, I may detect the hallmark of the anxious, nervous person—the cold, damp, and shaky hand.

Importance of the Trained Observer

The way you walk into the room is also revealing. Walking and standing are very complicated mechanisms which depend on the normal transmission and interpretation of nerve impulses going to and from the brain. In order for you not to fall over, or to walk normally, your feet must signal their position to the brain, which then controls their movement. In certain diseases, for example, pernicious anemia (a serious disorder which can be cured by injections of vitamin B_{12}), these nerve pathways are damaged. Such patients have a broad-based walk and their feet slap the ground to ensure stability. Someone with Parkinson's disease (a brain disorder usually found in older persons) has a characteristic gait. He moves with short steps, and his trunk is bent forward, as if he were chasing his own center of gravity. After a stroke, the affected leg may be dragged almost in a semicircle while the good one moves straight forward. Then there are the arthritics, crippled with hip and spine disease, and persons who have been hurt in various accidents or paralyzed with polio. Depending on the disease or injury, they may waddle, limp, or shuffle. Your gait tells me a great deal about you and may indicate disease of the brain, blood, bones, muscles, eyes, ears, and nerves—not to mention the alcoholic content of the blood.

Sizing Each Other Up

Now you sit down, and we appraise each other. The chemistry we develop is what the "doctor-patient relationship" is all about. In addition, some very important diagnostic clues may become apparent to me in that first little while and determine the emphasis of the examination to follow. You are being cheated if you are whisked from the waiting room directly onto an examining table, without being given the chance to tell your whole story to the doctor. The late Dr. Paul Dudley White, one of the world's great heart specialists, used to say that he knew just from talking with his patients whether or not they had heart disease—before examining them or taking an ECG. So be wary of checkups done only by computers or those in which you answer "yes-no" questions on printed forms which are then processed by a machine or a clerk.

Your assessment of me—am I arrogant and officious, or friendly and concerned—is important in determining the success or failure of our whole future relationship. The "vibes" I transmit and how you receive them will decide whether you will be candid, hostile, or evasive in answering my questions. ("What's the use of telling him my troubles? He couldn't care less.")

Attitudes and Reactions

As we begin to chat, I will also evaluate you in some important ways. Are you sad, anxious, suspicious, open, secretive, tired, alert, unduly animated, bored—or sick? These attitudes, personality characteristics, behavior patterns, and appearance all have an important bearing on, and indeed may be caused by, disease. For example, an overactive thyroid may make you fidgety; an unrecognized stroke may result in your speaking slowly or haltingly or saying the wrong word even though you know the right one.

I then look more closely at your appearance. Is your face florid and are your eyes bleary because you are an alcoholic? Have you lost a lot of weight? If you've had a stroke, your face may become distorted, your mouth may droop, and one eye may appear wider than the other. A similar appearance—sudden paralysis of one side of your face and one eye—can be caused, not by a stroke, but by *Bell's palsy*, an inflammation that affects the facial nerve. While a stroke is life-threatening, Bell's palsy usually only results in an unfortunate cosmetic effect and most cases clear up completely—as do many strokes. How can I distinguish between the benign Bell's palsy and a potentially dangerous stroke? If you are able to frown, it's probably a stroke. If you can't it's likely to be Bell's palsy. The reasons for this difference are complicated, but the observation itself is a simple one.

An early sign of *myasthenia gravis* (a disorder of nerve and muscle function) is drooping of one or both eyelids. This may be followed by weakness of other muscles, the tongue, and swallowing mechanisms.

"What a Tan"

There is a mistaken popular belief that to be pale is to be sick. How often have you heard the expression, "He looks terrible— he has no color." I have seen patients virtually at death's door with good color, while others in the bloom of health are pale. That's because complexion is largely determined by the amount of natural pigment in the skin, an individual characteristic.

Whether your skin pallor is due to anemia will, of course, soon be determined by a blood test. But I suspect it is, if your lips and tongue are also pale, the palms of your hands are white, and the inside of the lower eyelid (conjunctiva) has lost its red or pink color. In any event, the important thing is that looking pale is not necessarily significant. In fact, the opposite may well be the case. A ruddy appearance may indicate chronic alcoholism, liver disease, high blood pressure, or a serious disorder in which there are too many red blood cells so that the blood becomes thick (*polycythemia vera*). But just having an outdoor job, like the "Marlboro man" does, may confer a weather-beaten, rugged look in the absence of any disease.

Diagnosis at a Glance

A good doctor is a biological detective, using every clue that nature provides. Your appearance, complexion, and expression permit me to make a wide variety of diagnoses, virtually at a glance. For example, the way you breathe is revealing. Someone with advanced heart disease really has to work at breathing, puffing in short gasps. The asthmatic serenades me with a musical wheeze. The neurotic, anxious patient sits there sighing, or breathing rapidly and deeply but never able to take a deep enough breath—a nervous habit called hyperventilation. I can predict then and there that he will complain of dizziness, light-headedness and numbness and tingling of the hands and feet. These symptoms, as you will see later, may be due to the change in body gases produced by this type of breathing.

Do Old Friends Recognize You?

A disease may change your appearance so gradually over the years that neither you nor your family are aware of it. It may, however, be apparent to me the moment I first look at you. I was asked to examine a man before some minor surgery. As we chatted, I noted his head was unusually large, his jaw abnormally prominent, and his front teeth widely spaced. The tongue and nose were very big too, and his hands were thick. In short, he had the appearance of an *acromegalic*, due to a tumor in the pituitary, or "master gland," in the brain where growth hormone is produced. When healthy, this gland manufactures enough hormone for normal growth and development, and no more. The tumor, however, makes too much, so that over the years there is an insidious, gradual change in appearance as the bones get bigger and the tissue mass increases. In this particular instance, neither the man nor his wife was aware of his altered looks. Only when I specifically asked him did he realize that over the years his hat and shoe size had increased and that he was wearing bigger gloves. Friends he hadn't seen for years no longer recognized him.

The Interview

You may offer some interesting clues even in the "small talk" that precedes the targeted questions later in the history-taking. For example, the thermostat in my office is set at about 72°–74°. Most normal people are comfortable at this temperature. The first suggestion that your metabolism may be out of kilter could come from a simple statement like "How can you work in here doctor? It's so cold." Feeling cold when everyone around you is comfortable may be a subtle but important sign of underfunction of the thyroid gland (*hypothyroidism*). Medical texts describe patients with hypothyroidism as having a pudgy face, yellow-tinted and dry skin, swollen extremities, hoarse voice, slow speech, falling hair, low blood pressure, and slow pulse—and always complaining of constipation. But these are the full-blown signs of advanced disease. Any doctor and most patients can diagnose it at that stage. But the world is full of people who suffer from mild underfunction of the thyroid gland and don't know it. Their symptoms are fatigue (who isn't tired from time to time?), a decrease in the sexual appetite (who doesn't have that now and then?), and constant cold intolerance.

Alternatively, instead of complaining of the cold, you may ask, "Do you mind if I take off my tie (or undo my jacket)? It's so terribly warm in here." This alerts me to several diagnostic possibilities. It may mean that you are nervous or anxious about your examination; it may reflect overactivity of the thyroid gland, a low-grade fever, or evidence of the menopause, when women experience sudden attacks of heat, flushing, and sweats. In any event, feeling too warm or too cold when everyone else is comfortable is an important clue to be followed up carefully.

CHAPTER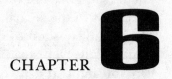

WHY ALL THE QUESTIONS?

I NOW ASK YOU specific questions calculated to uncover symptoms of which you may be unaware or which frighten you—so you don't volunteer them. How you answer will help me focus on "where the action is" in the rest of the examination. Every question has a specific purpose. Table 1 indicates how the history-taking is usually organized.

Table 1. Important Questions in the History-Taking

(1) *Age*   (2) *Occupation*   (3) *Marital Status*
(4) *Family Origin*   (5) *Recent Travels*
(6) *Family History*

—Stroke	—Diabetes mellitus
—High blood pressure	—Cancer
—Premature heart attacks	—Mental disorders
—High cholesterol and triglyceride	—Tuberculosis
	—Allergic diseases

(7) *Personal History and Habits*
    —Smoking
    —Drugs
    —Alcohol
    —Coffee and tea
    —Diet
    —Sleep
    —Exercise
    —Sex life
    —Fatigue
(8) *Medications*
    —Vitamins
    —Aspirin
    —Blood pressure pills
    —Cortisone
    —Cough medicine
    —Digitalis
    —Hormones
    —Iron
    —Laxatives
    —Thyroid pills
    —Tranquilizers
    —Appetite suppressants

    —Blood thinners
    —Water pills
    —Birth-control pills
    —Narcotics
    —Sleeping pills
(9) *Allergic History*
(10) *Past Health*
    —Diseases of childhood
    —Operations
    —Hospitalizations
(11) *Function of Body Systems*

How Old Are You?

Most patients admit their age to the doctor without any fuss. Others hesitate or give themselves the benefit of a few years, and some even insist they don't know how old they are. This latter situation has something to do with being born in a foreign country of illiterate parents ("In those days they didn't keep records," "The church burned down and so did my birth certificate," and finally, "I was born under a different calendar.") Whatever the reason, these people invariably look older than the stated age. Other patients will tell me how old they are, but not before they stall and play a little game. "Do you really have to know? Guess." I never do guess anymore because what these people are looking for is a compliment—not an honest answer. I once told a woman who asked me that I thought she was 56 years old. She turned out to be only 50, and countered my "insult" by looking at a photograph of my 13-year-old son and saying, "Doctor, I didn't know you had grandchildren."

I also try to avoid another kind of age estimate, this one more subtle. When a man and woman come in to see me together, I do not take their relationship for granted. For example, I never say, "Mr Smith, I want you and your daughter to know . . ." Invariably, she turns out to be his wife.

Whether or not I confide it to you, I do make a judgment as to whether you look older or younger than your age. Premature aging does not necessarily mean physical disease. It may be something that runs in your family or the result of chronic stress—personal, occupational, social, or economic—the toll of a tough, sad life. I also allow for wrinkling of the skin from too much exposure to the sun. On the other hand, if you are young-looking, it may be because you take good care of yourself and are in excellent health. Or these days it may simply reflect good cosmetic surgery.

What Kind of Work Do You Do?

Your occupation may make you vulnerable to specific diseases or symptoms. For example, miners and those working in a dusty environment are prone to lung disorders. Garage mechanics and workers in poorly ventilated tunnels may inhale toxic fumes, damaging their heart, blood, lungs, and nervous system. Musicians, blacksmiths, typists, and those who use one set of muscles over and over again may develop pain, spasm, and cramps, because of the excessive strain on the particular muscle group involved. Even being a doctor has distinct occupational hazards, since we are exposed to the whole gamut of infections. We're sneezed, coughed, and breathed on. We touch and are touched. We get hepatitis, even syphilis, by accidentally breaking our skin with a needle that has just drawn contaminated blood.

A long list of descriptive symptoms directly resulting from some specific work or play is to be found in the medical literature. You may have "housemaid's knee," "tennis elbow," or suffer from a group of allergic lung diseases due to inhaling mold from hay ("farmer's lung"), sugar cane, and bird droppings. For years I couldn't figure out "Baker's cyst," a painful swelling at the back of the knee. I was stymied. What repetitive maneuver performed in a bakery could possibly cause such swelling? Later I learned that Baker's cyst is named after Dr. W. M. Baker.

Repeated contact with a wide variety of substances to which you are allergic, like soaps, perfumes, and industrial chemicals, may cause mysterious skin rashes. Many of us are unknowingly allergic to pets at home, giving us symptoms that tax the ingenuity of the doctor. Nerve deafness (loss of hearing for high frequencies) used to be found mostly in boilermakers and artillery gunners, but now afflicts the "rock" generation, who spend hours in discos or playing their stereos loud enough to awaken the dead.

How Do You Cope?

Occupational hazards are not only physical in origin. Many of us work under more pressure, tension, frustration, or anxiety than we can handle. To the casual observer, we seem to cope with or even thrive on the fast pace. But inner tensions take their toll in the diarrhea and cramps of colitis, the pain of stomach ulcers, the cough and wheezing of asthma, skin rashes, high blood pressure, and probably premature heart attacks.

Two imaginative cardiologists, Ray H. Rosenman and Meyer Friedman, postulated, on the basis of certain psychological tests, that there are two main and differing personality types, designated A and B. Type A persons are driven, achievers, never satisfied, and chronically frustrated. They are always on a "tight schedule," either competing to reach the top or fighting to stay there. According to these doctors, the Type A's usually have higher cholesterol levels and are much more prone to heart attacks than are the Type B's. The latter individuals are easygoing, noncompetitive, don't fight the clock, perform at their own pace, are content with their lot in life, and are not overly concerned with their "image." This theory of personality types and vulnerability to heart disease is an attractive one, and many cardiologists believe it to define one, but only one, of the many risk factors that predispose to premature coronary disease.

Compulsory Retirement

There are also the stress and risk of no work at all. I appreciate the rationale for compulsory retirement—new blood, new ideas, new vigor, and opportunities for the young on the lower rungs of the ladder. But retirement ages were set in the early 1930's, when the average life span was only 60 years. Today it is over 70 years. Someone put out to pasture at 60 or 65 against his will may have too much life left, too much energy, and even some as yet unfulfilled dreams. The sudden transition from being busy, needed, wanted, and earning enough money to satisfy a certain life-style—to sitting around bored, without any more goals, deprived, because of the need to economize, of many pleasures once taken for granted may result in physical and emotional deterioration. Unless retirement has been fortified by a second career, a consuming hobby, or some other satisfying involvement, it accelerates the aging process. Unaccustomed inactivity—sitting out the rest of your life on a park bench, watching TV, or baby-sitting—encourages you to dwell on a host of complaints, real or imagined. The net result is depression—which in itself can cause such symptoms as fatigue, headache, loss of appetite, and weight loss, to list but a few of the more common ones.

It is interesting to observe the development of two opposite trends with respect to the question of retirement. On the one hand, several state legislatures have banned it from the civil sector. Employees are free to retire if they wish, but for most jobs they are now permitted to stay on as long as they are willing and able to do so. There is talk of extending this policy to industry. On the other hand, workers in their fifties who get no special pleasure or satisfaction from their job, who would rather work part-time or at something else, or do nothing at all, and who are able, because of some pension plan, are retiring earlier than they must, and this trend is increasing.

I am not opposed to leisure and pleasure. But I do believe

people should be allowed to work as long as they want to and can do so safely. Take them off the promotion ladder if you must, call them consultants, but keep them busy and involved. The healthy human body and mind were not designed to vegetate at any age.

Your Marital Status

Chronic anger, frustration, and suspicion, no matter where or why you experience them, can lead to ulcers, asthma, colitis, and heart attacks. The site of such stress is just as likely to be your home as where you work. An unhappy marriage, with constant fighting and accusations or guilt of marital infidelity, can result in a train of psychosomatic illnesses.

"No, Not Another Woman . . ."

Your sexual preferences are also of medical consequence. For example, there is a much higher incidence of venereal disease and hepatitis among "gays" than among heterosexuals. Almost half the number of new cases of syphilis in New York City occur in homosexuals. I remember very vividly one patient—a married man, devoted husband and father—who came to see me some time ago with an acutely inflamed knee. It didn't look like the usual arthritis or gout, and he denied injuring it. Gonorrhea occasionally manifests itself, not in the usual pus or discharge from the genital organs, but as an acute inflammation of one joint, usually a large one like the knee or elbow. When I had excluded other causes for his sore knee, the possibility that this might be gonorrhea occurred to me, but I didn't really believe he had it. So, as tactfully as I could, I asked my patient whether he had recently had sexual relations with some woman other than his wife, perhaps one whom he knew only casually. He vigorously denied it, and I did not pursue the matter. We finally removed some of the fluid from the hot, swollen knee in order to make the diagnosis. There, under the microscope, I saw the characteristic gonorrhea bacteria. I was puzzled. If he really hadn't had sexual contact with another woman, he must have gotten the infection from his wife. So she was the culprit, not he. She was playing around and infecting him. I was about to call her to come and be examined when one of my residents suggested yet another possibility. He asked the patient directly whether he had had a homosexual affair. The answer was "yes." He had not lied to me at all. He simply had not had sexual relations with another woman.

Infectious hepatitis, a viral disease of the liver which usually results in jaundice and a chronic, tiring illness is transmitted by close human contact. So we see a lot of it in schools, jails, and army camps. But since high concentrations of the virus are transmitted by way of the intestinal tract (mouth to anus), we are finding more and more of it among homosexuals.

Your Family Roots

Specific diseases are to be found in greater numbers in certain geographic areas. For example, the Japanese have a very high incidence of stomach cancer, as well as the world's highest stroke rate (presumably because of excessive salt in the diet and consequent high blood pressure). Chronic bronchitis is often called "English disease" because it is so common in the cold, damp climate of Britain. Thalassemia (also know as Mediterranean or Cooley's anemia) is a severe crippling disease of the blood that may result in early death. It occurs almost exclusively in people of Mediterranean origin—Greeks, Italians, and Middle Easterners. Émigrés from tropical and subtropical regions of Africa, the Middle East, the Orient, South America, and the Caribbean may harbor schistosomiasis (snail fever). At the time of the great influx of Puerto Ricans to the northeast United States, this disease often presented a difficult diagnostic problem. Doctors didn't always think of the possibility of snail fever in midtown Manhattan. And so, the dysentery and liver trouble caused by this infection went undiagnosed in many cases.

The thyroid gland needs iodine to make its hormone. When there is not enough in the diet, the gland enlarges and forms a *goiter*. Because of the low iodine content of the soil in parts of the northwest United States and in the region around the Great Lakes, whole families living in these areas were prone to develop

goiters. Today, with the availability of iodized salt and an awareness that such iodine deficiency can produce this disorder, goiter
is much less common, even in the "goiter belt."

Have You Traveled Anywhere Recently?— Infections Tourists Bring Back

Modern jet travel has made it possible for millions of tourists
to visit previously inaccessible areas—countries with different
standards of public health, and each with its own peculiar infectious diseases. Smallpox has been virtually eradicated from the
world, but other infections like cholera, malaria, typhoid fever,
and countless parasitic infestations caused by worms, insects, and
animals are brought back home by travelers in great numbers.
They're not always diagnosed quickly, either. Quite frankly, if
you have some fever and a few aches and pains, I'm more likely
to call it "flu" or a "virus" than dengue fever or tsutsugamushi
disease—unless, of course, you tell me you've just come back
from a vacation in the Caribbean, the Far East or Africa. Or if
you've had diarrhea for a few days, I may think of "stomach
virus," or something you ate that will clear up, maybe even colitis
or tumor—unless you tell me you've just come back from a remote part of Mexico or from Leningrad. In this latter city, the
water supply has been contaminated by a parasite known as *Giar-
dia lamblia,* which causes diarrhea. Analyzing the stool, identifying the infecting organism, and treating with the specific antibiotic may be all that is necessary in such cases—not an extensive,
expensive workup. So a travel history will alert me to "exotic"
disease possibilities and avoid a lot of unnecessary worry and
testing.

TELL ME ABOUT YOUR FAMILY

It's important that you and I know what diseases affect other
members of your immediate family, because "the apple does not
fall far from the tree." From a medical point of view, I don't
really care about your in-laws except for contagious disease. I am
concerned mainly with your blood relatives—grandparents, par-

ents, brothers, and sisters, with an aunt or uncle or two thrown in. Are they alive? At what ages did they die and from what? The important diseases that run in families are stroke and high blood pressure, premature heart attacks, diabetes mellitus and blood fat disorders, cancer, mental disorders, and allergy.

In addition to inherited traits, you may share certain disorders with others in your family by virtue of common exposure to social and environmental factors like housing conditions, chronic infections, hygiene, eating, drinking, and smoking habits.

Do Your Relatives Have Stroke and High Blood Pressure (Hypertension)?

The term *stroke* refers to brain damage following an interruption, usually sudden, of its blood supply. This can happen in several ways. A clot may form in one of the arteries of the brain (thrombosis) or lodge there after having traveled in the bloodstream from another part of the body (embolus). Or an artery whose walls have previously been weakened by untreated high blood pressure may rupture and hemorrhage directly into the brain.

If your parents or any of your brothers and sisters have suffered a stroke, your blood pressure must be checked throughout your lifetime. One or two normal readings are not enough, because hypertension can appear at any time from childhood on.

Have There Been Many Heart Attacks in Your Family?

The commonest cause of death in most Western countries is the heart attack, killing more than 600,000 people each year in the United States alone. If your parents died from this disease before they were 65, or if any of your brothers and sisters had a coronary attack, I will want to know about it to try to protect you from the same fate. I may not always be able to do so, but it's worth a vigorous effort. There's no magic pill or guaranteed regimen. We simply have to work together trying to reduce or eliminate all the known risk factors that may increase your vulnerability. I will urge you to give up smoking, keep your weight and blood pressure down, eat a "prudent" diet low in cholesterol, and exercise regularly throughout your life.

"Do As I Say, Not As I Do"

The amount of sympathy—or censure—the uncooperative patient gets from a doctor will depend on the doctor's own habits. For example, the physician who smokes, usually "understands" your inability to stop. It would be embarrassing for him to sit there, cigarette in hand, and tell you how bad it is for your health—and that you (but not he) must stop. The doctor who "ties one on now and then" is sympathetic to your occasional "need to unwind" with a drink or two—or more. The fat doctor appreciates that "life is too short to deprive yourself of things you love to eat," or that it's not so easy to lose weight, even if you "really try." A few years ago, I determined with iron resolve to lose weight—and I did take off some twenty pounds. My tailor and I were delighted. But, oh, those poor fat people who came to my office at the height of my dietary success. "You're weak-willed and spineless. How dare you say you can't lose weight? Don't insult my intelligence by telling me you're starving but can't take off a single pound. You want a diet pill? Absolutely not. Go home and use some willpower—and don't come back until you've lost at least ten pounds."

But then, in a year or two, my own resolve weakened. My clothes mysteriously began to shrink, the collars on my shirts became tight for some reason, and finally my double chin returned. My patients were embarrassed for me, and generously told me I was looking well, that I had lost my gaunt appearance. Only my wife and my scale were honest with me. I had regained most of the twenty pounds. And then, when a fat patient came to see me, of course I understood the problem. "You want something to control your appetite? Well, these pills aren't really effective over the long term, but why don't you try this one for a couple of weeks? It may help you start. You want the name of a hypnotist? That's not a bad idea. Who knows, he may help you. Don't feel guilty. It's not all your fault, and it certainly isn't easy."

Are You Cancer Prone?

Cancer of the lung, stomach, prostate, breast, cervix, or bowel may occur with frightening frequency in a given family. This may be due to genetic factors, transmission of some viruses we haven't yet identified, or even common exposure to harmful environmental factors. We just don't know. But we are making progress in controlling some forms of cancer because of earlier detection (largely owing to public education and self-examination, especially of the breast, and to Pap smears), improved diagnostic techniques (sonar, body scanner x-rays, special blood tests), and more effective treatment (selective, powerful forms of radiation, better surgery, combinations of new drugs, and more recently immunotherapy—by means of which the defenses of the body are strengthened against malignant tumors). Hopefully, we will one day have vaccines against different kinds of cancers much as we now have against various infections.

Despite all these efforts, cancer remains the second most important cause of death. In 1976, about 360,000 people died of it in the United States. So, if when we discuss the health of other members of your family you tell me that several of your blood relatives had cancer, I will be especially careful to examine you for early evidence of the disease. Unfortunately, a strong family history of cancer sometimes causes a phobia about malignancy in some patients who can never be really convinced that they are free of the disease. They go from doctor to doctor requesting uncomfortable and expensive diagnostic procedures in their constant search for reassurance.

Are Mental Disorders Common Among Your Relatives?

Mental disease in various forms—"nervous breakdown," suicide, epilepsy—may run in families. Such disorders may be genetic, like Huntington's chorea, an uncommon mental disease which develops very gradually and becomes full-blown after age 40. Before the successful treatment of early syphilis with penicillin, brain damage in the late form of this disease was an important cause of mental disorder in adult life. However, more important today are the various forms of schizophrenia and manic-depressive states which may be found in more than one member of a family. They are probably due to some as yet undefined chemical disorder in the body, and impressive advances have been made in their treatment.

Hundreds of thousands of persons, previously destined to lifetime incarceration in mental hospitals, are now successfully treated by a wide variety of medications and backup psychiatric care. The impact of lithium, thorazine, and other psychoactive drugs is only in part reflected in the decline of the state mental hospital population in the United States from 550,000 in 1953 to fewer than 200,000 in 1976.

As our techniques to identify and measure more and more substances in the blood and urine improve, so will we recognize that much of what we call "mental disease" today is due to an excess or a deficiency of some vital body chemical. When corrected, presto, "instant mental health." That will leave the rest of us, with our fears, obsessions, compulsions, and complexes, fair game for the psychiatrist.

Are Any of Your Relatives Diabetic?

Diabetes is a disorder of sugar metabolism. It runs in families, so if any of your blood relatives are affected, you should be regularly tested throughout life with urinalysis and blood tests. When the disease begins in adult life, it is called *chemical* or *maturity-onset diabetes*. It does not usually cause the severe disease of arteries seen in children, in whom the eyes, brain, legs, kidney, and heart are so often affected.

Do You Come From an Allergic Family?

Asthma and hay fever, as well as sensitivity to certain foods and drugs, often run in families. If you or any of your close relatives are allergic, I will be very careful about giving you any new medication, no matter how simple or how widely it is used. I once had to resuscitate from an acute allergic attack an asthmatic who took two aspirin tablets.

These, then, are the main diseases I ask about in taking your family history. Such detailed questioning, while very productive, can sometimes be a waste of time. Once, I spent fifteen minutes asking a patient about his parents and the diseases that ran in his family, only to learn later that he was an adopted child, and knew nothing about his "real" parents.

PERSONAL HABITS

Do You Still Smoke?

Although there are still a few dyed-in-the-wool reactionaries around who don't think cigarettes are all that bad, most doctors, scientists, and government agencies consider cigarette smoking hazardous.

The health establishment is committed to getting you to stop smoking. The dangers of tobacco scream out at you from subway, bus, and highway signs—and even on the cigarette packages themselves: "The Surgeon General has determined that cigarette smoking is dangerous to your health." This campaign has had some impact, but not enough. Fewer adults in the United States are smoking cigarettes. There is a greater demand for a smoke-free environment among the traveling public. At medical meetings, particularly, the conference rooms just aren't smoke-filled anymore. In this country 100,000 doctors are said to have given up cigarettes. In England, reduced smoking is thought to be the reason for the drop in the death rate among medical men. So as a profession, we really practice what we preach. What is so disappointing is the fact that our teen-agers, especially girls, are taking up the habit in growing numbers. No one really knows why.

"Do you smoke regularly? Cigarettes, pipe, or cigars? How much and for how many years have you done so?" Heavy smokers are very much like addicts of any kind: they feel guilty about the habit and sometimes try to mask or minimize its extent. For example, a patient may deny that he smokes. If I then ask, "Have you ever smoked?" he may answer, "Yes." "When did you stop?" "Last week."

When cigarettes were shown to increase your chances of getting lung cancer or dying from heart disease, many smokers switched to pipes and cigars. But recent studies have shown that even these are not harmless, especially if the smoking is heavy and the tobacco is inhaled. What's more, pipe smokers may develop cancer of the lip or tongue due to irritation from the stem and heat from the smoke.

One Way to Stop Smoking

The most effective way to get you to stop smoking is to demonstrate what harm the habit is actually causing you. My personal experience in this regard is a case in point. I used to smoke cigarettes. I knew all about why I shouldn't, but so do you—so does everybody—and too many still smoke. Then, one day, about fifteen years ago I was demonstrating a new radioelectrocardiograph at a scientific meeting. I was wearing the device, walking about a large auditorium, smoking—and transmitting my electrocardiogram to an oscilloscope several hundred yards away. Some doctors looking at the screen noticed irregularities of the heart rhythm. When they asked the technician who the subject was, she pointed to me. I came back to the oscilloscope and to my dismay saw on the screen my electrocardiogram with several "extra beats," increasing in number every time I inhaled the cigarette smoke. I had been totally unaware of them. While it's true that such cardiac irregularities are almost always innocent in otherwise healthy persons, they can, on occasion, be the forerunner of sudden death. That was all the information I needed about me and tobacco. What I had known all along was now supported by hard evidence, and I quit, then and there. I have not smoked cigarettes since. I wish more people could have that kind of experience and understand it as I did.

The mechanism by which cigarettes cause lung cancer (irritant—tars, resins, heat?) and heart disease (by accelerating arteriosclerosis—nicotine) is not clear. Any or all of these factors or others not yet identified may be responsible.

What's the best way to stop? It varies. First, you have to be convinced—and a little frightened—as I was. Some people (about 50 percent) have had success for varying periods of time at special clinics and group meetings with similarly motivated friends. Others go to hypnotists (occasionally successful) or use various commercially available substances which give you an awful taste when you smoke. But in the final analysis, it requires a resolute emotional and intellectual commitment. Once you have that, it's easy.

What About "Pot"?

As long as we're on the subject of your smoking habits, I will also ask about marijuana. Despite the legal constraints on its use, "pot" smoking is widespread, and not only among teen-agers and college students. Adults, often sophisticated, who should know better also indulge quite regularly. It is estimated that at least forty million people in the United States have smoked marijuana at one time or another, and 13 million continue to do so.

Whether or not the chronic use of marijuana causes any physical disease is not yet established. Some researchers think it may produce impotence, chronic mental problems, and, when used by pregnant women, birth defects. Like alcohol, "pot" will impair coordination while driving, and like tobacco, it can aggravate bronchitis. On the other hand, there is some evidence that, when used under medical supervision, marijuana is helpful in the management of glaucoma (increased pressure in the eye which can lead to blindness), relief of pain in cancer, and the treatment of certain psychiatric disorders.

At the present time, the greatest known risk from "grass" is neither physical nor psychological, but getting caught. Many lives and careers have been ruined, not by the biological consequences of marijuana, but as the result of unduly harsh punishment for its use. The campaign to decriminalize marijuana is gaining momentum, but it would be a pity if society were to equate this legal move with a belief that the substance is harmless. All the data are not yet in, and those who smoke marijuana regularly are experimenting with a potentially hazardous agent.

Are You Much of a Drinker?

Don't confuse social drinking with alcoholism. A cocktail before dinner, or some wine with it, a little brandy or port after dessert, afford a pleasure and relaxation that few of us would easily give up. Nor should we. *Alcoholism,* on the other hand, is a disease. No one knows why some of us are satisfied with and enjoy a couple of drinks, while others feel the need to drink themselves into a stupor, often at the risk of their personal happiness, careers, and health. Part of the problem is no doubt psychiatric, but the rest of it must be physical—probably some chemical imbalance or malfunction within the body.

With respect to social drinking, there are no figures concerning what is "too much." Each of us has, and usually knows, his own limit. How well you tolerate a given amount of alcohol depends on its concentration (percentage or proof), how you take it (wine, beer, whiskey—and diluted, "straight," or in soda), and whether your stomach is empty (permitting rapid absorption into the bloodstream) or full (giving a more gradual effect).

The "Alcohol Is Good for You" Legend

There are certain myths about alcohol that persist and are widely accepted. We hear about them all the time—at cocktail parties, in the movies, or on TV. For example:

Scene: A battlefield. His best buddy has been badly wounded. While waiting for the paramedics, our hero raises the partially conscious victim's head, and pours some whiskey down his throat. *Comment:* That's bad. The injured man may be too weak to swallow, so that the whiskey may go down the windpipe into the lung—and give him pneumonia. Or his gut may be perforated, and the liquor will leak all over his insides, giving him peritonitis.

Scene: The North Pole. The rescue party finds the lost explorer. He's got frostbite—feet, hands, ears are frozen and painful. Out comes the flask—in goes the whiskey. *Comment:* Bad. The St. Bernard dog with the flask around his neck doesn't know any better, but you should. The alcohol, a dilator of blood vessels, will open arteries other than those in the frozen limbs, shunting blood away from the areas that need it most.

Scene: Your friend has just sustained what appears to be a heart attack—is barely conscious, complaining of chest pain. Here comes the flask again—poured into or swallowed by the victim. *Comment:* Wrong thing to do. Why? First of all, your diagnosis may not be correct. Your friend may have a perforated ulcer in the stomach and not a heart attack at all. Anything taken by mouth in this situation, especially alcohol, is dangerous. And even if it is a heart attack, you're better off calling for help, keeping the patient warm, and watching that he doesn't choke on his own secretions. Don't burden him with the additional work of swallowing and digesting whiskey, which under these circumstances can cause a disturbance of heart rhythm and make the heart work less efficiently.

And finally—*Scene:* Some friends chatting about their health one evening. "You have heart trouble? You should be taking brandy regularly. It's good for your heart." *Comment:* Wrong. Alcohol is, for the most part, a cardiac depressant. There is even a form of heart disease called "alcohol cardiomyopathy" (*myo* means muscle, *pathy* means disease). Also, if the rhythm of the heart is out of whack, alcohol can make it worse. The commonest symptom of heart trouble is angina pectoris—chest pain, pressure, or tightness usually brought on by some form of exertion or emotional stress. Even though alcohol has a sedative or tranquilizing effect, it sometimes aggravates angina pectoris.

All this adds up to one conclusion. If you enjoy social drinking—fine. But don't pretend that you're taking a medicine you need.

One of the few possibly legitimate medical uses of alcohol is in the treatment of arterial disease—when the blood vessels in the legs are narrowed, giving you pain when you walk. An ounce or two of whiskey before exercise may improve these symptoms.

Too Much Alcohol—Big Breasts, Small Testicles

Aside from the social and legal difficulties resulting from alcoholism (being identified as a drunk, inability to keep a job, poor work performance, absenteeism, automobile and other accidents, domestic strife), alcoholism also causes specific diseases. An observation made in 1973, and of great concern to the Food and Drug Administration is that alcohol in any form (liquor, beer, or wine) consumed regularly by a pregnant woman can cause birth defects in her child. Because of this, the possibility of labeling alcohol as being hazardous during pregnancy is now under consideration.

Other more common toxic effects of alcohol include personality changes due to the direct toxic effect of alcohol on the brain and heart, nutritional disturbances and liver disease (cirrhosis, with all its terrible consequences). When the liver becomes congested and scarred from chronic alcoholic abuse, many of its vital mechanisms become impaired. One of these is to eliminate female hormone (estrogen) from the body, small amounts of which are present even in normal men. When the liver is damaged, it can no longer deactivate the estrogen, which then accumulates in the bloodstream. If the subject is a male, he now has too high a level of female hormones in his body. The result is a hairless face, which needs to be shaved only every few days, loss of the typical male distribution of body hair, decreased sex drive, and the unhappy combination of big breasts and small testicles.

Another serious late effect of alcoholism and cirrhosis of the liver is massive hemorrhage. Blood that normally flows through the liver is prevented from doing so by scar tissue which forms in the cells damaged by the alcohol. So the blood backs up from the liver into the veins of the stomach and esophagus (the food pipe) and the lower bowel, engorging them with blood until the blood vessels finally burst. The patient may then bleed to death through the mouth or, less commonly, from the rectum.

Once I have established that you are an alcoholic, I will also look for evidence of venereal disease, even though you may not remember the contact. A common triad of symptoms in the alcoholic is cirrhosis, venereal disease, and a tattooed skin—acquired during a stuporous debauch.

Are You a Coffee Addict?

How much coffee, cola, tea and, to a lesser extent, chocolate you take every day is important because the caffeine in these substances is a stimulant of the heart and nervous system. In excess, it will cause insomnia, jitters, tremor, and palpitations (rapid, irregular, or forceful beating of the heart). That's why I usually advise persons with cardiac disorders, particularly those with irregular heart action, to take decaffeinated beverages wherever possible. Recent reports suggesting that coffee may cause heart disease, cancer of the bladder, and various other disorders, have proven to be unfounded.

Diet, the Game People Play

Losing weight is a national pastime. Everyone's doing it—the fat and the thin, the sick and the healthy, the young and the old. After a few weeks of dedication to some grueling regimen, we're down ten pounds, and off we go to the tailor or dressmaker—happy, proud, and delighted to pay for the necessary alterations. A few weeks later, we're back to where we were, maybe even a little heavier, and now can't get into our clothes. So it's off to the tailor again, this time ashamed and resentful. If you're one of those who go through life up and down the weight yo-yo, take my advice, buy two wardrobes—one for when you're fat, the other for when you're thin. It's cheaper than the alterations.

The world is full of authorities on how to lose weight. They write books and magazine articles about it, we see them on TV, or they show up in our homes full of great ideas. "You want to lose weight? Eat grapefruit, or all the fat you want, or drink sixteen glasses of water a day, or get that marvelous liquid protein supplement at the health store." Everyone is an expert and will guarantee you'll lose weight—everyone, that is, except your doctor. All he can do is assess the energy requirements in your daily activities and plan a no-fun, no-nonsense diet in which you simply consume fewer calories than you expend. Follow that concept, and you'll not only lose weight, but keep it off. The trouble is that it requires discipline and commitment for a lifetime, not just a few days.

Unfortunately, the preoccupation with weight loss is not to be found among those who need it most—the 250- or 300-pounders. They're already usually numb to the situation and became discouraged a long time ago. The fanatics are those who want to lose a little purely for cosmetic reasons—like dropping from 119 to 116 pounds. "Doctor, I feel so bloated at this weight. If I could only lose four pounds." They're the ones most likely to take "water pills," adopt food fads and bizarre eating habits which, if continued for long enough, can lead to trouble in the form of vitamin or other nutritional deficiencies. For example, most of us can tolerate the so-called water diet for a while. But if you have heart failure or kidney disease, excessive fluids can be harmful. The macrobiotic diet is fraught with the danger of vitamin and protein deficiencies. Any eating fad that emphasizes a given substance to the exclusion of other nutrients is probably harmful over the long term. So I will always ask if you're on some "miracle" diet. If you're a vegetarian and exclude meat but eat eggs, milk, vegetables and carbohydrates, you're safe. I have never seen any deficiency disease in people following such diets even for a lifetime.

The Semistarvation Protein Diet:

Where substantial weight reduction is not only cosmetically desirable, but important from a medical point of view, it can be achieved by the use of a semistarvation protein supplemental diet. The candidate for such a regimen is someone who is massively obese—50 or more pounds overweight and who has heart trouble, high blood pressure, diabetes, lung disease, or painful arthritis. In each of these conditions, weight loss is extremely important. For example, in every extra pound of fat there are miles of tiny blood vessels through which the blood must be pumped. This can be an embarrassment to a sick heart. In very fat people high blood pressure requires much more medication, and fat diabetics need more insulin. A person with chronic bronchitis or emphysema breathes more easily when he is thin, and in arthritics, weight-bearing joints, such as the knees and back, are under less strain when the extra pounds are lost.

Unfortunately, "liquid protein diets" have been available in supermarkets and drug stores to anyone who wanted them. Thousands and thousands of overweight people, or those who thought they were, went on crash diets using this supplement— without supervision. Not surprisingly, several deaths occurred. Any drastic manipulation of the body chemistry is fraught with danger and must be very carefully managed. In my opinion, access to this material should be forbidden except by prescription.

One such preparation, consisting of the protein from egg

white (which, unlike the yolk, does not raise cholesterol), is availble to doctors only. When *taken under strict control,* it will result in an average weight loss of four to five pounds a week for as long as it is continued. It should be supplemented by the appropriate vitamins, minerals and enough potassium—but it *must* be done only under your doctor's guidance, and even then, not everyone can take it safely.

But one of the effects of this and other high-protein diets is a profound water loss in the first few days—almost as if you were taking a diuretic. This causes not only dehydration but loss of potassium as well—a combination of effects which can be fatal in patients with certain forms of heart disease and other disorders.

Over the long term, sustained weight loss requires "behavior modification," a drastic and permanent change in your diet philosophy. And that's the hardest part.

Your Sleeping Habits

Some of us need less sleep than others, especially as we get older. A famous older heart surgeon I know functions very well with only four or five hours' sleep. While the rest of the world is dreaming at 4:30 A.M., he is up, reviewing charts and preparing for his first operation at 7:00 A.M. Other equally energetic people have a "big head" the next day unless they get their full nine hours.

Trouble falling asleep may be due to simple anxiety, worry, depression, or exhilaration and intense pleasure. In many cases there is no apparent reason for the insomnia. Appetite depressants (anorexiants) can also keep you awake because of their stimulant effect, despite advertising claims to the contrary, as can strong tea or coffee, or food taken near bedtime.

Another cause of insomnia is too much thyroid hormone entering your bloodstream, either from an overactive thyroid gland or in pill form. You may be taking thyroid without knowing it, usually in some "diet" pill.

Some of us have no trouble falling asleep, but wake up a couple of hours later and toss and turn the rest of the night. A "nightcap" may help you get to sleep, but you may awaken a little later when the effect of the alcohol wears off—a kind of "withdrawal" reaction.

Some of us have slipped into a life-style in which we do not get as much sleep as we need, not because of insomnia, but because we go to bed too late and get up too early. So many people consult the doctor because they're always tired. After a time-consuming and expensive examination, we often find all they need is a little more sleep.

Do You Exercise Regularly?

If you are physically active at work or at play, you have a better outlook with respect to heart attacks and longevity than does someone who leads a sedentary life.

Survival of the Fittest

The most important study confirming the benefit of regular *strenuous* exercise was reported late in 1977 by a group of medical researchers at Harvard. They analyzed the daily physical activity of 17,000 men over the years since graduation. Those who did not burn up at least 2,000 calories a week in some form of strenuous exercise had a 64 percent higher incidence of heart attacks than those who did. How can you expend this number of calories? Here are some examples: Biking eleven miles in an hour or walking five miles in an hour takes 420 to 480 calories. If you pedal just a little faster—twelve miles in an hour—you will use up 480 to 600 calories. Running more than six miles an hour or playing squash or handball requires more than 660 calories in one hour.

Of greater importance than the number of calories expended is the manner in which you expend them. The more rigorous and strenuous the effort, the greater the protection. Unfortunately, if you exercise only modestly, or use up fewer than 2,000 calories per week, the benefit is apparently not obvious, according to this Harvard study.

Earlier reports had also suggested that exercise is good for you, but not so dramatically. For example, it was shown that in England the drivers on the double-decker buses, sitting at the wheel without much physical exertion, had a higher incidence of heart disease than did the conductors who ran up and down the stairs all day collecting fares. In another survey by a group of British doctors, some 16,000 people ages 40 to 64 were questioned about their exercise habits. Among those who exercised vigorously and regularly the incidence of coronary heart disease was only one third that among those in the group who either did not exercise at all or did so only lightly. There is also some convincing evidence that when persons who are physically fit do suffer a heart attack, their chances of living through it are better than those for the sedentary and physically deconditioned. Regular exercise makes it possible for you to perform the same work at a slower heart rate and less shortness of breath.

A Great Tranquilizer

The benefits of regular exercise are now being widely popularized. Every morning, winter and summer, rain or shine, joggers fill our streets and parks. Most doctors agree that exercise is "good for you"—some types of exercise better than others. For example, bowling, golf, and weight lifting have very little effect on increasing your cardiac fitness. But jogging, cross-country skiing, and biking do improve the efficiency of your heart, as judged in terms of pulse-rate and blood-pressure response.

Regardless of its effect in preventing or modifying the severity of heart attacks, there is no question that a vigorous workout makes you feel good. Exercise is a great tranquilizer. Keep physically fit and active by exercising regularly unless there is some compelling reason not to. For example, if your heart muscle is weak (congestive heart failure), or you have angina pectoris or suffered a heart attack at some time, do not join any "rehabilitation" program without an exercise prescription from your doctor and skilled supervision. We now have ways of determining how much and what kind of exercise is good for you, and at what rate it should be performed and increased.

Prescribed Like a Medicine

Exercise is not good for everyone. It must be prescribed as carefully as a medicine, especially for the sick or elderly. No one above 40 years of age should embark on a vigorous training program without first undergoing a thorough cardiac examination including an electrocardiographic stress test (to be discussed later). Also, if you have back problems or arthritis, check with your orthopedist or internist to make sure the exercise won't throw you into painful spasm. No matter your age and health status, whatever fitness regimen you choose to follow should be done on an ongoing basis, not in fits and starts. If you've worked up to a certain level, and then stop exercising for a week or two, don't begin again where you left off. Work your way back from some intermediate point.

How's Your Sex Life?

Has your doctor ever discussed your sex life with you? I recently reviewed several printed questionnaires used by physicians and hospitals to get base-line health information from their patients. These included one prepared by the American Society of Internal Medicine, an organization of qualified internists in the United States. Nowhere was the vital question of sexual activity in women referred to—only in men.

Difficult though it is for me to greet you (especially if you're a new patient) with "How do you do, come in, sit down, I'm happy to meet you, and how's your sex life?" some time in the interview the matter should come up.

Impotent or Impudent?

A very frequent complaint among men, and also their wives, especially when I ask about it, is *impotence.* (Recently, a very agitated gentleman complained that he was "impudent.") I'm surprised at the number of apparently virile, healthy, well-adjusted men who, when given the opportunity, describe great anxiety or dissatisfaction with their sexual performance. They always have some excuse to explain it: "My prostate is getting larger." "I work under tremendous tension. My boss wears me out." "I get very tired commuting." "I had a heart attack ten years ago." In reality, there is no correlation between impotence and an enlarged prostate, your boss, or even your old heart attack. Some men attribute impaired sexual performance to various medications they are taking, only a few of which may actually have this effect. The ones that sometimes do include rauwolfia products (reserpine, Serpasil, Raudixin), used in the treatment of high blood pressure or anxiety; Aldomet (a blood-pressure-lowering pill; Atromid-S (a cholesterol-lowering agent); various tranquilizers; and Aldactone (a water pill or diuretic). Other diuretics and drugs used in the treatment of high blood pressure do not have this side effect.

A Sexual Emergency

I have known problems of sexual performance sometimes to constitute an emergency. A vigorous 84-year-old man phoned me demanding an appointment that very day because of an "urgent matter." He arrived distraught, to tell me that for the last two nights he had been unable to have an erection. Another gent, he 89 years old, found himself impotent after a stroke some months earlier. After several unsuccessful attempts, he called, indignant, asking when he would fully recover. I told him I could not be certain, but hoped he would remain optimistic and keep trying. Thereafter he called every few days to complain that despite my reassurance, "nothing has happened yet." (By the way, he's still trying—and calling.) I mention these cases to emphasize that age in itself is not as important a factor in sexual prowess or interest as you may think.

Impotence may take the form, not only of difficulty in obtaining and maintaining an erection, but more commonly, of premature ejaculation. This is especially true among younger men, in whom erection is prompt and adequate, but short-lived. This is often due to anxiety. Another common complaint among teenagers and young adults is that the penis is too small.

More Imagined than Real?

Whatever its presenting form, impotence is a relative matter and may be more imagined than real. Many men who perform quite normally (by your standards and mine) are dissatisfied because they have heard too many tall stories, or insist on comparing their "endowment" with that displayed by "stars" in pornographic movies. They simply expect too much, and perhaps so do their mates. (In reality, penis size is probably the least important factor in female sexual satisfaction.)

Impotence does not have a physical cause in the majority of cases, and is more apt to be due to psychological factors—depression, anxiety, boredom, or fear of aging. One of my patients went on and on about his impotence, how depressed he was about it and how sad it made his wife. Well into the physical examination, I suddenly asked him, "Are you impotent away from home?" He replied with an incredulous "Of course not." Under these circumstances, psychiatry or marriage counseling may be effective.

Sometimes, however, impotence is actually due to some physical disorder like a decrease in blood supply to the penis because of narrowing and arteriosclerosis of the arteries that supply it, any chronic debilitating disease, diabetes, anemia, or low thyroid function. Some decrease in male hormone (testosterone) does occur with aging or with disease of the glands that make it (testicles and adrenals) or of the pituitary gland, which stimulates its production. The usual prostatectomy (removal of the prostate) done to relieve the symptoms of simple enlargement of the prostate will not usually cause impotence. But various treatments for cancer of the prostate—for example, administration of female hormone, removal of the testicles (and thus of male hormone), extensive surgical procedures necessary to control the malignancy—can result in true impotence. For such men there are now several kinds of prosthetic devices that make intercourse mechanically possible. If you fall into this group, discuss the problem with your urologist.

In any event, a sudden decrease in sexual interest or performance warrants a careful examination to exclude treatable physical and emotional causes.

The Frigid Woman

When a man becomes impotent, he prefers to believe it's because of a specific reason beyond his control—a pill he has to take, a disease somewhere in his body, or some severe emotional stress. Whatever the reason, it's not his fault. The psychiatrist is the last person he wants to see about it, although that's where he's most likely to be helped. But when his wife is "frigid," disinterested, or unresponsive (curious how it's almost never the "girlfriend"), that's where she's sent first.

A poorly functioning sexual partner, whether it's due to his own impotence or because the woman is "cold," is a blow to the ego as well as a challenge to the male. None of us likes to be confronted with the fact that we are, after all, "resistible."

A woman's dissatisfaction with her sexual life may be due to physical reasons, but they have much more to do with her relationship to her man. She simply may not love or even like him. Add to that his poor sexual technique, lack of consideration, or some form of impotence, and you have the classic setup for "frigidity." And even if she likes him, his insistence on hasty penetration before adequate vaginal lubrication will cause pain and reduce enjoyment. Ignorance of the female anatomy, especially the role of the clitoris in heightening a woman's enjoyment and climax, will also cause chronic dissatisfaction. Recurrent premature ejaculation may result in conditioned frustration in the female, and only rare climax. Insistence on sexual variations which some women find objectionable can also produce hostility and consequently frigidity.

Among the more common purely physical bases for a woman's not enjoying lovemaking are infection, irritation, tumors and structural abnormalities of the vagina that cause pain. Common chronic vaginal infections are viral sores (herpes), *Trichomonas* (an organism frequently encountered in men and women, which causes a persistent vaginal discharge), yeast or fungal overgrowth (usually a complication of some antibiotic therapy), and the different venereal diseases. In older women, as female hormone production declines, the lining inside the vagina becomes dry and thin, like parchment. Penetration causes pain and bleeding. This is easily treated with hormones (cream, pills or injections). Common structural disorders which interfere with normal intercourse include a tight hymen that has not been adequately distended or stretched. Finally, when there is a decrease in female hormone, such as occurs in the menopause or when there is a disease of the pituitary gland in the brain, of the thyroid, or of the ovary itself, sexual desire is sometimes diminished. But in actual fact, many women have a paradoxical increase in their libido after the menopause.

Do You Tire Easily?

"I used to come home from work and go out on the town, to the theater, bowl, play tennis, or make love. Now, I go straight to bed (alone) after dinner, or just fall asleep at the television set." Although feeling tired is usually due to boredom, depression, emotional stress, overwork, or chronic lack of exercise, it may also reflect some underlying infection, anemia, low thyroid function, heart trouble, or a back problem. It is what we call a "nonspecific" symptom—because it can be due to virtually "anything"—and, as such, taxes the diagnostic ingenuity of the doctor. Fatigue due to depression or emotional upset is usually present the moment you awaken, even after a good night's sleep. However, when some disease is making you tired, you feel progressively worse as the day wears on.

If you're tired enough to make a special trip to the doctor about it, that warrants serious interest and investigation on his part. Fatigue may be nature's tip-off that something is wrong. For example, when we carefully question persons who have survived heart attacks, unusual fatigue days and weeks before the attack itself emerges as one of the most important warning symptoms. Unfortunately, feeling tired is such a common complaint, and so often psychological, it is often ignored as a serious signal. Many people accept it as the norm, instead of checking it out. They ask for pep pills, stimulants such as the amphetamines, to increase their energy. This is dangerous, because these agents mask what may be an important indicator of disease. They are a crutch that does not solve the underlying problem. Such drugs are habituating, so that eventually you come to depend on them and can't function satisfactorily without them. Finally, in older persons or those with heart disease, high blood pressure, or disturbance of heart rhythm, stimulants may be dangerous.

DRUG HISTORY

Are You a Pill-Popper?

We are a pill-taking culture. We swallow tablets to put us to sleep and to keep us awake, to make us happier or to tranquilize us, to stimulate the appetite or to depress it. Because we're too busy to take the time to develop regular bowel habits, we rely on "stool softeners" and laxatives to "keep us going." Pills have become so much a way of life that we tend to forget the old adage: "In every medicine there is a little poison." Medications not only have effects we want but have side effects we don't want.

Vitamins Are Not Candy

Vitamin pills are medicines. Vitamin supplements, when taken in recommended dosages, rarely have any adverse side effects. But do you need them? Should those of us who eat a "normal" diet, who are not "food faddists" or sick and undernourished, and who are not constantly on some crash program to lose weight take a "multivitamin" every morning? The billions of dollars of sales each year attest to the fact that millions of us do. Are the benefits real or imagined? I don't know, nor do I think it matters very much—if you feel better taking them. And many people do, despite the fact that there is no hard, scientific evidence that vitamin supplements are required to maintain health in the presence of an adequate diet. Although such a diet is hard to define, if each day you are taking some protein in the form of meat, fish, fowl, eggs, or milk, eat green vegetables, fruit, and carbohydrates—and are maintaining your weight—your diet is probably balanced.

The usual capsule is made up of various members of the vitamin B group, vitamin C, small amounts of vitamins A, D and E, and a smattering of minerals like calcium, zinc, magnesium, and sometimes iron.

How do the drug companies determine the amount of each of

these to include? In experiments on humans and animals, scientists have been able to determine for most of these vitamins an amount below which we will develop symptoms of deficiency. This value is called the MDR (minimum daily requirement). The MDR is so low, and so easily attained in the usual Western diet, that the pharmaceutical houses arbitrarily multiply it by ten or more times in their capsule. That amount will certainly prevent you from actually being deficient in these vitamins. But preventing deficiency is not quite the same as providing a sense of well-being. It may be that feeling really well, something we cannot measure in animals or humans, requires these higher vitamin levels. It is this assumption that makes patients ask for and doctors prescribe vitamin supplements.

Carrying this theory one step farther, some people mistakenly think that the more vitamins you take, the better off you are. But too much of the vitamin B family may cause nausea, and vitamin B_1 in excess, like thyroid, can make you nervous and excitable. Vitamins A and D are necessary for healthy skin and bone, but when taken in excess may produce calcium disorders, kidney and bone disease. The Food and Drug Administration protects you from overdose of these substances by requiring a prescription before you can get them in high dosage. Generally speaking, if you follow the directions on the bottle, you won't have any side effects from vitamins. But remember, just because one is good, don't take ten.

The Vitamin C Controversy

Do massive doses of vitamin C protect against colds? The theory that they do has been popularized by a very distinguished scientist who has won two Nobel prizes, Dr. Linus Pauling. He believes that we don't have enough vitamin C, since it cannot be stored by the body. What we eat is utilized but really insufficient to meet our needs, and we are all deficient in it. *I don't know whether Dr. Pauling is right or wrong,* but his theory cannot be casually dismissed and should be tested to arrive at a definitive answer. At this time, I am not aware of any conclusive evidence that has confirmed or denied his hypothesis. However, certain studies suggest that in schoolchildren, massive doses of vitamin C in the thousands of units have been effective against the common cold.

I have seen some side effects even from usual doses of vitamins. In some patients, as little as 200 units of vitamin E may result in "extra beats" and elevated blood pressure. Vitamin E is said by many to be good for whatever ails you—heart trouble, skin disease, diabetes, arthritis, and aging. Very few, if any, of these claims have been documented.

If your vitamin capsule contains "high-potency" B complex, don't be alarmed by the deep-yellow discoloration and strong odor it imparts to your urine.

Aspirin (and Other Headache Pills)

Aspirin is probably the most useful and widely used drug there is. I doubt there is anyone in the civilized world who doesn't always keep some at home. Some 35 million tablets are taken every day in the United States alone. It helps control pain, fever, and even insomnia. (Incidentally, nobody is really sure how it works.) Now you know why, when you call your doctor at 2:00 A.M. with complaints of feeling "lousy," he tells you to take two aspirin and call him in the morning. Unless you're having a heart attack, stroke or some other catastrophe, he couldn't give you better advice. Fortunately, there have been so many jokes about "take two aspirin and call me in the morning," most doctors have become sensitive about giving this advice . . . and patients consider it a nocturnal "cop-out."

A very exciting clinical observation suggests that two or three aspirin tablets a day may protect against heart attacks and strokes by preventing the formation of clots within the blood vessels of the heart and brain. Large-scale studies to test this theory, sponsored by the U.S. government, are currently being carried out in several medical centers.

As useful as it is, aspirin also has serious side effects when taken for long periods of time. The most important of these is bleeding from the upper intestinal tract (stomach, esophagus) due to erosion of its lining This is true not only of plain aspirin but, despite advertisements to the contrary, of the buffered product as well. Such blood loss is often insidious and gradual. I have seen several older persons who were on aspirin for months, usually for control of arthritic pain, develop anemia severe enough to require blood transfusions—yet they were unaware of it.

Aspirin can also cause stomach irritation and pain, without bleeding, and some persons are frankly allergic to it. So remember—aspirin is a medicine. You should not take it continuously without medical supervision. If for one reason or another you are taking aspirin every day you should have stool specimens tested for blood every few weeks.

Never take aspirin and anticoagulants together unless your doctor knows about it. Since aspirin has some "blood-thinning" properties of its own, when used with anticoagulants the two drugs together may cause dangerous bleeding. So if you are on anticoagulants and need mild pain relief or something to reduce fever, an aspirin substitute like Tylenol should be used.

Are You Taking Any Blood-Pressure Pills?

The control of high blood pressure is vital. Fortunately most of the drugs used for that purpose are well tolerated. Sometimes, however, they cause side effects like skin rashes (any of them), psychological depression (the rauwolfia group), impotence (Aldomet, Inderal, Aldactone, rauwolfia), very low heart rate (Inderal), fatigue, muscle weakness, and disturbances of heart action due to the loss of potassium from the body by the way of the urine (diuretic or "water pills"). Finally, antihypertension medications may cause your blood pressure to drop suddenly and too much, especially when you change position abruptly, like jumping out of bed. This may result in dizziness, light-headedness, fainting, or excessive fatigue. If you are receiving treatment for high blood pressure, always avoid getting up quickly from the lying or sitting position. All these side effects disappear with simple adjustment in dosage or switching to another drug.

Cortisone—the "Miracle" Drug

Arthritis is a very common and important disorder which afflicts millions of people throughout the world. In most cases, its symptoms can be controlled by aspirin or other antiinflammatory drugs (Indocin, Motrin). Sometimes, however, when the arthritis is very severe, doctor and patient resort to the cortisone family of drugs (steroids) for relief, especially during a flare-up of symptoms. Chronic use of these agents in high doses can be hazardous. *Never keep taking cortisone unless your doctor knows about it.* If there is no other way to lessen your pain and you must have a steroid, your doctor will determine an optimal dose—one that is both effective and reasonably safe. Larger amounts may give you a "moonface," thinning of the bones which then break easily, retention of salt causing swelling of the feet and elevation of the blood pressure, changes in hair distribution on the face, stomach ulcers, and behavioral changes. If you have had TB or have an old scar on your chest x-ray, you may even be given antituberculosis medicines if cortisone is prescribed, because it can cause a flare-up of old tubercular infection.

Stopping Suddenly Is Dangerous

Even more dangerous than the chronic use of too much cortisone is stopping it abruptly. Cortisone is a life-regulating hormone. It is produced by two small glands—the adrenals, which also make epinephrine (adrenaline)—one situated on top of each kidney. When they have made enough cortisone, and the level of this drug in the blood is normal, the adrenals get "turned off," much as a thermostat controls a heating system. But this regulating or feedback mechanism can't tell whether you got the cortisone naturally from the gland or from the drugstore. When a certain concentration is reached, regardless of its origin, the gland stops making any more. As long as you are getting cortisone the easy way—by pills—the adrenal glands don't have to make any of their own and so stop working. If this goes on long enough, the glands virtually wither from disuse. At that point, with the adrenals inactive, should you suddenly stop taking the cortisone pills, the blood level drops sharply because its only supply has been cut off. The body needs it, but the gland can't respond quickly enough—and you may go into shock. On the other hand, if the cortisone dosage is reduced gradually rather than stopped abruptly, the gland has the time to resume its function, especially if it has not been suppressed for too long.

Do You Take Cough Medicines All the Time?

If you are one of those persons who go through life taking cough medicines to suppress a chronic cough, it's important that I know it. A persistent cough may be due to some underlying lung disease which needs proper treatment and eradication, not just masking. You may be coughing because of something as trivial as a postnasal drip or mild bronchitis, or as serious as a lung tumor or heart failure, with water in the lungs. Also, some of the cough remedies that are still occasionally available "over the counter," that is, without a prescription, contain codeine. Codeine is made from opium and is an addicting narcotic. I have seen several patients who have become codeine addicts simply from chronic use of cough syrup. By the way, codeine is also constipating, and the cough syrup has sugar in it—something you should know if you're diabetic.

Has Digitalis Been Prescribed for You?

Digitalis is the most widely used drug for the treatment of heart trouble. It acts in two ways. First, it actually strengthens the heart muscle, so that every contraction or beat is stronger and expels more blood. When the heart muscle is weak and doesn't pump efficiently, the result is heart failure. Digitalis, then, is the number-one agent to treat such failure. Another action of digitalis is to regulate certain disturbances of cardiac rhythm. Rapid heart rates due to irritability of the heart or weakness are controlled by digitalis.

In order for this drug to be effective, a critical concentration must be maintained in the blood at all times. This means that the pill has to be taken regularly, and for most people that means every day. But if you have been on this agent for weeks, months or years, too much of it may accumulate in the blood, especially if you also have kidney or liver disease. These are the organs that excrete the digitalis so that it doesn't build up in the body. If they are not working perfectly, you may become toxic from too much digitalis. Also, older people need less of the drug, as do thin, small individuals. When higher than necessary concentrations of the drug circulate in your bloodstream, you become sick and dangerously so. One type of digitalis agent is called lanatoside. To emphasize the risks of its overdosage, we were taught as medical students that "lanatoside takes more lives than homicide." That's true only if you are unaware of its potential side effects. Therefore, if when taking digitalis for any reason, you gradually notice loss of appetite and weight, nausea, vomiting, headaches visual disturbances, or mental confusion, think of excessive digitalis in your system as a possible explanation.

A Dangerous Appetite Suppressant

Because too much digitalis has such a profound effect on the appetite, it is sometimes included along with thyroid in "secret" preparations given for weight reduction by disreputable practitioners. The U.S. Food and Drug Administration and the medical profession have condemned such practices. But since digitalis is so readily available for legitimate use in the treatment of heart disorders, there is no effective way to control its unethical administration for weight control other than by patient and doctor education. Whenever you are given a drug to lose weight, insist on knowing all its constituents. Make sure to ask specifically whether it contains digitalis, thyroid, or amphetamines ("uppers"). If it does, refuse to take it.

Another reason I must know whether you're taking any digitalis preparation is to help me evaluate your electrocardiogram. Even in normal persons, this drug produces certain changes in the ECG which look very much like those due to heart disease. That doesn't mean digitalis makes your heart sick—on the contrary. But it does change the appearance of the tracing, and unless I know about it, we will both worry unnecessarily.

Many years ago, in the early days of electrocardiography, a few unscrupulous insurance agents, using the knowledge that digitalis distorts the ECG, defrauded the insurance industry of millions of dollars. Their scheme was to take out large disability policies on derelicts, feed them small amounts of digitalis, arrange to have them complain of cardiac symptoms, and then submit the "abnormal" ECG as evidence of heart trouble.

One final warning about digitalis. Chances for toxicity with this drug are greatly increased if your body levels of potassium are low. Most people never have to worry about that. But diuretic or water pills cause the kidney to excrete potassium along with the water. Be very careful about this possibility if you're taking digitalis.

Sex Hormones—by Needle and Pill

Some men and women take sex hormones "on the side"—that is, they're not formally prescribed. Someone has told them they are good for your sex or keep you young. Female hormones (estrogen) are generally believed to eliminate the hot flushes of the menopause, prolong youthful appearance, improve sex drive, and increase the feeling of general well-being.

Hot Flushes—Physical or Psychological?

As their periods become irregular and finally stop, some women begin to experience "hot flushes." Others, probably the majority, do not. We cannot predict who will and who won't. Measuring hormone levels doesn't help either.

The cause of hot flushes is not fully understood, and there is now even some question whether estrogen replacement really prevents them. For example, a study was recently done with a large number of women who had menopausal symptoms. They were all given pills which they were told contained female hormones. But only half actually received the active prescription. The rest were taking an identical-looking pill which was blank (placebo). The response of both groups were analyzed. To everyone's surprise, those getting the blank had the same reduction in symptoms as did the estrogen-treated group.

Perhaps the lift so many women feel when they take estrogen is psychological, but it is my impression that these hormones do have a beneficial effect. On the negative side, estrogens are strongly suspected of contributing to cancer of the uterus. This, of course, is of no concern to the woman who has had a hysterectomy. Most doctors, however, continue to prescribe replacement female hormone therapy when there is proof that it is needed. The most direct way of obtaining such proof is to get a scraping of the lining of the vagina (it doesn't hurt at all) and to look at it under the microscope. If there is a deficiency of hormone, the vaginal cells have a characteristic appearance. Blood tests can also be used, but these are more expensive and not really necessary for this purpose. If you are taking an estrogen product for any reason, try to make do with the lowest effective dose. Also use it intermittently, stopping for a few days each month. This withdrawal permits shedding of the lining of the uterus, and may theoretically reduce the risk of uterine cancer.

Male Hormones for Potency?

Men take hormones too, usually *testosterone,* to improve sexual performance. Whatever effect this substance has is often psychological, except when levels of male hormone can be shown to be abnormally low. This occurs when the testicles fail to develop owing to an uncommon glandular disorder, or where they have been surgically removed because of tumor or to control cancer of the prostate. But usually, when we actually measure the levels of testosterone, we find them normal in patients complaining of impotence.

Even so, when additional hormone is given to these subjects, some of them improve. How can we explain this if the hormone level was adequate to begin with? Testosterone, in addition to being a male sex hormone, is also a tissue "builder." It improves the appetite, raises the energy level, and so confers a sense of "well-being." This, in itself, can enhance sexual desire and performance quite apart from any direct action on the organs of sex. Also, a "normal" testosterone level is, after all, a matter of statistics. The books tell us the "normal range" of testosterone is 4 to 6 units. This figure was arrived at by testing thousands of apparently normal adult males. Supposing I find the content in your blood is 4.5 Is that normal—for you? Maybe it used to be 5.8 without our knowing it, and then, for some reason, dropped to 4.5 That's still theoretically "within normal limits," but possibly too low for you.

Despite the foregoing, I believe that the action of testosterone in most cases is mainly psychological—a "placebo" effect—and I discourage my own patients from taking it. I do so for several reasons. If a man's impotence is psychological, he ought to try to find out why and work it out. Any benefit from testosterone in such cases will only be temporary. Also, prolonged administration of this hormone means that your own glands will make less, so that ultimately they "atrophy" or wither, and you become dependent on the needle or pill. Finally, many urologists believe that even though testosterone doesn't actually cause cancer of the prostate, taking it may activate a small, dormant tumor which may be present there. Even tumors of the liver (happily, so far nonmalignant) have been reported in men using the male hormone. So, *if you have decided to take testosterone for whatever reason, make sure your prostate is examined every six months.*

The Power of a Placebo

A placebo is an inert substance. Doctors use it when they think your complaints are not "real," but you insist on being treated anyway. Instead of giving you a drug that may hurt you, they give you a blank and tell you it's potent. A patient improving with such "medication" is said to demonstrate the "placebo effect." The power of suggestion is so great, the doctor-patient relationship so special, the will to improve so strong, that under many circumstances such an inert tablet prescribed with enough enthusiasm will produce miraculous "cures."

I remember very vividly one experience I had several years ago. It dramatizes the power of the placebo. A leading drug company had developed a drug reported to be effective in preventing angina pectoris (heart pain on exertion). Our cardiac clinic was asked to evaluate it. A study was designed to eliminate all bias on the part of the doctors and the patients involved. The "medication" was to consist of pills. These were labeled A, B, C, and D. They all looked and tasted identical, but only two contained the active ingredients. The other two were placebos. None of the doctors or patients knew the contents of any of the tablets. One elderly gentleman with severe angina volunteered for the study. He continued taking all his usual medication, but in addition was given tablet C. Ten days later, he returned to the clinic—ecstatic. "You won't believe this," he literally shouted. "I haven't had a single chest pain this last week. It used to hit me at least ten times a day. Now I can walk—even dance. Your new pill is a miracle, doctor."

Of course, I wasn't supposed to be influenced by his story, in order not to affect my scientific neutrality. But I couldn't help conclude that tablet C must contain the active principle. As I interviewed the other patients, it seemed to me that all those getting C were responding, perhaps not as dramatically, but to some extent. The old gentleman continued to improve for the twelve weeks of the study. As we neared the end of the test period, he became concerned that, after it was over, he wouldn't get any more of his "magic" new medicine. I assured him that because of his dramatic response, we would make it available to him one way or another.

When the research project ended, the participating doctors in the clinic met to assess the efficacy of each of the pills (A, B, C, and D) in every patient. We did so before the code was broken. I stated that on the basis of my observations, preparation C was very effective. I wasn't so sure about the three others. Then we opened the sealed envelope. I was wrong. Tablet C was inert. I was stunned. I simply refused to believe it. Convinced the manufacturer had made an error in labeling the various pills, I had them analyzed independently. Sure enough, C was blank. As it turned out, the active substance under study was found not to have any beneficial effect in angina, and never reached the pharmaceutical marketplace. So my old friend really didn't lose out by getting the inert form all those weeks, after all. He had improved dramatically because he hoped and expected to respond well—because he had confidence in his doctors. He not only fooled himself. He fooled me too, perhaps because I was just as anxious for him to get better and was delighted that he did.

Are You Taking Iron for "Tired Blood"?

If you use iron preparations for "tired blood," "bad blood," or "poor blood," you may develop gastric irritation, stomach cramps, constipation, or diarrhea. What's more, you may not even know you're taking it, because so many vitamins also contain iron. Iron turns the stool black—but so does blood in the intestinal tract. (Blood changes in color from red to black as it moves from the stomach all the way down through and out the rectum.) So unless I know you are taking iron, a black stool means you're bleeding somewhere in the gut. But nature can be tricky. I have seen patients with black stools on iron pills who, in addition, are bleeding. So whenever your stools are black, we check them anyway to make sure they don't contain blood.

More serious than the color confusion, taking iron to "perk up tired blood" may mask underlying anemia, just as a cough medicine can obscure serious causes of cough. Anemia is a symptom, not a disease. It means that for one reason or another you're deficient in blood. Instead of simply treating the "low blood," we should first determine what's causing it—malnutrition, chronic blood loss in the stool, an infection somewhere, a malignant tumor, or a disorder in the bone marrow that makes the blood. Do not pay any attention to the advertising that would have you take iron in a certain product because you're "tired" or "anemic." If you feel that way, find out why from your doctor. Temporary masking of such important symptoms may be lethal.

Women tend to be slightly anemic because of a combination of poor dietary iron intake and excessive blood loss during their menstrual periods. They require iron supplements. Men who eat the "normal" Western diet are rarely anemic.

A common source of insidious blood loss in men and women is bleeding hemorrhoids ("piles"). These are dilated veins in the rectum much like the varicose veins you see in legs. They bleed from the irritation and friction of hard stools. After weeks or months, a low-grade anemia develops. Additional iron is prescribed, while the hemorrhoids are treated with stool softeners, suppositories, or some form of surgical intervention.

Are You a Laxative "Junkie"?

It's unfortunate that laxative advertising is permitted—and is so widespread. Turn on the TV and you're likely to see a somber-faced announcer, wearing a white coat to make him look like a doctor, or a movie star (also obviously well qualified) ask you and thirty million others very confidentially if you've moved your bowels today. If not, he's got the answer for you—delicious brand X or Y.

The best way to ensure normal elimination is not to make your bowel dependent on drugs, but to drink enough water, eat plenty of bulk (bran, raw fruit, raw vegetables, potato skins) in your food, and take the time for elimination. So many of us choose the purgative shortcut because we're in too much of a hurry to take a few extra minutes each day to "wait for nature." We end up becoming chronically addicted to laxatives or enemas—a habit that once established is not easy to break.

The sudden need for laxatives may be an important sign of some obstruction in the bowel, usually a growth. Such tumors make their presence known by causing alternating constipation and diarrhea. First you take "something" for the constipation and then attribute the subsequent diarrhea to the laxative.

I have never understood why government regulatory agencies forbid radio and TV advertising of liquor and tobacco, yet permit the sales pitch for iron and laxatives, whose use can delay diagnosis of cancer or other serious disorders.

Are You Taking Thyroid Pills?

If your thyroid gland is sick, diseased, or "sluggish," and not making enough hormone, then you need thyroid supplement. But I'm afraid that most people taking this medication are diet faddists or those with normal thyroid function who wish to become thin. *Such indiscriminate use of thyroid hormone, especially in people with underlying heart disease, can cause heart attacks or serious disturbances of heart rhythm.* If you're taking thyroid not prescribed by your doctor but because a friend recommended it to keep your figure trim, now is a good time to check whether you really need it. Remember that every one of our hormone-producing glands operates on a feedback system. They produce and release their substances when the blood concentration is low. If you take the active principle by mouth, there is a high blood level, and so the gland gets turned off. After a while, it withers from disuse. So never take any hormone—be it thyroid, testosterone, or cortisone—unless you've been tested and told you really need it.

Tranquilizers—"the Road to Miltown"

If you're under an acute emotional stress because of bereavement of a loved one or because of some temporary economic or other personal problem, tranquilizers are helpful. However, don't become dependent on such drugs in order to help you cope over the long term. It's an "escape to nowhere." It's like breaking a leg, then using a crutch or wearing a cast forever. I know that such advice is easier to give than to take, but do try to get some help in understanding and perhaps modifying your life situation—rather than relying on tranquilizers. They not only "hook" you emotionally but can also cause various allergic reactions, usually skin rashes. Some drugs, notably Librium, produce serious side effects when taken in conjunction with alcohol. Others make you sick when you eat cheese. Certain agents like Valium can result in depression, which is then attributed to the emotional disorder for which the tranquilizer was taken in the first place. It's a sad commentary on our times and culture that so many of us need to take "mood modifiers" to function effectively in our environment. As far as I am concerned, the ongoing need for and use of tranquilizers have the same underlying psychological significance as alcoholism and even addiction to "illegal" drugs.

Are You "Artificially" Thin?

If you ask me for an appetite suppressant, chances are I'm going to refuse to give it to you—not because I'm mean or unsympathetic. Pills to reduce your appetite are of limited value, because you will develop a tolerance to them in a few weeks. And that's not worth it, because they can cause nervousness and irritability, insomnia, lack of coordination, increase in blood pressure, and heart palpitations. So they should be especially avoided if you have a nervous disorder, high blood pressure, or heart disease. Most of the appetite suppressants belong to the amphetamine family ("speed") and may be habit-forming or addicting. Sometimes, I weaken and prescribe them for a few weeks to give psychological support and encouragement to fat people trying to lose weight. In my view, however, they have no place in any long-range program of weight reduction.

Are You Taking "Blood Thinners" (Anticoagulants)?

Anticoagulants are prescribed for two major reasons: (1) If you have had open-heart surgery, and are the proud owner of an artificial valve or two, you need an anticoagulant (Coumadin) to keep the blood from clotting on it. (Newer valves may not require anticoagulants indefinitely, but it's too early to be sure.) (2) If you have a tendency to form clots somewhere in your vascular tree (heart, veins, or arteries) and these break up (embolism), sending little pieces where they can do a lot of damage (to the brain, kidneys, lungs, legs), you will need blood thinners for weeks, months, or years.

You're Taking Rat Poison?

Anticoagulants interfere with the normal clotting mechanisms in the blood. In small amounts, they can save your life. Too much can kill you. These agents are so effective they are used as rat poison. The animal bleeds to death from eating too much. *So, if you are taking anticoagulants, you must be closely supervised.*

This involves testing your blood at frequent intervals (usually every three to four weeks) to make sure it's not too thin and not too thick—but just right. If it is too thin you will bleed too easily and can develop internal hemorrhages even after a trivial injury. If not thin enough, the purpose of the treatment is defeated, and then the clot or embolism may recur.

You may wonder why a fixed dose of the anticoagulant can't be given so as to eliminate the bother and expense of frequent checking. There are many reasons. The drug may accumulate. You may develop other disorders, for example, liver disease, which also interfere with blood clotting, giving a summation effect and the risk of hemorrhage. Changes in temperature and the foods you eat may affect the stability of the treatment. Other medications, for example, aspirin, sleeping pills, or antibiotics, can alter the action of the anticoagulant so as to render it either inert or too potent, with the risk of clot or hemorrhage, respectively.

To Thin or Not to Thin, That Is the Question

Whether or not anticoagulants should be used in the treatment of heart attacks was at one time a matter of great controversy. Some doctors felt that they should be administered without exception and be continued indefinitely. Others believed that anticoagulation should be effected for only a few weeks, and then stopped. A third group insisted these drugs should virtually never be given, except perhaps in the most serious cases.

The controversy is by no means over. A few diehards remain in each of the camps. Most cardiologists, however, prescribe anticoagulants in acute heart attacks only when you appear to be at special risk for developing blood clots in the veins for example, if you are fat or have heart failure, or your heart rhythm is very irregular, so that confinement to bed may lead to sludging of blood and clot formation in the legs.

There is a new and very interesting use for anticoagulants you should know about. It involves small amounts of a short-acting blood thinner called heparin. One of the major risks of surgery, especially in the elderly, is the risk of clot formation and embolism. It has been found that when very small doses of heparin are given—not so much as to cause bleeding, but enough to slow down the clotting tendency just a little—the incidence of such embolism is reduced.

Are You Taking Water Pills, and Why?

Diuretics, or "water pills," as they are popularly called, may be prescribed for several reasons—to eliminate excessive fluid which accumulates in heart, liver, or kidney disease; to lower high blood pressure; and to decrease the pressure within the eyes in glaucoma. They are also useful in eliminating some of the fluid retained prior to the menstrual period. If you are taking diuretics regularly to lose weight, you're only kidding yourself. Even though you may in fact drop three or four pounds, that's only tissue water. The real culprit in obesity is fat, on which diuretics have no effect. The tissue fluid soon reaccumulates, and you regain the weight. So you take a diuretic again, and the seesaw pattern recurs. This whole up-and-down exercise is not only fruitless, it may also present problems. The water that leaves the body as urine takes with it potassium, so that chronic use of diuretics can cause potassium deficiency. This in turn may lead to muscle weakness, leg cramps, lethargy, and cardiac rhythm disorders. If you happen to be taking digitalis, you may become toxic to that drug as well.

Diuretics, Diabetes, and Gout

Chronic and frequent use of diuretics, especially in high dosage, may cause other problems as well. The water you lose when you take one of these pills is due to its action on the kidney. As you will see later, one of the most important functions of the kidney is to regulate water and salt balance in the body. It decides what volume of fluid is to be retained, and how much should be excreted in the urine. Diuretics interfere with this process, paralyzing salt and water reabsorption. They also raise the uric acid level in the blood, which occasionally will produce acute attacks of *gout* (a form of arthritis which causes severe pain of a joint such as the big toe, heel, elbow, wrist). So it's important that I know whether you are using or abusing diuretics.

One final side effect of water pills you should know about is their potential for raising blood sugar, causing a chemical type of *diabetes*. This becomes important if you already have this disorder or suddenly develop it.

Are You Taking the "Pill"—and Should You Be?

Few discoveries in medicine have had a greater impact on the human race than the "pill," introduced in 1955 (at about the same time as the miniskirt). It has emancipated women from the constant fear of and the social, economic, and physical risks of unwanted pregnancies and from clumsy, less esthetic and less effective methods of contraception. It has made population control a reality, revolutionized our sexual mores, and constitutes a cornerstone of the women's "liberation" movement.

A woman's main interest in the "pill" is whether it is effective and safe. With respect to its efficacy, you need not worry. When taken properly, it is virtually foolproof—close to 100 percent sure. Of course, those who cannot understand or follow instructions should use other forms of contraception, for example, an intrauterine device or a diaphragm.

How Does the "Pill" Work?

Despite what you may read or hear about its dangers and side effects, the "pill" is safe, inexpensive, and the most easily transportable, desirable form of contraception available. And how it does the job is fascinating too. The oral contraceptive is composed basically of two different female hormones. These operate on the same kind of feedback principle as do other hormones like thyroid, insulin, or cortisone. The sex and reproductive hormones have an axis with the brain, which controls how much female hormone is made and its function. For a baby to be conceived and born, certain requirements have to be met. First of all, an egg has to be released by the ovary. Then the sperm must be able to get into the tube to fertilize it. Finally, the egg must have a suitable place within the uterus to settle down and grow.

The "pill" interferes with all three requirements. One of its ingredients gets into the blood and turns on the feedback mechanism which then stops the brain from making the hormone that will release the egg. So the prime requirement of pregnancy is not met—no egg. But should that not work, the hormone in the "pill" makes the cervix very sticky with mucus, so the sperm has a hard time getting in even if there were an egg. Finally, in the very unlikely event that fertilization should occur, the hormones act directly on the lining of the uterus, where the fertilized egg develops. It makes it barren and unable to sustain growth and development of the embryo. All in all, a triple whammy.

Hazards of the "Pill"

Fifteen million women in the United States take oral contraceptives. What are the hazards, and how commonly do they occur? The "pill" can cause high blood pressure. It can induce blood clotting, usually in the veins of the leg (*phlebitis*). If a piece of this clot breaks off and travels to the lung (embolism), serious illness or death may result. But the overall incidence of phlebitis among women taking low-estrogen oral contraceptives is only 81 for every 100,000, as compared with 50 per 100,000 in non-users—not much difference. Between the ages of 20 and 34, one death due to phlebitis occurs in every 50,000 women taking the "pill."

So much for the "pill" and its effects on veins. It can also involve the arteries, so that its use is associated with a higher risk for developing a stroke (especially if you have migraine headaches) or a heart attack (if your blood pressure is high, if you smoke cigarettes, or if you're over 40 years of age). *But if you don't have migraine and your blood pressure is normal, if you don't smoke and are under 40, the danger of the "pill" is so small it is not even statistically definable—and certainly can in no way be compared with the many risks of an unwanted pregnancy.*

Despite the fact that oral contraceptives contain estrogen, which is under some suspicion for causing cancer of the uterus and possibly the breast, there have been no cases of cancer thus far attributed to the "pill" among the millions of women who use it. Several instances of benign liver tumors have been observed, but these are not life-threatening.

Side Effects of the "Pill"

There are some possible side effects you should know about which are uncomfortable or objectionable, but are not dangerous to you. For example, the "pill" can cause weight gain (a benefit to some very thin women) and fluid retention so that you may feel bloated taking it. Certain preparations containing a male type of hormone like testosterone in addition to the usual female hormones may cause hair loss and growth of hair on the face. Occasionally, when you're ready to have children and no longer use contraceptives, the normal cycle does not return for several months and you may then need hormonal treatment to restore fertility. Oral contraceptives may cause chronic nausea and vomiting. Enlargement of the breasts may be troublesome but some "Twiggy-like" women are delighted with this secondary effect. A common and subtle side effect is mental depression and impaired sexual drive (but in some women there is the reverse effect). Some women develop a brownish pigmentation on the upper lip (the moustache area) or on the cheekbones, similar to the discoloration sometimes seen during pregnancy. Most of these side effects clear up when you switch to another brand.

The pill is here to stay. No matter the nausea or other side effects—most women prefer it to any other form of contraception. It's the only form of birth control that's transferable from one woman to the next. Most of the preparations marketed today are very similar and work the same way. So if you've lost your pills somewhere or left them at home on a holiday, or your dog has eaten them, or your maid has accidentally flushed them down the toilet, you can always borrow enough to tide you over from a neighbor or friend.

Incidentally, the pill has uses other than birth control. It helps regulate the cycle, shortens the flow, and often does away with menstrual cramps. It also makes it possible for you to schedule and reschedule your period for whatever reason—marriages and holidays need not be planned so rigidly anymore by today's emancipated woman.

What does all this add up to in terms of whether you should use the pill or some other contraceptive method? My advice is that if you are forty years of age or older, you should not use oral contraceptives. Below forty, if you have no vascular disease or high blood pressure, it is the preferred technique—safe, effective and esthetic. *At any age, if you are on the pill, you should have regular examinations, at least twice a year by your gynecologist.*

Narcotics, and the Problem of Drug Addiction

The illegal use of hard drugs (cocaine, codeine, heroin, morphine, demerol) is a serious, widespread, and apparently growing problem. Its management is, for the most part, beyond the capability of the medical profession. The basis of any solution requires action by government for more effective prevention of the distribution and sale of narcotics, the establishment of drug withdrawal clinics and rehabilitation centers, and the elimination of social conditions that breed the need for drugs. Doctors can help in the education process, especially among the young, emphasizing and publicizing all the medical hazards of addiction. These range from behavioral abnormalities (living one's life on a constant "trip") to blood and liver poisoning, coma, and death.

Doctors themselves can and sometimes do create addicts unwittingly by prescribing narcotic pain-killers for chronic conditions. For example, suppose you have a "bad back," arthritis, or recurrent tension headaches. It takes much less time and involvement with your problem to prescribe some codeine or Demerol or Talwin than to arrange for physiotherapy, orthopedic support, or psychiatric consultation. You begin to depend on these narcotic agents more and more, until finally you're hooked. Potent pain-killers have an important role in short-term situations, such as the first few days after an operation, or in the management of the pain of advanced cancer where addiction will present no problem, but not in a chronic disorder which may continue for years.

How to Get to Sleep

Most of us, from time to time, have trouble getting to sleep because of some acute problem, worry, pain, anxiety, illness, or exhilaration and excitement. Under these special circumstances, we may take "something." But *dependence* on sleeping pills, taking them by force of habit every night of your life, can create difficulties. Most of these drugs are habituating; are not very well tolerated in the elderly, in whom they can cause depression of brain function with resulting confusion and "senility"; are associated with hangovers the next day; and carry the risk of unintentional overdosage. Every now and then we hear about someone found dead in bed, beside an empty bottle of sleeping pills—presumably a suicide. Although most of these cases are due to a deliberate overdose, some are not. Death may be the result of a phenomenon called "automatism." You are restless, can't get to sleep, so you take a sleeping pill. You wait, impatiently, and still awake, you take another tablet. In a little while, you are groggy, but not quite asleep. You can't remember how many pills you've taken, so you reach out to take just one more—perhaps, one too many. We know about this mechanism from thousands of people who have been resuscitated and who have been able to tell us how it all happened. *So if you are in the habit of taking something to help you sleep, keep only one extra pill on your night table—and the bottle in the medicine cabinet.*

All Sleeping Pills Are Not the Same

There are several types of sleeping pills, the commonest of which are the *barbiturates* (Seconal, phenobarbital, Nembutal, Tuinal, Amytal). They vary in how fast they get you to sleep and for how long they keep you asleep ("short-acting" and "long-act-ing"). Barbiturates may have a paradoxical effect in older persons, who then become excitable or irritable rather than sleepy.

As with so many other agents, the body has a mechanism for getting rid of these medications. That's what makes it possible to take one or two pills every day. If we didn't "metabolize" or ex-crete these preparations, one pill would last a lifetime, and we'd be sleeping through all of it. The kidneys and liver are responsi-ble for eliminating sleeping pills once they've served their pur-pose. But when these organs are not working well, the drug ac-cumulates in the body, resulting in drowsiness the next day, a chronic hangover, or constant fatigue.

There are *nonbarbiturate* sleeping pills that are relatively safe and well tolerated in most age groups, the best known of which are chloral hydrate and Dalmane. I avoid prescribing Doriden, another synthetic, because a relatively modest overdose may be serious.

Many drugs not generally classed as sleeping pills can also re-lax you and help you fall asleep. These include commonly used tranquilizers like meprobamate (Equanil, Miltown), Librium, and Valium. Antihistamines (Phenergan, Benadryl) will help you sleep too, with less risk of dangerous overdose and none of ha-bituation.

A source of friction between doctor and patient used to be the number of sleeping pills dispensed. "C'mon, doc, let me have at least two hundred. Nothing's going to happen to me. I hate to bother you every month for a new prescription. You're not worried about me committing suicide, are you?" And you were generally offended if I refused—which I always did. But now the government has helped both of us out of this quandary by limiting to one month's supply the number of sleeping pills and tranquilizers I am allowed to give you. That's still enough to hurt you were you to take them all at once, but not quite as bad as the full bottle of one or two hundred.

ALLERGIES

Food and Drug Allergies

Be sure to tell me, if I don't ask you first, about any drugs and foods to which you are sensitive. It is vital that I have this information. Should an emergency situation arise, when you may need important or lifesaving drugs in a hurry and are not in a position to indicate such sensitivity, the results can be disastrous.

Substances most likely to give you a sensitivity reaction are the antibiotics and tranquilizers. *But remember, you can be allergic to any medicine.* I have reported in the medical literature the case of a woman with asthma who nearly died after she took a single aspirin tablet. This is not to imply that all people with asthma are sensitive to aspirin, but if you are generally allergic, you should be very careful about any drug you take.

An allergic response may be mild and chronic, giving us ample time to recognize the symptoms and discontinue the drug. However, it may also be sudden and life-threatening. Examples of reversible and usually harmless reactions are skin rash, hives, or itching. However, allergic responses are not limited to the skin. They may affect the lungs (asthma), the gut (diarrhea), the blood (bleeding), the liver (jaundice)—and so on. Quinidine, commonly used for the treatment of an irregular heartbeat, can cause a host of side effects and allergic reactions. These include fever, diarrhea, skin rashes, disturbances of the blood count, and noises in the ears. The diarrhea may be so subtle that you may not associate it with the drug.

Certain x-rays of the kidney, gallbladder, brain, or heart require that you be given dyes by injection in order for us to be able to visualize the organ being studied. Because these dyes occasionally cause a massive, potentially life-threatening reaction, you will always be questioned for sensitivity to the dye before receiving it. If you have previously had an untoward reaction, you will be given antihistamines and cortisone-type drugs to prevent an acute allergic reaction.

Cross-Sensitization (Two-Way Allergy)

"Cross-sensitivity" means that if you are allergic to one agent, you may also be sensitive to another which has similar but not identical chemical properties. For example, if penicillin gives you a rash or asthma, you may also react badly to related antibiotics like Ampicillin or Keflin.

Medication is not the only cause of allergy. You may be allergic to substances in the air you breathe (molds, pollen, and other pollutants); the clothes you wear (wool, nylon, fur); the foods you eat (shellfish, strawberries, milk, wheat, eggs, pork, and many others); your cosmetics (perfumes, soaps, deodorants, hair dyes); and the animals in your home (dogs, cats, birds).

Defense Systems

The phenomenon of *allergy* is an example of how your body wastes one of its defense mechanisms against a harmless substance. Man is endowed with several complicated systems of defense, which help overcome real dangers in our environment—usually infections. When a noxious agent attacks us—for example, a bacteria, virus, or environmental poison of some kind—the body forms "antibodies." These take up positions in the blood and other organs in order to neutralize the invader. When these antibodies come in contact with the attacking substance, a chemical called a "mediator" is released. It is the mediator that causes allergic symptoms—the tearing eyes, stuffy nose, skin rash, narrowed airways which cause wheezing. The best-known mediator is histamine. There is no apparent reason for the body to mount such a spirited defensive reaction against most of the things to which we are allergic. What possible harm can come of a strawberry or a shrimp? And why some of us react this way to some challenge and others don't remains a mystery.

Allergic Symptoms—Subtle or Obvious

When a cause-and-effect relationship is obvious, we know we are allergic. Suppose you eat a lobster and later in the evening break out in hives; the association is clear. Or if you put on some perfume and hours later begin to itch, that's also pretty easy to figure out. But there are allergic responses so mild and delayed as to go unrecognized as such. For example, a perpetually "nervous stomach" or chronic diarrhea may mean you are allergic to some food. If you always seem to have a "cold," you may have an allergy to an inhalant. If you're a "sniffer" with a permanently stuffy nose and dry cough, before blaming "sinus trouble," "air pollution," or "born that way," make sure you are not in contact with a bird, cat, dog, hamster, or horse—at home or at work.

If you're allergic to something in your environment, but aren't quite sure what it is, you can be skin-tested to find out. Unfortunately, allergic persons often react positively to almost every substance they're tested for, so that limits the usefulness of these tests. If we think something you're eating is the culprit, we stop your regular diet—and reintroduce one food at a time until we hit upon the one that's giving you the trouble.

Treating Your Allergies

The treatment of an allergic response can be either simple or complicated. For example, if the offending material is a specific hair wash, soap, dye, or perfume, you just avoid it. If you can't wear wool, wear synthetics. If you can't eat crabmeat, eat chicken. If you're allergic to your dog, much as it hurts, you'll have to find another home for him. But if you are allergic to something you can't avoid—like the air you breathe—then you may need pills (antihistamines) and drugs to break the spasm in your bronchial tubes (bronchodilators such as Tedral, Quibron, aminophylline). If the acute allergic reaction swells your vocal cords, you may suddenly have difficulty breathing, and that may require an emergency injection of adrenaline or cortisone to save your life. Some allergic persons require desensitizing shots, the principle of which is to keep challenging you with tiny amounts of the allergic material. You are given too little to make you sick, yet enough for your body to get used to, so that hopefully it will stop trying to defend itself against a really harmless substance. These treatments are long, costly, and not always effective.

REVIEWING YOUR GENERAL HEALTH

Your *past medical history*—what illnesses you had as a child, whether you were ever sick enough to be in hospital, a list of your operations or serious injuries—has an important bearing on your current health assessment, as you will see below.

Diseases It's Better to Have When You're Young

Some of the diseases you had as a child can cause complications later in life. Equally important, the ones you didn't have leave you vulnerable to contracting them in adult life, when they are usually more serious. For example, the symptoms of measles and mumps in the young are almost always fairly mild. Once you've had these infections, you become immune to them. But should you get them as an adult, you may suffer serious complications involving the brain and lungs (measles) or the testicles (mumps), causing sterility. Fortunately, immunization against both infections is now available, and should be part of the routine immunization schedule of all children. When a little girl gets German measles, all she has is a fever, a faint rash, and some painful glands in the back of the neck. But if she contracts this illness as a pregnant adult, she may very well give birth to a deformed child.

Rheumatic Fever Licks the Joints and Bites the Heart

Rheumatic fever is a childhood disease that can produce important symptoms later in life. The villain of the piece is a germ called *streptococcus*, which first strikes the throat, making it very sore—the famous "strep throat." But this is only a diversionary tactic. The real damage is done later, as a result of the heart and joints becoming allergic to some substance in the streptococcus. A few weeks after the throat is all better, the joints become tender and swollen. These symptoms last a few days or weeks, and are sometimes mistaken for "growing pains" or a "charley-horse," so that if you're asked whether you had rheumatic fever during childhood, you may deny it, not knowing that you did.

Along with the throat and joints, the heart is also involved. This may not be as obvious as a swollen knee or elbow, and may be undetected early in the disease. Years later, long after the sore throats and joint pains have been forgotten, the result of the allergic process which has been smoldering all along in the heart becomes apparent as a heart murmur due to a deformity of one or more heart valves. So rheumatic fever "licks the joints and bites the heart."

The diseased valves, in addition to affecting the way the heart functions (as you will see later, they leak and/or get stuck), are also very vulnerable to infection. A germ anywhere in the body, harmless under normal circumstances, can find a home in these valves and cause a very serious disease called *acute* or *subacute infective endocarditis* (we used to call it "bacterial" until we discovered that fungi can also attack the valves). This was almost always fatal before the availability of antibiotics, but can now usually be prevented or, if it occurs, cured. Trivial dental procedures, especially those involving the gums, can result in the usually innocent germs in the mouth getting into the bloodstream, traveling to and infecting a deformed valve. That's why a child who has had rheumatic fever must undergo very careful annual examinations to see whether a murmur has appeared. If it has, he must then be started on continuous antibiotics, usualiy penicillin (unless he is allergic to it), which are continued into adult life. In addition, any unexplained infection, fever, sore throat, or any operation (including simple dental work) must be covered with additional antibiotics to prevent infection of the rheumatic heart valves.

Unlike measles, mumps, German measles, diphtheria, and the other important diseases of childhood, there is no vaccine against rheumatic fever. But there is penicillin, as a result of which the incidence of this disease is dropping dramatically. All it takes is early recognition of the strep throat and its prompt eradication with penicillin.

Your Previous Operations

I want to know what previous surgery you've had. Why don't I wait until I examine you? Because not all operations leave a scar. Suppose you complain of "gas" or a feeling of fullness after eating. My first suspicion is gallbladder disease. But if your gallbladder has been removed, it makes this diagnosis less likely. Not impossible, mind you, because even though the gallbladder itself has been removed, the ducts that carry the bile from the liver to the gut are left intact. Years after the operation, they may form gravel or stones and give symptoms identical with those of an acute gallbladder attack.

Whether or not your appendix has been removed is important too, because right lower abdominal pain is a common symptom of chronic appendicitis. If the appendix has been taken out, this diagnosis is no longer tenable, and I will have to look elsewhere for an explanation of your symptoms. Adhesions, the formation of scar tissue after the operation, sometimes causes such pain.

If your uterus has been taken out (hysterectomy), it is important to know whether the ovaries have been removed as well. If they were spared, your "femininity" is unchanged, since female hormone is produced by the ovaries, not the uterus. If you have only one ovary left, or even a small portion of one, you still have enough female hormone to prevent you from becoming menopausal. If, however, both ovaries have been taken out, you will abruptly undergo "change of life" (surgical menopause). You now become vulnerable not only to the "hot flushes" but also to the arteriosclerotic heart disease (hardening of the arteries) which is uncommon in women before the menopause.

HOW WELL YOUR BODY SYSTEMS FUNCTION

We now systematically go through a series of questions together. These are designed and organized to assess the function of all the major systems of your body—the heart and circulation, lungs, glands, bones and joints, skin, nervous system, digestive tract, and reproductive system. I will be probing for symptoms of which either you are unaware until asked, or you think are of no significance, and so don't volunteer them. I will be asking you about things that I can't see, feel, or hear for myself—like pain, cough, shortness of breath, change in bowel habits, or intermittent bleeding.

That which troubles you is called a *symptom;* what I observe is a *sign.* Symptoms usually develop long before signs become apparent. *For every diagnosis based on physical examination and tests, ten are made first by a careful history-taking.* A classical example is angina pectoris, which may be present for years before the clinical examination or even the electrocardiogram become abnormal. In cancer of the bowel, a change in your bowel habits which only you can tell me about often precedes the weight loss, bloody stool, and abdominal pain which are the late—maybe too late— evidences of the disease.

ALL ABOUT THE SKIN

Itching

There is no point asking you if you have a rash because in a few minutes, during the physical examination, I will see for myself. And even though an itch is not visible, the scratch marks are. If you do itch, chances are it's because you're reacting to your body soap or laundry detergent, the clothes you wear, your cosmetics, something you're eating, or a medication. It may be that you're bathing too often and drying your skin too much. (I have not seen patients itch from dirty skin.) There is also a serious disorder in which the flow of bile from the liver to the intestines is blocked. The retained bile backs up into the blood (jaundice) and makes the skin feel very itchy. Also, when the kidneys are severely damaged, waste products retained in the body (uremia) cause itching.

You may not itch all over, but just in one area—for example, in the vagina (often caused by anxiety but also by certain ointments or lotions, infections, or diabetes), around the anus (again possibly from nervousness but also from piles, worms, fungi or the irritation of chronic diarrhea), in the armpits (from your deodorant), or the face (due to the soap or cosmetic you're using). Some people are sensitive to light and develop itching on the face or other areas exposed to the sun.

Do You Perspire Easily?

The key word here is "easily." All of us sweat, depending on where we are, what we're doing, the temperature of our environment, and how we're dressed. But is your sweating appropriate? Do you have beads of perspiration on your face when everyone else in the room is bone dry?

Excessive perspiration occurs in those areas of the body that are most richly endowed with sweat glands—namely, the palms, the soles, the armpits, and the genital area. Its commonest cause, even in a cold room, is nervous tension—the "cold sweat." An overactive thyroid gland also makes you perspire, but then you feel warm. If you're a menopausal woman with too little female hormone, or a man with too much (because you have cancer of the prostate and are being given estrogens), you may have attacks of "hot flushes." But unlike hyperthyroidism, in which the skin is always hot and wet, it remains normally dry and cool between flushes. Other causes of excessive sweating are fever, an infection somewhere, alcohol, and drugs. Sweating that occurs mostly at night raises the suspicion of active tuberculosis.

If you sweat in only one side of the body, like an arm, hand, or leg, the cause is probably some kind of brain disease, spinal cord damage, or an injured nerve. In leprosy there are local areas of decreased sweating.

For every characteristic of man, there is always some neurosis—and sweating is no exception. There is a psychiatric disorder in which the unfortunate patient is convinced that his perspiration is foul-smelling, even when it actually is not—and nothing will convince him otherwise. When the sweat does smell bad, review your diet. Been eating too much garlic and too many onions?

THE HEAD

Do You Suffer from Headaches?

The most common cause of *recurring headache*, especially in the back of the head and neck, is muscle spasm due to nervous tension. This is often aggravated by, or the result of, underlying arthritis of the spine high up in the neck. Heat, rest, tranquilizers, and aspirin usually give relief.

Even though the great majority of headaches are nothing to worry about, if they have come on abruptly without apparent reason and persist for more than a few days, they should be investigated. "Eyestrain," contrary to popular belief, is not a common source of headache although it can be. I haven't seen many of the symptoms disappear with a change of glasses. Another popular misconception is that high blood pressure always causes headache. That's not so. Hypertension often produces no symptoms but may give headache. And that's important for you to know. If you mistakenly believe that just because you don't have headaches, your pressure can't be high, you may not have it checked as often as you should.

The Many Faces of Headache

I can usually tell from your description whether or not your headache reflects something serious. For example, if it is relieved in just a few minutes by a couple of aspirin tablets, the chances are it's due to *tension*. If it is situated above one eye, it's probably from *sinusitis*. *Stomach upset* may give you a throbbing head pain which gets better when you lie down. If the headache comes on suddenly, it may be due to *neuralgia* (inflammation or irritation of the nerves in the skull), but if it is worsened with movement of the eyes, the cause may be either *eyestrain* or perhaps *glaucoma* (increased pressure within the eyeball—a serious disorder which, if untreated, can lead to blindness). Headache due to *high blood pressure* is apt to be throbbing. If the pain awakens you or becomes worse at night or when you're lying down, we have to consider the possibility of a *brain tumor*. In that event, the area of the skull overlying the tumor is frequently tender. Headache in the morning just after you awaken is often due to an overheated or poorly ventilated bedroom.

Migraine, a Special Kind of Headache

Women are more susceptible than men to migraine headache. This disorder quite commonly runs in families, and starts fairly early in life, usually between 10 and 35 years of age. The typical attack affects one side of the head and lasts several hours, but may continue for days. If severe, it is accompanied by nausea and vomiting. The onset of a migraine headache is very characteristic. Before the pain, there is usually some visual phenomenon, like flashing or bright lights, photophobia (sensitivity to light), even transient blindness. This is the warning, or "prodrome," and is followed hours later by the headache itself.

The prevention and treatment of migraine are not one of medicine's success stories. We think the headache results from spasm and narrowing of the arteries inside the brain and dilation or widening of the external vessels in the scalp. Drugs like ergotamine (Cafergot), if taken the moment symptoms appear, may abort the attack or make it less painful. Sansert, specifically developed for the prevention but not the treatment of migraine, is often effective, but over the long term it may cause serious side effects. Its use is therefore limited to the most severe cases. Breathing high concentrations of oxygen, taking tranquilizers, using the drug Inderal, have all been reported to help. But like so many other maladies for which everyone has his own "cure," treatment is really not effective.

If you've been suffering from migraine all these years, and are in your forties, I have good news for you. Most attacks begin to taper and stop after 50 years of age.

Importance of the Unimportant Head Injury

A serious and not uncommon cause of headache, especially in older persons or those taking anticoagulants, is a slight blow on the head. This may result in oozing from a blood vessel inside the skull, but outside the brain. The blood gradually forms a pocket called a *subdural hematoma,* which gets bigger and bigger, and then presses on the brain. Headache is the first symptom, but later there may be lack of coordination, personality change, and other neurological consequences. Unless we think about this possibility, such patients may simply be diagnosed as having a stroke or "mental condition"—especially if they're old—and that's that. A great pity too, because when the cause is recognized, the patient can be cured by simply sucking up the old blood through a small hole in the skull.

During my medical internship, I worked in a mental hospital for a few months. One of the inmates, a previously successful businessman, had been committed as psychotic because of a gradual deterioration in his behavior. After several years he died. At autopsy, he was found to have a subdural hematoma, which, had it been correctly diagnosed, could easily have been cured.

My questions to you about headaches are therefore likely to include the following: Are they accompanied by visual changes? (Possible migraine.) Are they one-sided? (May be due to migraine, localized tumor or other abnormalities within the brain, or sinusitis.) Do they throb? (Suggests elevated blood pressure.) Do they awaken you at night? (May reflect a serious rather than a trivial cause.) Do they hurt most in the back of the head and neck, and does aspirin relieve them? (Very likely anxiety, nervous tension, or arthritis of the spine.)

Do You Have Fainting Spells, Attacks of Dizziness, or Vertigo?

All of us feel dizzy, light-headed, or giddy from time to time, usually because of emotional stress, fatigue, hot weather, something we ate or drank, or a "virus." *Vertigo* (the feeling the room is rotating around you or that you are spinning around some object in it) is less common, and not quite the same symptom as *dizziness*, although it may have similar underlying causes. *Fainting* (syncope), a temporary loss of consciousness, is the most dramatic of this group of complaints. Its significance depends on the circumstances under which it occurs, your age, and whether or not you are known to have an underlying disorder of the heart or brain.

Dizziness, vertigo, and fainting are usually due to trouble in the inner ear, to brain disease like epilepsy or tumor, or to the fact that the brain is not getting enough blood, usually because of hardening of its arteries.

Structures in the inner ear called the *labyrinths* regulate posture by sending signals to the brain indicating our position in space from moment to moment. When the labyrinths are not functioning properly, because of a virus (viral labyrinthitis) or other infection, or because their blood supply is reduced by arteriosclerosis of the arteries feeding them, the result is dizziness or vertigo. Such an attack is often so sudden and severe you may not even be able to raise your head off the pillow. The viral variety usually follows a cold and clears up in a few days.

The Danger of Lowering Blood Pressure Fast

There are several different ways in which blood supply to the brain may be so reduced as to cause temporary dizziness or loss of consciousness. One of these is an abrupt drop in blood pressure. This is more apt to happen in older people, especially those with narrowed arteries supplying the brain.

If you are taking pills to control high blood pressure, they may sometimes lower it too much and too fast, especially when you change position quickly, as from lying to standing or sitting. This will leave you dizzy or make you faint. Even without medication, if your pressure is low, sudden postural changes may also induce fainting. This does not necessarily mean you are sick. Neither is the Grenadier Guard outside Buckingham Palace (or any other healthy soldier on ceremonial duty) who, standing rigidly at attention for several hours, finally keels over in a dead faint. In this case, blood that should be returning up to the brain is being kept down in the motionless legs by gravity. Why all the heroines in Victorian novels fainted, I'm not sure. In those days, it was considered "feminine" to swoon, part of the myth of the delicate female. It was, in fact, probably due to the tight girdle and bodice, constricting the veins and preventing the return of blood to the heart and brain.

If you have angina pectoris and take nitroglycerine (the little tablet you see some people putting under the tongue), you may faint because of a sharp drop in pressure caused by the tablet. That's why you should always sit down before taking a "nitro."

Another serious cause of decreased blood supply to the brain is disease of the aortic valve, which opens every time the heart contracts, permitting the blood to exit. When this valve is distorted and narrowed for any reason (one of the most common being chronic rheumatic fever), so that it does not open widely enough, too little blood leaves the heart. The supply is now inadequate to sustain the muscles and brain during exercise—and such patients "faint" too.

There are other interesting circumstances in which fainting may occur. In persons with chronic bronchitis, a paroxysm of cough suddenly shifts enough blood away from the brain and induces loss of consciousness ("cough syncope"). "Micturition syncope" occurs in men who have been lying in bed and who have a full bladder. When they stand and start to void, they faint.

How Your Heart Rate Affects Your Brain

The brain may also be deprived of blood when your heart abruptly beats too fast, too slowly, or not at all. The normal heart contracts rhythmically 60 to 90 times a minute. If it suddenly slows to 40 per minute or less, there is a decrease of blood to the brain—and dizziness. A further drop will make you unconscious. For example, if there is no flow of blood to the brain for three to six seconds, you will feel faint; in only eight to ten seconds, you will lose consciousness. Permanent brain damage occurs after four or five minutes, and death thereafter.

If the heart suddenly speeds up to a very rapid rate, so that there isn't enough time for it to fill with blood between beats, the net result is the same as too slow a rate. The brain is deprived of oxygen, and dizziness or loss of consciousness may occur, depending on how fast the heart is actually beating.

Why Some People Faint at the Sight of Blood

Chronic "fainters" usually have an exaggerated response to emotional or stressful situations, sometimes as trivial as the sight of blood, especially their own. The stimulus, whatever it may be, drops the blood pressure suddenly. The patient faints. As soon as the body hits the floor, neutralizing the effect of gravity so that blood flows once more from the legs to the brain, the faint ends. Many such attacks occur in relation to meals, especially if the dining room or restaurant is warm and stuffy, with a lot of tobacco smoke in the air and alcohol in the stomach. Doctors call it "vasovagal syncope."

It May Not Be a Heart Attack at All

The "fainter" presents a frightening picture—especially these days when we're all conditioned to expect the worst. He is pale, cold, and clammy. His pulse is slow, less than 60 per minute. It really does look like a heart attack. The greatest danger today of such a harmless faint is that it will happen in the presence of someone who is very anxious to do a little cardiac resuscitation. Instead of being allowed to recover spontaneously in a couple of minutes, the helpless victim is pounced upon by the vigorous and well-meaning "lifesaver," who will pound the chest, do mouth-to-mouth breathing, and perform other maneuvers. If the victim survives all this, he may well be left with a few unnecessarily broken ribs—an example of how the road to hell is paved with good intentions. But it could be worse. In the 1700's a popular technique of resuscitation was to fill an animal bladder with smoke and blow it into the victim's rectum.

If you witness someone collapsing in a public place, before you do anything dramatic, first check the pulse and look to see if the "victim" is breathing. If you can count the pulse at the neck (or anywhere else that's convenient, like the wrist) and you see the chest rise and fall—leave him alone. He'll come to.

Remember then that dizziness and fainting may be trivial or serious. As I question you, I will usually be able to determine the cause. As a rule, however, the onset of these symptoms after age 40 often requires a series of diagnostic tests to be described later.

Do You Have Ringing or Buzzing in the Ears?

Noise in the ears (*tinnitus*) is a common complaint, especially among persons 60 years of age or older. You may perceive it as a hissing, banging, roaring, buzzing, ringing, or clicking. It may be constant or intermittent; you may have some loss of hearing with it or vertigo; it may not bother you very much or it may "drive you crazy."

Tinnitus has several causes. Before I get you involved in a costly diagnostic workup, I'll first make sure you don't have some local disease of the ear or wax in your ear canals, which gives a bubbling or crackling sound. On rare occasions, noise in the head is due to a brain tumor. If that's the case, it's usually heard in only one ear and accompanied by rapid loss of hearing on the affected side. Tinnitus may be caused by drugs like quinidine, aspirin, or streptomycin. If your blood pressure is very high, you may hear a rhythmic pounding, synchronous with each heartbeat, when you are lying down. Patients with anemia sometimes hear such noises. They clear up when the anemia is treated. All these possibilities have to be considered, but when all's said and done, the garden variety of tinnitus is due either to Ménière's disease (an inner ear disorder) or to hardening of the arteries in and around the ear. This does not necessarily mean that the arteriosclerosis is widespread or that you are going to have a stroke.

Persons with tinnitus are so troubled and worried about it they go from doctor to doctor (usually ear specialists or neurologists) looking for a cure. Take my advice. Avoid fruitless, expensive redundant consultations. All you need is one good examination to tell you where the trouble is—and isn't. Don't waste your money on medication. There is none that will stop these noises. They either clear up spontaneously, become intermittent or, if due to blood vessel disease, remain chronic. If that happens, you will finally adjust to it so that you are no longer aware of the noise.

Do You Ever Have Double Vision (Diplopia)?

You may see double out of one or both eyes, especially when you're so tired your eye muscles are too weak to focus. This symptom may also be due to local disease of the eye, like a cataract. From time to time it occurs in patients who have a generalized muscle problem like myasthenia gravis, in which the eye muscles are simply too weak to focus properly. Migraine attacks may cause double vision, as can any form of brain disease. *But the most ominous cause of diplopia is narrowing of the blood vessels somewhere in the brain. Strokes are often preceded weeks or months by attacks of double vision which usually last only for seconds or minutes.* Such a developing stroke may cause other neurological symptoms, so I will ask whether in addition to the double vision you also have loss of sensation or temporary weakness in an arm or leg, or transient slurring of speech. If you do, we will try to prevent the impending stroke with anticoagulants or surgery.

Is Your Memory Deteriorating?

The ability to recall recent events or names is sometimes gradually and insidiously lost with advancing age. We don't understand why it strikes some people relatively early in life and others hardly at all.

Memory loss in older persons is due to a change in brain function. This can occur in several ways. Its arteries may become narrowed and carry less blood to the oxygen-dependent nervous tissue. Perhaps some small strokes went unrecognized. There may even be chemical changes within the brain, either drug-induced or associated with aging ("degenerative process"). Whatever the reason, the memory defect may not be striking at first and progresses so slowly that it is not immediately apparent to the casual observer. Characteristically, events in the distant past are well remembered, while something that happened a day or two ago is forgotten.

Grace Kelly Is Not the President

The subject will typically reminisce with great accuracy and detail about how he knew Teddy Roosevelt or Woodrow Wilson, what they looked like and said. But ask him the name of the U.S. President today, and he may well tell you, as did one of my patients, it's Grace Kelly.

Sometimes a younger person will complain that his memory is not as good as it used to be. This is usually a sign of depression and inability to concentrate, rather than trouble within the brain. The forgotten fact or name may not have been assimilated into the thought process in the first place. When challenged, the failure to remember generates additional anxiety, and soon the subject fears he is losing his mind. Reassurance, explanation, antidepressive agents, or psychotherapy usually help this particular situation, which is almost always short-lived.

In the medical interview, memory loss makes itself apparent very quickly. The patient repeats the same complaints or asks the same question several times. He may forget what has been done to him in the physical exam. "Aren't you taking my blood pressure today?" is a favorite question, usually after it's been recorded in both arms in the sitting, standing, and recumbent positions.

How to Handle It

Despite the large number of drugs purporting to help, I have never seen any successful treatment for memory loss, even inhalation of high concentrations of oxygen or large doses of vitamins. However, its management on a social and interpersonal level is important. For example, when you observe that a parent, husband, or wife is clearly beginning to forget things, the temptation is to insist they remember. You want to shake them. "Of course you saw the Smiths last week. We were at their house together." At first this will generate insistent denial. But, in time, the patient comes to realize that he doesn't remember recent events. He begins to worry and be depressed about it, and that further impairs his memory. He is no longer secure in his environment. He becomes defensive and decides to go along with whatever is alleged to have happened, or he makes things up in order to answer a question (confabulation).

The best way to handle the situation is by reassurance. If you notice memory loss in some older person, don't harp on it, never insist he "should" remember. Instead, try this approach. "You don't remember meeting Mrs. Smith? Well, that's not surprising, she was only here for a few minutes." While this doesn't actually help the patient's memory, it does prevent the overlay of fear and depression that can aggravate the situation and in some older individuals renders them paranoid (persecution complex).

Memory loss not only is frustrating to the patient and those around him, but can be dangerous as well. Where medication whose dosage is critical has been prescribed (digitalis, insulin, antihypertensive drugs, antibiotics, sleeping pills, tranquilizers), too much may be taken, or not enough. In providing care for the elderly, we not only have to ensure such basic needs as housing, food, and medical care. We must also establish some way of supervising any drug therapy prescribed.

Do You Have Nosebleeds?

High blood pressure is one of the most important causes of *nosebleeds* in middle-aged or older people. (The most frequent one is nose-picking.) But if the pressure is normal, we look for other causes. Dry, overheated rooms, especially in winter, cause crusts to form in the nose, so that we pick it or blow it and make it bleed. An outburst of coughing due to food going down "the wrong passage," a blow to the nose, or violent exercise, especially in youngsters, can start up a bleed. Chronic sinus trouble or allergy, with inflamed, swollen or irritated nasal passages, will make you prone to nosebleeds. There is also an inherited disorder in which the blood vessels throughout the body have very thin walls. When these are irritated (in the nose by fingers, in the stomach by food), they bleed easily and sometimes profusely. Finally, the sudden occurrence of nasal hemorrhage in someone with a normal blood pressure, and no local factors in the nose to account for it, may be evidence of leukemia or other disorders which affect the clotting mechanism in the blood. If you're taking anti-coagulants, the first thing to do when you have a nosebleed is to have your blood checked (prothrombin time).

Is Your Tongue Sore?

It's a wonder that more of us don't have a sore tongue just from biting it. Haven't you marveled at how nature protects us from injury during the chewing process? How do the teeth know exactly where to come together when the tongue is mixing up the food, and not bite off part of it?

I don't mind if you go directly to the dentist when your tongue is sore—especially if you wear braces or dentures, or have had recent dental work done. But if he finds nothing, please tell me too. Although pain in the tongue may be due to mechanical problems in the mouth like braces and dentures, it may also reflect disease elsewhere in the body. Incidentally, if you've recently been in the hospital and had any operation requiring you be put to sleep, a painful tongue may be the result of manipulation. While you are asleep, the anesthetist puts a tube over your tongue and into your throat, to keep open the airway into your lungs (intubation). This procedure can sometimes injure the tongue and leave it sore for days.

The first question I ask if you complain of a sore tongue is about smoking. Cigarettes and pipes will make the tongue feel (and look) raw. Very hot or spicy foods can also irritate the tongue. Other causes of pain, irritation, or swelling are chronic infection, tumors, stings and bites, nutritional and vitamin deficiency, allergic reactions and many drugs, including aspirin.

Do Your Gums Bleed Easily?

Bleeding gums are of as much interest to me as to your dentist. The most frequent causes are a very hard toothbrush, excessive tartar on the teeth due to poor dental hygiene, and anticoagulants. But, as with painful tongue, there are specific diseases that can do it too, like blood disorders (leukemia, especially in children), nutritional deficiencies, and infection.

THROAT AND CHEST

Do You Have Any Problems with Your Throat?

As I proceed with the inquiry about various systems of the body, I want the answers to more key questions. "Are you intermittently hoarse? Do you have any difficulty swallowing?" If you are a singer, auctioneer, politician, and use your voice a great deal, or are a heavy smoker, the reason for your hoarseness (swelling and irritation of the vocal cords) is obvious. Decreased function of the thyroid gland may also cause swelling of the vocal cords and hoarseness, as can heart failure. Tuberculosis, when it was more common than it is today, was another important cause. A child is sometimes brought to the doctor because he has suddenly become hoarse. We may find a peanut or a piece of a toy lodged in the larnyx or upper esophagus. Finally, if it is none of the above, we have to consider the possibility of a growth on the vocal cords.

Whatever the suspected cause, we have to look at the cords directly whenever persistent hoarseness develops. It is fairly easy to do and painless. If, on direct examination, no tumor is seen, and the cords themselves look normal, we note how well they open and close. Vocal cord movement is controlled by branches of the vagus nerve which passes down from the brain behind the heart. Any pressure on that nerve—as, for example, by an enlarged heart, a big thyroid, swollen lymph glands surrounding a cancer of the lung, or enlargement (aneurysm) of the aorta—may interfere with the mechanics of the vocal cords and cause hoarseness.

There is a form of neurotic hysteria in which a patient suddenly loses his voice for no apparent reason. This diagnosis is generally made when all the other important causes have been ruled out.

Do You Have Trouble Swallowing?

Dysphagia, or difficulty in swallowing, is a common complaint, especially among nervous women who are otherwise healthy but who have an iron-deficiency anemia (the "tired blood" of the TV ads). It disappears with treatment of the anemia and reassurance. I don't know why men are less prone to this symptom, even when they too are anemic. But difficulty in swallowing is not always neurotic or nutritional, and can be caused by actual mechanical interference with the passage of food and water down the food pipe (esophagus), such as is caused by a growth there or in the upper stomach.

The act of swallowing is a complicated mechanism controlled

by nerve impulses to and from the brain. The various reflexes involved ensure that food will move from the mouth into the stomach and not into the lungs by way of the windpipe. Vomiting shifts this swallowing mechanism into "reverse gear." When the muscles that are used in swallowing are diseased (myasthenia gravis, stroke), or weak (severe illness), or when the nerves that activate them are injured (stroke, polio), swallowing may become difficult or impossible.

Are You Always Coughing?

Chronic *cough* is common at any age. Like headache, it may represent something trivial or life-threatening, and so demands very careful consideration. The history alone will often tell me why you are coughing.

The *cough reflex* is an important defense mechanism. You cough to expel a foreign substance from the lungs and throat— solid (something you are choking on), liquid (mucus, pus, or blood anywhere in the respiratory tree), or even gaseous (fumes or irritants in your environment). Although cough is a reflex, it is also under voluntary control, unlike the knee jerk, which you can't stop even if you want to. When you feel like coughing, you can suppress it. A good example of mass cough control is evident at a concert. During the performance, there is complete silence. Then, as the orchestra retools between movements, the air is punctuated by a cacophony of coughs, which are stilled once the music resumes.

The Nerve That Controls the Cough

The *vagus nerve*, which controls the cough reflex, sends little branches to the respiratory tract—the larynx, trachea (windpipe), and lungs. Here, these small nerve endings may be stimulated by infection, inflammation, or the pressure of a tumor, making you cough. One important branch of the vagus called Arnold's nerve must have gotten lost in the shuffle, because instead of going down the larynx to the bronchial tubes and into the lungs, it somehow got diverted to the outer ear canal, of all places. This branch is not only interesting but important too, because trouble in the outer ear can stimulate it—and make you cough. For example, impacted wax in the canal, a jelly bean put there by a child, irritation or infection of the skin within the ear can all cause such a chronic cough. If in the course of my examination I find no other reason for your cough, remind me to look in your ears.

Since Arnold's branch comes off the large vagus nerve that also serves the gut, its stimulation may have gastrointestinal effects too. The next time you feel bloated after eating, put a cold cloth over your ear. You may experience relief of your symptoms.

The Cough That Disappears During Sleep

A recurrent dry cough or constant clearing of the throat may be due to a nervous habit and worsen under duress. Like so many other habits, it disappears during sleep.

If you look down someone's throat, you will see hanging in the midline a small piece of tissue, like a mini-tongue. It's called the *uvula.* In some people, it is a little longer than it should be, tickles the back of the throat, and gives a chronic cough, occasionally troublesome enough to require removal.

A Symphony of Coughs

We can classify coughs in terms of what causes them—trouble in the respiratory system (anywhere from the sinuses to the lungs), heart disease, or some disorder elsewhere in the chest.

In the *respiratory system,* a postnasal drip from your sinuses down to your throat will make you cough. A cold, any irritation or infection of the lining of your air passages (as from chronic smoking, laryngitis, or bronchitis), or trouble within the lung itself (pneumonia, TB, or cancer) will make you cough.

If your heart is weak, causing extra fluid to accumulate in the lungs, you will have a "nonproductive" cough—that is, one without sputum. Something pressing on the vagus nerve, like an aneurysm of the aorta or some large lymph gland in the chest, will also result in a dry cough.

Certain characteristics of the cough—for example, is it recent or long-standing, is it worse in the morning or at night, is it accompanied by sputum (how much, what color, and is there any blood with it), are you more apt to get it lying down—will help me decide where to look and how further to investigate.

If a youngster develops a persistent cough, we think of an allergic condition, or if he is living in a crowded household with someone else who has the disease, of TB. When a middle-aged person, especially one who smokes, has a persistent cough, he or she may have cancer of the lung.

Chronic morning cough in heavy cigarette smokers is often assumed to be a "natural" consequence of that habit. It usually is, but such long-standing coughs may signal the onset of chronic bronchitis. I am also wary about a "smoker's cough" because the cigarettes may be a "red herring," and the real reason may be heart failure or lung cancer.

If you cough only in the morning on awakening and are fine the rest of the day, mucus secretions may be accumulating during the night from infected sinuses. If you go to bed feeling well but are awakened at night by paroxysms of cough that force you to sit up for relief, you may have a weak heart. Cough on exertion suggests either heart trouble or lung disease.

If the cough is dry, so that you don't bring anything up, it is likely due to some irritant, allergy, heart failure, pressure on the vagus nerve, or anxiety.

Many "coughers" don't spit up because small amounts of mucus or blood reaching the throat on their way up from the lungs are often swallowed reflexly. That's why, when we suspect someone who can't raise phlegm of having active TB, and are looking for the bug that causes it, we may wash out the stomach.

Blood in the sputum may come from the nose, throat, bronchial passages or lungs, and it's important that we determine the source accurately. Yellow or green sputum means infection, which may originate anywhere from up in the sinuses to down in the air passages. Later, we'll smell it (abscesses and severe infections in the lung produce putrid pus), look at it under a microscope, and send it to the lab to identify the infecting agent.

So cough is an important and complicated symptom. In the

following chapters you will read how we actually pursue its investigation.

Are You Unduly Short of Breath?

Normal breathing is automatic and unlabored. You're no more conscious of it than you are of the heartbeat. Being short of breath means you are aware of your breathing. It becomes work.

No matter how fit you are, if you run long enough and hard enough, you will be short of breath. But if suddenly things you were able to do quite easily now cause difficulty in breathing, and this huffing and puffing lasts longer and doesn't disappear as quickly as it used to with rest—that's important. This decrease in exercise tolerance may simply reflect the fact that you're "out of shape"—physically deconditioned owing to chronic underactivity. You may not have been aware of it before because you just didn't have occasion to exert yourself. If you spend your life sitting in a chair, taking the elevator instead of walking up a flight or two, never going by foot when you can ride, engaging in no physical activity whatsoever, you will not be able to produce, on demand, a burst of power and energy without becoming breathless. What's more, if, in addition to being totally sedentary, you also gain weight, even a little more effort than usual will almost always produce shortness of breath.

Another cause of "lack of air" is chronic and excessive cigarette smoking. *I know no heavy smoker who has enough "wind."*

Trying to Get a "Satisfying" Breath

There is one symptom that feels like shortness of breath but is not—the inability to take a deep breath even at rest. This is a nervous habit called *hyperventilation,* which most of us have experienced at some time or another. It can be the source of worry because it is mistaken for evidence of heart or lung trouble. Hyperventilation is frequent among anxious, high-strung people, usually young or menopausal women, or those with chronic psychological stress. As they keep trying to get a "satisfying" breath, they breathe more deeply, inhale more oxygen, and blow out more carbon dioxide from the lungs. This changes the balance of gases and other chemicals in the blood and sets in motion a train of other symptoms—numbness and tingling of the hands and feet, light-headedness, and in some cases actual fainting. If I think you are hyperventilating, when I examine you later I will have you breathe deeply and rapidly for 30 to 45 seconds as you sit on the examining table. Your symptoms will be reproduced, you will be satisfied that we've made the right diagnosis, you will be reassured, and perhaps together we may be able to eliminate the habit.

Shortness of Breath Due to Heart Trouble

If you complain of being short of breath, I will ask you a few more questions to be sure that it is indeed due to impaired physical fitness, obesity, cigarette smoking, or neurotic breathing habits, and not a reflection of heart or lung disease. Are you short of breath when you lie down? If the heart muscle is strained and weak, it cannot pump out all the blood within it every time it contracts. After a while, blood begins to back up into the lungs, causing them to become congested or filled with blood, which replaces the air in your lungs. This makes you short of breath, since the lungs are less compliant. Furthermore, when you lie flat, the blood in your legs, normally pulled down by gravity, returns to the heart, increasing the load or volume that has to be squeezed out, and causing even more to accumulate in the lungs. This is why shortness of breath due to heart disease is worsened by the recumbent position. Such patients feel more comfortable sleeping propped up in bed.

When lung trouble rather than heart disease is the cause, the shortness of breath is not as position-dependent and is accompanied by a chronic cough.

Angina pectoris the designation for "heart pain" (*angina* meaning pain and *pectoris* meaning the chest), usually occurs on exertion and is due to an inadequate amount of blood to the heart muscle. Often the earliest symptom of angina is not pain in the chest but shortness of breath. It ceases as soon as you stop what you are doing.

Various respiratory disorders, including bronchitis (with or without asthma) and a disease called emphysema, cause breathlessness. *Emphysema* results from recurrent or chronic bronchitis. Long-standing infection of the bronchial tubes narrows them so that the air in the lungs is not completely exhaled. After a while, because of the large volume of retained air, the chest becomes permanently overinflated and larger than normal (barrel chest). For some reason, I have found patients with the worst emphysema to be the hardest to persuade to quit smoking cigarettes.

Do You Have Pain or Tightness in the Chest?

We come now to a very important series of questions, especially for the middle-aged man or postmenopausal woman. Your answers may provide the first clue to narrowing of the coronary arteries within the heart.

Symptoms of *coronary artery disease* may precede any electrocardiographic changes by months or years, so it's no use depending on the ECG to make the diagnosis.

Many people have angina pectoris and don't know it. They attribute discomfort in the chest to "gas," arthritis, rheumatism, indigestion, hiatus hernia, neuralgia, "spasm," and a host of other incorrect sources. Patients with angina may not worry because "the pain isn't sharp like a knife." But cardiac pain is rarely sharp; it's more like a heaviness, constriction or pressure, "as if I had a weight, an elephant, sitting on my chest," as some patients describe it. They are also falsely encouraged when the distress is of short duration. "It's really nothing, doctor, it goes right away. It's not as if it lasted for hours."

Angina pectoris never persists longer than a few minutes—unless you're having a full-blown heart attack. It does not occur at rest, except in advanced stages. It is more likely to come on when you are walking against the wind, or up a hill, especially after a heavy meal. It can radiate down either arm, more commonly but not only the left, to the jaw, the ears, and through to the back. Sometimes it occurs when you are having an argument or in other emotional situations such as watching an exciting sports event or movie. When the precipitating effort or stress ends, the angina stops. It is almost always aggravated by cold weather, hence the exodus of patients with this symptom to warmer climates during the winter months. The other interesting fact is that it is often relieved by belching, for which reason patients with angina believe their symptoms are digestive.

Before we recognized the symptoms and mechanisms of angina pectoris, many death certificates were signed naming the cause as a gastric disorder. Ask an older person how some of his relatives died. He may well tell you that it was from "acute indigestion." This is because just before he died, the victim complained of pain or pressure behind the breastbone, accompanied by "gas" and temporarily relieved by belching.

So it isn't enough for me to limit my question to "Do you have pain in the chest," as you may say, "No." I follow it up with "Do you feel a heaviness, pressure, awareness or a shortness of breath on exertion or emotional upset which disappears when you rest?" A "yes" answer strongly suggests angina pectoris.

Thyroid Function: How Well Is Your Thermostat Regulated?

I will ask you a series of questions designed to find out whether your thyroid gland is functioning normally. Earlier, you read how your response to temperature changes may indicate the condition of your thyroid. "Does hot or cold weather bother you?" If you answer "no" and I suspect from previous clues or from your appearance that the matter should be pursued a little further, there are several ways of rephrasing the question. For example, I may ask whether you and your spouse agree about keeping the windows open at night in cold weather. Do you find the room too cold while he is quite comfortable? If you sleep together in one bed, do you use the same number of blankets, or do you prefer an extra one or two? Do you disagree about the need for air conditioning in the summertime or the amount of heat in winter? I diagnosed my wife's underfunctioning thyroid when I found her wrapped in a woolen blanket in front of a fire while the rest of us were virtually "well done."

Other evidences of low thyroid function are unusual fatigue, inability to lose weight despite dedicated dieting, dryness of the skin, muscle cramps, coarsening or loss of hair, change in the menstrual characteristics (heavy, prolonged flow), constipation and, in the late stages, swelling or puffiness of the face and a pasty tint to the skin. By the same token, in hyperthyroidism (overactive thyroid), apart from heat intolerance (always sweating), you may note palpitations, tremor, nervousness, emotional instability with crying episodes, unexplained weight loss despite a good appetite, and falling out of the hair, which has become fine and silky.

THE DIGESTIVE TRACT

How Well Do You Handle Your Food?

I now listen for symptoms which may indicate peptic ulcer, gallbladder trouble, hiatus hernia, cancer, or nervous irritability of the gut.

It is very important to distinguish pain and discomfort caused by gas and indigestion from that due to heart disease. But remember that *intestinal and cardiac disorders can exist together.* If you have pressure and are distended after eating, and we find you have gallstones, that doesn't necessarily mean that you don't also have heart disease. The final diagnosis, as you will see later, will depend on the physical examination, x-rays of the intestinal tract, and the electrocardiogram.

Pain with swallowing may be due to a scratch in the lining of the food pipe by a bone, a pill, or some abrasive food eaten earlier. Distress *immediately* after eating indicates a disorder high up in the intestinal tract—that is, somewhere in the esophagus or stomach. Cancer in its late stages is one cause. Its pain is continuous, but worsened by eating. *Ulcer pain,* on the other hand, is gnawing and hungerlike, temporarily relieved by food, especially one with antacid properties like milk, not caused by it.

Pain, bloating, or a feeling of fullness, not immediately, but one or two hours after eating is likely due to gallbladder disease, especially if you had fried, fatty, or gas-forming foods like cabbage. But such an attack may also follow a plain meal.

Hiatus hernia (not "high anus hernia," as one patient called it) refers to a weakness of the diaphragm (the muscular wall that separates the abdomen from the chest), permitting the upper stomach to bulge into the chest cavity. Chronic irritation of the esophagus by the acid regurgitating into it from the stomach causes pain, which most people call "heartburn." This is a very common disorder, especially after age 50, and unlike other hernias rarely needs surgical correction. It is distinguishable from gall-bladder disease in that it produces a feeling of fullness *immediately* after eating, especially if you're lying down, and is partially relieved by belching or sitting up.

If you have a hiatus hernia, you must eat small meals frequently and take antacids one half to one hour after meals. Also, sleeping at night with the head of the bed elevated minimizes the chances for a reflux or regurgitation of food from the stomach into the chest.

Burping or Belching

A very common symptom, one that is baffling to many patients, and whose simple explanation they almost always refuse to accept, is a constant burping or belching. They can't wait to demonstrate their gaseous prowess. "Why does my stomach make so much gas? Look, I haven't even eaten anything, and I'm all distended. Listen—Oh, I beg your pardon, I'm so embarrassed, but there's nothing I can do. There—here's more." Belching is never a symptom of disease. It's just a habit. An empty stomach doesn't produce gas. All the burping and intestinal commotion are air, which is being constantly swallowed. This is a habit most frequently seen in nervous people or those who eat too quickly. It's not easy to treat either. We sometimes prescribe charcoal, simethicone (Mylicon), or other substances which bind the air, but these are not effective when the problem is air gulping. Putting something between the teeth, like a cigarette holder, eraser, or pencil, may reduce the amount of air swallowed.

So the key questions with respect to the upper intestinal tract are (1) have you recently had pain in the upper abdomen that occurs one to two hours after eating (suggests gallbladder disease); (2) awakens you at night (may mean ulcer because at that time, the stomach is empty and not able to buffer the acid which is constantly produced); (3) is relieved by antacid medications such as Rolaids, Gelusil, Maalox (suggests stomach ulcers because these preparations neutralize excessive acids); (4) is relieved by milk or eating (again suggests ulcer); (5) occurs during a meal or immediately after (suggests cancer of the stomach or hiatus hernia)? (6) Does food ever get stuck when you swallow? (Suggests an inflammation or tumor of the esophagus or food pipe.)

Is Your Appetite Poor?

The fat, neurotic, compulsive eater invariably insists he has no appetite. "That's what's so surprising, doctor. I'm never hungry, but I still can't lose weight." Of course, you and I know he's "never hungry" because his stomach is never empty, what with all the nibbling and eating between meals.

Altered food intake and eating habits (too much or too little) are largely psychological, and range from compulsive overeating to profound aversion to food.

We really don't understand why some people are fat and others, who apparently eat as much or more, are not. However, most weight problems result from poor eating habits, excessive food intake, or glandular imbalance (usually underfunction of the thyroid). By bad eating habits I mean eating more and large portions of the wrong foods, then sitting around—not burning it off. Our custom of taking the heaviest meal in the evening, and then letting it settle while we sit around watching TV, accounts for some of our national obesity. Most Europeans have their big meal at lunch. They then go back to work, where they can burn off some of the calories consumed. The final repast is a light supper. The key here is the chance to expend energy and calories after the main meal. Remember, no matter what you may read in advertisements or diet books, *net weight reflects the balance between the energy you take in (food) and the energy you burn (exercise).* Constant nibbling, eating between meals and before going to bed will make you fat, especially if you don't exercise regularly.

Unexplained Weight Loss

If weight loss is not the result of dieting, it is potentially more serious than overweight. It may be due to emotional depression, which is often accompanied by poor appetite and decreased food intake. There is a serious psychiatric disorder called *anorexia nervosa,* difficult to treat and sometimes fatal, in which the patient, usually a young woman, simply does not eat. It is very sad to observe her eating habits. Sometimes, instead of leaving the food alone, she goes at it with gusto. She cuts it, mashes it, moves it around the plate, does everything to it but eat it. By the time she's "finished the meal," even though not a morsel has been swallowed, the appearance of the plate suggests a hearty appetite.

If you are too thin or have lost weight, I must think of overactivity of the thyroid gland (energy from the food you eat is too rapidly burned up), a cancer somewhere (usually ruins the appetite), a chronic disease like diabetes mellitus (sugar is being excreted in the urine instead of being utilized for conversion to protein and fat), or a chronic infection somewhere (TB, infectious hepatitis). Weight loss may also be due to the effect of a medicine you are taking for the treatment of some unrelated condition. For example, patients with heart disease who are given digitalis may lose weight because an excessive amount of this drug can depress the appetite. This is especially true in older persons.

A deliberate attempt to lose weight that is too successful (too much, too soon, and continuing even after the regimen is abandoned) is suspicious. Every now and then some underlying disease begins coincidentally with the weight reduction program, and its presence is masked by the fact that you actually were trying to lose weight at one point.

Have There Been Any Changes in Your Bowel Movements?

In our culture, especially among the elderly, there is a preoccupation with bowel movements, "regular" evacuation being considered of prime importance. When I ask patients about their "BM's," I get some very different answers. Some are enraptured with theirs, maintaining that they're "beautiful, just beautiful." But others are totally disinterested, and never look in the toilet bowl, or at least are unwilling to admit to it. And when I ask them, "Have you ever noticed blood or mucus in your stool?"

I'm given a very haughty "I wouldn't know." I have visited patients in the coronary care unit, hovering between life and death after a heart attack, whose main concern is not with their heart but whether or not they "enjoyed" a good evacuation that morning.

Bad Bowel Habits

TV commercials notwithstanding, daily bowel movements are not a necessity. Whether or not your evacuations are regular is largely a matter of habit, the kind of diet you eat, and the particular characteristics of your bowel function and structure. When I was in medical school, a female was defined as "a chronically constipated biped with low back pain." Many women and some men are constipated because of their distaste for water. If you drink enough water (six to eight glasses a day), you're much less likely to be constipated.

Other causes of constipation are lack of bulk in the diet and failure to set aside a certain time each day for evacuation. Curiously, despite our preoccupation with our bowels, we do very little to regularize them. Other commitments come first, and we ignore the urge to defecate. It soon passes, and we have to wait for the next signal. Such chronic delay predisposes to chronic constipation.

Another cause of constipation is low thyroid function, in which the tempo of the gut slows down in keeping with the diminished metabolism throughout the body.

I ask about your bowels because I want to make sure you don't have a malignancy there. Constipation and diarrhea are important symptoms. The latter may reflect infection (enteritis), be the result of a trip to some distant land, or be caused by inflammation of the bowel (colitis). It may also result from some medication (quinidine, antibiotics) or be due to food allergy. It may be caused by a deficiency of a certain enzyme (lactase) which breaks down the sugars in milk and milk products. We are finding an increasing number of people born with this lactase deficiency who have had chronic diarrhea all their lives. When they stop taking milk, cheese, and ice cream, their stools become normal.

Constipation may be due to mechanical blockage by a tumor somewhere in the bowel, the laxative habit, dehydration, or hypothyroidism.

Blood in Your Stool

Blood in the stool may either be bright red, if it originates low down in the bowel (possibly from hemorrhoids, a polyp, or a tumor), or be black, if the site of the bleeding is higher up in the intestinal tract. It takes several hours for blood to pass through the thirty feet of gut on its way out, during which time it turns black—jet black, with the color and consistency of tar. Remember that iron pills, and Pepto-Bismol can also cause black stools indistinguishable to the naked eye from those due to bleeding. However, we have chemical tests to distinguish between the digested blood and these substances.

A Critical Question

"Have your bowel habits changed recently?" For example, if you have been constipated as long as you can remember, and now suddenly have episodes of diarrhea interspersed with periods of constipation, we have to be on the alert for a tumor or cancer. It is also important to establish whether you have noticed any change in the caliber of the stool. Movements that have become thinner or ribbonlike may indicate either a growth somewhere in the lower bowel or spasm. Other danger signals include abdominal cramping, bleeding, diarrhea alternating with constipation, or any "redness" in the stool. One of my patients who had been bleeding for weeks didn't tell me about it because she thought it was due to the borscht she had been eating. Mucus in the stool by itself is usually innocent, a sign of irritability. But when the mucus is mixed with pus and blood, it always points to a serious condition—either infection, inflammation, or cancer of the large bowel.

GYNECOLOGICAL HISTORY

All About Your Periods

The characteristics of your menstrual flow are very revealing, and may indicate disorders ranging from glandular disease to infection to pelvic tumors. At what age did your periods start? How old were you when they stopped? If you're still menstruating, are you regular? Is there a change in the character of the flow? Are your periods less or more frequent than they used to be? Are they shorter or longer? Do you bleed more or less?

The duration of the period is quite variable among normal women. Although 28 days is usually considered standard, the cycle may be as short as 24–25 days or as prolonged as 33 days. Whereas most healthy women are usually regular, others, free of disease, are always irregular. Menstruation usually lasts 5 days, but it may be as short as 2 or 3 or as long as 7.

Your Cycle

Even if your cycle is regular, there may be significant changes in your menstrual pattern. For example, you may bleed, stain or spot between periods. *Any bleeding between periods must always be investigated, because, although it may be hormonal due to pregnancy or from the "pill," it is presumed due to a benign or malignant tumor until proven otherwise.* You may also become aware of a change in the amount of flow. You should not normally use more than 18 pads during the entire period. Unusually heavy bleeding reflects disease of the uterus (fibroids, polyps, cancer) or ovaries; a change in your thyroid function (if the thyroid gland is underfunctioning, the menstrual periods last longer and are heavier; if it is overactive, the periods are shorter and the amount of flow decreases); or something wrong in the way your blood clots.

Sometimes, your menstrual periods will stop long before the menopause is due. In addition to pregnancy, sometimes unsuspected, other conditions that will cause such premature termination of menstruation are a profound emotional shock (like the death of a loved one), diabetes, severe anemia or leukemia, high fevers, severe malnutrition, and other illnesses.

The Menopause ("The Pause That Depresses")

More has been made of menopausal symptoms than is probably justified. Most women finish with their menstrual periods without any significant side effects. A year or two before they end, you will note a change in their characteristics. The amount of flow varies, the cycles become irregular, and you begin to miss one or two months. We consider all this "normal" because it occurs so often. However, *you must see your gynecologist right away if there is any spotting, bleeding between periods, or excessive flow at any time.* Although the most likely cause of these symptoms is diminishing function of the ovaries and reduced hormone production, tumors of the cervix and uterus can also be responsible.

The *menopause* may give you the hot flushes referred to earlier, make you nervous, depressed and irritable, and cause you to swallow air without even knowing it so that you're constantly belching. But some symptoms, especially depression, are often at least partly due to real or imagined personal problems occurring at that time in life, rather than measurable hormonal deficiencies.

One commonly accepted myth is that a woman's sexual desires drop sharply with the menopause. The reverse is often true. Liberated from the need to engage in contraceptive practices, many women adjust to the menopause with a newfound sense of sexual freedom.

Screening for Cancer

Do you regularly have "Pap" tests (Papanicolaou smears) for early detection of cancer of the cervix? The first "Pap" test should be done after the onset of sexual relations and should be repeated annually. Some gynecologists advise testing twice a year after the late thirties.

Have You Felt a Lump in Your Breast?

At this point I ask whether you have ever noticed any lumps in your breasts. At least 90 percent of breast tumors are found by women themselves. A very small lump may be missed by the doctor, especially if the breasts are large and the examination cursory. So I encourage you to double-check once a month. Later, in the section on the physical examination of the chest, you will read how to do it.

THE GENITOURINARY TRACT (KIDNEYS, BLADDER, PROSTATE)

How often you urinate, the volume, color, odor, force of the stream, and whether or not it burns or hurts—all indicate whether you have any problems with your kidney, bladder, or prostate (*not* prostrate) gland.

Do You Have to Get Up Every Night to Urinate?

If you are in the habit of taking a beer at bedtime, or wine with dinner, you may expect to be awakened sometime during the night. That's normal. But when you've had no liquids after dinner and still have to "go" two or three times, then something's wrong. You may have a urinary infection, you may be diabetic, or, if you're a middle-aged man, your prostate may be enlarged.

It's Probably Your Prostate

After the urine is formed in the kidneys, it passes down two tubes (ureters), one from each kidney, into the bladder, where it is stored for a while, until it is convenient for you to eliminate it. Nerve endings situated in the bladder wall are stimulated as the urine fills and distends it. These nerves signal the brain that it is time for you to urinate. But for a long time this message is only a suggestion, not a command. You can comfortably ignore it and void at your convenience. But after a while, as more and more urine drips in, you've "got to go." The urethra then carries the urine from the bladder out of the body.

Normally the size of a walnut, the prostate lies behind the urethra, the channel that carries the urine from the bladder out of the body. In women, there is nothing to obstruct the urethra, but in men, an enlarged prostate presses on it, causing the urine to back up in the bladder. So now, not only does it keep coming in, but it has trouble getting out. Because of the obstruction, it can only be eliminated when the pressure really builds up in the bladder. Because of this obstruction by the prostate, there is always some urine left in the bladder. The nerve endings there stop signaling the need to void this residual amount, so even though there is urine in the bladder, you are not aware of it. But when more forms, you have to void again. This happens because your bladder has become irritable secondary to the retained urine; therefore you have to "go" each time a little more urine is added to the basic amount. That's why if your prostate is enlarged, you need to relieve yourself much more frequently than if you were able to empty your bladder completely each time.

Since the urethra is pressed on by the enlarged prostate, the stream of urine is narrowed and its force is decreased, so that the ability to "pee over a fence" is lost. The flow may also be split (something that can cause embarrassment in the men's room. If your prostate is big, keep two urinals clear on each side).

What Goes In Must Come Out

Apart from the enlargement of the prostate, which is easily confirmed by a rectal examination with the finger, there is another cause of increased urination—drinking too much water. Several conditions may make you thirsty, the most common of which is *diabetes mellitus*. Diabetics do not produce the amount of insulin needed to burn up sugar, and so it accumulates in the blood. The body tries to get rid of the excess sugar in the urine. Since the kidneys can't excrete solid sugar, they have to draw on the body water to dissolve it. This loss of water in turn makes you thirsty, so you drink more and void large volumes. Furthermore, because the sugar is excreted instead of being made available to the body for energy, you lose weight. A combination, then, of *weight loss, increased thirst, and increased urination indicates diabetes mellitus.*

In women, *vaginal itching* is another clue to diabetes. It results from the heavy concentration of sugar in the urine around the vagina which provides a good place for fungus to grow.

Does It Burn When You Urinate?

A burning sensation or a sense of warmth when urinating usually means infection in the bladder (cystitis), prostate (prostatitis), or urethra (urethritis). Aside from venereal disease, the commonest cause of urinary infection in men is prostatitis.

Is There Blood in Your Urine?

Although blood in the urine and in the ejaculate in men may be due to engorgement of the veins in the prostate gland or seminal vesicles, and, in women, easy to confuse with menstrual flow, *bloody urine demands meticulous investigation.* It may reflect tumor or infection of the kidney, ureter, urinary bladder, prostate or urethra. This is one area that doesn't lend itself particularly to physical examination, so if you do have blood in the urine, you're in for a lot of testing.

THE LEGS

Do You Have Leg Cramps?

We think of *arteriosclerosis,* or hardening of the arteries, as mainly involving the heart and brain. And so it does. But it can affect arteries anywhere—including those going to the legs. When they are narrowed, the blood supply to the leg muscles is diminished. At rest, this reduced amount of blood is usually adequate, but when you walk or run, the need for more blood by the muscles cannot be met and you develop a cramp—usually in the calf. This pain is to the legs what angina pectoris is to the heart. When you stop walking, it disappears. *Leg pain due to vascular disease almost always occurs on effort.*

Most of us at some time or another have *leg cramps at night.* Often they are severe enough to awaken us, and there we are hopping about, rubbing the muscle in spasm, straightening out the toes—anything to get relief. The cause is not clear, but contrary to popular belief it is not usually circulatory. These cramps may occur in patients who take diuretics, which cause the excretion not only of water but also of certain salts like sodium, magnesium, and potassium. Their deficiency may account for the nocturnal pain. I think leg cramps happen more often when the feet are uncovered and cool. So if you are prone to such cramps, try wearing socks at night. There is one theory that these symptoms are due to pooling of the blood in the veins of the legs and that elevating them with a pillow may help. Try it, and if it doesn't help, quinine taken at bedtime often appears to give relief by some unknown action.

Do You Have Pain in the Big Toe?

This is almost always a sign of gout, but it may also be due to poorly fitting or narrow shoes. The pain of gout is very characteristic. In addition to the ache in the bone, the overlying skin is extremely sensitive. During an attack, even the lightest pressure, like a bed sheet touching the affected part, produces pain.

Do Your Ankles Swell?

Most people's ankles do swell at times, especially if they are fat, those who stand a great deal, have varicose veins, or have been on a long airplane trip. Leg veins are very interesting structures. They are not simple tubes that carry used or deoxygenated blood back to the heart (arteries carry oxygenated blood from the heart to the various organs of the body). Veins enable blood flow to defy the laws of gravity when you are standing. How do they do this? First of all, the heart itself squeezes out the blood with such force that it travels down the body and up again by virtue of this strong head of pressure. What is so special about the veins is they have little valves in them which allow the blood to move up toward the heart, but not down. When these valves are defective the veins become varicosed because this one-way flow is not maintained. As a result, blood pools in the distended veins, and fluid in the blood seeps out through the vein walls into the tissues of the legs, making them swell.

Heart failure also gives you swollen ankles and feet. This is partly due to the fact that the cardiac contraction which normally keeps the blood circulating is weakened when the heart is strained. So the force, while enough to squeeze the blood out of the heart, is not great enough to keep it going full circle back to the heart against the pull of gravity. The blood then pools in the legs. There is another mechanism responsible for swollen ankles in heart failure. The weakened heart muscle cannot expel all the blood returning to it. The amount in excess of what it can handle backs up into the circulation, and ends up in the legs.

THE WRAP-UP

It takes much longer to read about the key questions in a checkup than it does to ask them. We will spend about fifteen or twenty minutes talking before the physical examination itself—mostly about the subjects I've covered here. You can have other questions and complaints of your own which I have not discussed in these pages. My questions may generate others. When you answer "Yes" to a query, I may have to follow it up with other pertinent questions. The purpose of all this is to help me decide where to focus my efforts in the next stage of your evaluation—the actual physical examination.

CHAPTER **7**

THE PHYSICAL EXAMINATION—
FINALLY

WELL, we've looked at each other, discussed all manner of things, and decided whether we have anything going between us. If we do, then you're probably a little less nervous now about getting your physical, and I'm likely to have a fairly good idea of what to concentrate on in the remainder of our session together. You now come into the examining room for the physical part of the checkup.

Just as each doctor will phrase questions in his own way, with different nuances and emphases, so will he approach the physical examination in his particular style and sequence. In the following pages, you will read how I perform a physical examination. It's not necessarily better than the one your doctor does, and it's similar enough so that you will understand what is happening in your own exam.

I will not undertake a complete physical with you wearing

134

clothes. (That is not to say you've got to sit there stark naked if all you've come for is to get a prescription refilled, have me look briefly at your sore throat, or deliver a telegram.) To make this point with my patients, I have a small figurine in my office. Years ago, in China, when women's modesty and not women's lib was the vogue, a female patient would not expose her body. She would simply point out on the model the area troubling her. We (and they) don't do it like that anymore. I insist on a state of complete undress under an examining gown. I will not listen to your heart and lungs through a shirt or blouse, examine your breasts under a bra, or feel your abdomen through a slip or shorts.

You'd be surprised at some of the contortions patients go through with the gown in order to conceal those parts of the body not actually being examined. I prefer not to uncover one area at a time because the body is more than the sum of its parts. It is important that I first assess it as a whole, noting any loss of symmetry, the distribution of hair, fat and muscle, skin rashes, nutritional state and proportions. We can then cover up what I'm not looking at.

Weighing You: Either My Scale or Yours Is Wrong

After you have undressed, we weigh and measure you. I have already determined in our interview how many pounds you've lost or gained in recent months. I'm always surprised at the variations between my scale and yours. Patients will express shock at how much they weigh in my office. "Isn't that funny? At home this morning I weighed six pounds less."

Ideal weight is not easily defined. Whether you weigh too much or too little depends to some extent on your bone structure and body build. I don't rely on the formal height-weight tables. I prefer to form an overall impression of whether you're too fat or too thin, and then use a simple rule of thumb to guide me. It works best in men. I start with a base of 115 pounds. Then for every inch above 5 feet, I add 5 pounds. So that if you are 5'8" tall, a good weight for you should roughly be 115 lb + (8 × 5) or 40 = 155 lb. If you are 6 feet, it would be 115 lb + (12 × 5) or

60 = 175 lb. This formula doesn't apply to women in whom cosmetic considerations are overriding. Here, I simply determine whether you're too heavy or too thin, and hope you'll agree.

Because weight varies during the day—largely due to the changes in the amount of body fluid—if you want to keep an accurate record, weigh yourself at the same time every day, preferably in the morning, after emptying your bladder and bowels and before having breakfast.

How to Take Your Temperature

When are they going to make a thermometer you and I can read? Electronic ones are available but are not yet in widespread use.

The most reliable way to take temperature is rectally, and it's also safest in children, who can harm themselves by cracking the thermometer in the mouth. Rectal temperatures are about a half degree higher than oral readings, so that if you are recording rectally, subtract 0.5 to 0.7 degrees. In some European countries, the thermometer is put in the armpit. These readings are about one degree lower than those taken by mouth.

Although temperature is usually recorded in degrees Fahrenheit in the United States, it is measured in centigrade almost everywhere else. You should learn the metric system anyway, because it will soon be universally used. As a guide in the meantime, note the following: 99.5°F = 37.5°C, 100.5°F = 38°C, 96°F = 35.5°C.

Before taking your temperature, make sure you haven't just consumed something hot or cold. There was once a very nice, thoughtful nurse working with me who, without my knowledge, was preparing hot coffee for patients sitting in the waiting room. For a long time I couldn't understand why so many of them had high fever on routine examination.

What's High and What's Low?

Ideal temperature is popularly thought to be 98.6°F (or 37°C)—exactly—and anything above or below that figure is suspect. A simple experiment will show you the real variations that may occur in healthy people. Take your temperature at various times during a 24-hour period when you're in good health. You'll probably find a low near 96°F during sleep (when your body metabolism is slowest) to a high of 99.5°F at about eight or nine o'clock in the evening (when your body processes are at their peak).

Body temperature is a reflection of many complicated chemical processes—the burning of calories, the generation of energy, and the dissipation of heat. Add to this dynamic situation the impact of variable outside temperatures, different clothing, eating hot and cold foods, your sweating characteristics—and you can well appreciate why normal temperature fluctuates as it does. But patients still call to tell me that their temperature is just about 99°F, "and for me, that's fever." Or "my temperature is below 98°, "and for me, that's low." With the possible exception of significant underfunction of the thyroid, there is no such thing as abnormally low temperature. If yours is less than you think it should be, the possibilities include (a) you've been out in very cold weather, (b) you've had a cold drink before the thermometer was put in the mouth, (c) it has been deliberately lowered by artificial means to slow the heart and body metabolism during cardiac surgery (hypothermia), (d) you're dead.

When your temperature during the day is 99.5° or higher, and if you tell me that you have been feeling tired, aching all over, and have a slight headache, then you do have fever.

Fever and Sympathy

Fever may be quite welcome when you're feeling sick. It makes it "official" to everyone around you that you're not malingering. Children, especially, are delighted with one or two degrees above normal, since this assures them a day or two home from school. If you call a friend for a little sympathy when you're feeling sick, he'll almost always ask if you have any fever. Tell him "No," and that's the end of that. Or when you want your doctor to make a house-call, his first question will also be "Do you have a fever?" If you say "No," he won't come. If you say "Yes," he'll tell you to get into a cab and come right over.

Different Kinds of Fever

We can make some interesting observations with fever. For example, the pulse rate usually goes up about 10 beats per minute above your usual rate with each degree of temperature elevation. If you have an infection with fever and your pulse is not increased, the possibilities include typhoid fever (pretty rare these days), hepatitis, or a viral (as opposed to a bacterial) infection.

Years ago, before all the sophisticated diagnostic technology available today, doctors depended a great deal on every scrap of information obtained at the bedside. Patients used to run fevers for weeks because we had no antibiotics with which to treat them. Hospital charts were carefully studied for characteristic temperature curves. Was the elevation constant or intermittent; did it spike in the evening; did it ever drop to normal? Today, fevers don't usually persist for weeks without diagnosis and treatment, so that kind of information is considered much less important. Temperature elevation is considered a "nonspecific sign," signaling that something somewhere is wrong but offering no clue as to what it is.

It may be due to a host of different disorders—infection somewhere in the body (kidneys, bowel, teeth, throat, chest, skin) or even cancer. A fever without apparent cause persisting for more than two weeks, is called FUO (fever of unknown origin), a favorite admitting diagnosis for the hospital. Sometimes even after extensive testing to determine the cause, we find no abnormalities and the temperature just simply goes away. Thank goodness for the expression, "It was probably a virus." How much ignorance on our part that covers up.

SIZING YOU UP

I now assess the symmetry of your body and whether you are normally proportioned: There is an easy way to tell. With your arms outstretched at the level of your shoulders, the span between your fingertips should equal your total height. Also, if you are a normally developed adult, the distance from the top of your head to the groin is half the total body height, as is, of course, the distance from the groin to the soles of the feet.

I then look for obvious deformities or asymmetry in your body, such as curvature of the spine or "hunchback," and for signs of paralysis, evidence of a stroke, or the tremor, expressionless face, and drooling mouth of Parkinson's disease.

The "Strong Man" Physique

Characteristic abnormalities of body shape offer important clues to disease. For example, overactivity of the adrenal gland (or taking too much cortisone by mouth) gives a characteristic fat distribution over the back of the neck, called a "buffalo hump." There is a congenital disease called *coarctation of the aorta* (coarctation means narrowing), which alters body build. The aorta, the large artery that comes out of the heart, first sends branches up to the brain, then to the arms, and finally to the trunk and lower part of the body. In coarctation, a segment of the aorta going to the lower part of the body is narrowed or constricted. As a result, most of the blood coming out of the heart goes to the head, upper chest and arms, while too little flows to the legs. As you might expect, there is high blood pressure in the arms (one of the unusual forms that are curable by surgery) and low pressure in the legs, the only disease in which this is so. (Coarctation of the aorta is the reason we always measure the blood pressure in the legs of anyone who has hypertension.) If this constriction is not recognized and corrected surgically at an early age, the patient grows up looking like a strong man at the circus—with a striking chest, broad shoulders, and powerful arms. But when he takes his trousers off, we see puny legs and a small lower torso.

Your Hair Distribution

How your hair is distributed may tell me whether or not you have a glandular disturbance. For example, a woman who regularly needs to shave her face may have a tumor of the ovary or the adrenal glands. A man who needs to shave only every two or three days (and is not a eunuch) may have liver trouble (often caused by alcoholism) or is receiving female hormone (usually for cancer of the prostate). Persons with low thyroid function have sparse eyebrows, without hair in the outer third or half. In normal women, the genital hair line is horizontal. In men, it is less well defined, and tapers toward the belly button. Young adolescent males are often embarrassed by the fact that long after they consider themselves fully developed, they continue to have the female distribution of hair in the pubic (genital) area. If you have such anxiety, let me assure you that the typical change may not take place for several years after puberty, and there is nothing wrong with you on that account.

BLOOD PRESSURE

Virtually everyone agrees that blood pressure readings should be taken routinely and regularly, that high blood pressure is dangerous and must be lowered to normal values.

Blood pressure testing—the act of having the cuff placed on the arm and inflated—makes people anxious, and this alone may elevate the reading above what it would "normally" be. In order to minimize this fear, especially among new patients, I leave the cuff on for a while before I inflate it. This permits you to become accustomed to it—while I casually putter around, straighten my examination tray, step out of the room for a moment, or in some other way "defuse" the situation. I then measure the blood pressure in the right arm in the sitting position first. I pump up the cuff around your arm, compressing the artery beneath it. When I now listen with my stethoscope over the artery in the angle between the arm and the forearm, I hear no sound because there is no blood flowing through due to the inflated cuff. I then slowly release the air in the cuff, decompressing the underlying artery and allowing blood to flow through it once more. The point at which I first hear a pulse or beat coming through is called the *systolic blood pressure*. As the air continues to leave the cuff, the point at which the pulse is no longer heard is called the *diastolic pressure*.

Blood pressure is expressed as the systolic pressure (the top figure) over the diastolic pressure (or lower number). A typical blood pressure reading is 130 (systolic) over 80 (diastolic) and is written as 130/80 mm Hg. The *mm Hg* part simply means millimeters of mercury—the height in millimeters to which the pressure in the cuff will raise mercury in a column. Some blood pressure machines use a column of mercury, others have a gauge.

Why It Varies

Blood pressure varies with different positions of the body, so I record it with you sitting and standing. What's more, I take it in both arms. Normally there is very little difference between the right and the left side (no more than 5 to 10 "points" or millimeters). A greater variation may indicate disease of the aorta interfering with the delivery of blood to the arteries in the arm where the pressure is lower.

If I find your blood pressure high (greater than 160/95 in an adult), I will take it again later in the examination. Even if it is low the second time, I don't ignore the first high reading. It tells me that you react to stress by raising your pressure. The examination in my office is not the worst stress you're apt to experience in the course of your life. Chances are that from time to time you're aggravated at work or at home, or are worried, frightened, or tense. Some of us respond to such threatening circumstances, be they psychological or physical, real or imagined, by developing asthma, diarrhea, skin rashes, or palpitations; others respond by raising the blood pressure. In any event, if I've found elevated readings at this first visit, I'll have you come back several times to check your pressure. This will give me some idea whether the pressure is truly high or only "labile"—that is, up and down—and whether the initial elevation was real or simply an overreaction to the threat of the physical examination.

If the Readings Are High

If the readings are really high, like 200/120 then that's a different ball game. I chart the range only over the next day or two because that kind of pressure is dangerous and should be evaluated and treated without delay.

I could never understand the rationale of making a secret of your blood pressure. You're entitled to know it. A normal pressure is good news we should share. If it's high, I'm going to need your cooperation, probably for the rest of your life, and the better informed you are, the more likely I am to get it. If you want to buy a cuff and follow the course of the treatment, that's perfectly reasonable too. You should do whatever is comfortable for you.

Common Patient Reactions to the Blood Pressure Cuff

Sometimes while I'm taking blood pressure, a patient will turn his head to look at the gauge on the wall and is shocked to see the needle go to 200 or more. Relax. That's not necessarily your blood pressure. Since I don't know how much air it will take to obliterate the artery under my stethoscope, I inflate the cuff until the dial registers a high reading, and then let it down slowly. Regardless of where we started on the dial, the point at which the pulse becomes audible is your systolic pressure.

Instead of looking at the gauge, other patients scrutinize my face—trying to get some clues about their pressure from my expression. Sometimes, when I'm tired, feeling out of sorts myself, or have a dour expression, they are alarmed. "My goodness, what's the matter? Is the pressure too high?" If I keep a poker face, a matter-of-fact expression, even that generates anxiety. "You're really mysterious today. Is the pressure too high?" And if I decide to be jovial, and smile as I squeeze the bulb, they'll say, "What's so funny about my blood pressure?"

I remember one day sending a very religious old Jewish man to the hospital. After he arrived, he performed a traditional prayer ritual in which a small black box containing religious documents is placed on the forehead, and some leather strips are very slowly wound around the arm as the prayers are said. An Irish patient in the next bed watched this performance with great admiration. When I visited later in the morning, the Irishman said to me, "Doc, you've got to hand it to the Jews. That guy only came here last night, and he's already taking his own pressure this morning."

What's Normal?

What are the normal pressure limits? Although there is no universal agreement, most doctors feel that in adults systolic pressures consistently above 160 and diastolic pressures greater than 95 are abnormal.

Sometimes, when I tell a patient his pressure is very good, like 110/80, he's worried it's too low. Statistics show that the lower the pressure, the longer you'll live. You may not have as much energy as the rest of us and may become a little light-headed when you change position suddenly, but you'll go on forever. We rarely treat or raise pressure that is naturally low in people who are up and about. Count your blessings, and leave it alone. But if the very low reading (below 100 systolic) is due to overly vigorous treatment for high blood pressure, to hypothyroidism or other glandular disorder, or to severe heart disease, then we do intervene by removing the responsible cause.

If you're taking medication for control of your blood pressure, you'll be coming back at regular intervals to see whether it's effective. For some reason, patients occasionally stop their pills before the visit "just to see if I still need them." This is frustrating to the doctor who has asked you to come back specifically to determine the effect of the drug. If you've not been taking it as directed right up to the visit, it's a waste of time for both of us.

Every now and then, someone receiving treatment for high blood pressure, when told his readings have become normal, asks whether he can now stop the medication. The answer is usually "no." High blood pressure control is a lifetime affair. While we can often reduce the number and dosage of the drugs you're taking, especially if you lose weight, discontinuation almost always results in prompt return of the elevated pressure.

Follow Orders on Medication

And that brings me to one other point about drugs generally. When you have an acute problem, like a sore throat, a bad cold, or a sprained back, you will be given a supply of medicine for a few days. But if you have a chronic disorder which lasts for years, like coronary artery disease with angina, high blood pressure, or diabetes, treatment is an ongoing affair. Never stop taking the pills you've been given simply because you've run out of them. After all, I can't prescribe enough of any drug to last you a lifetime. If you have exhausted your supply before your next visit, don't just take nothing. Phone for a prescription renewal to last you until the next visit. This is very important, because (a) many chronic disorders require continuous treatment and (b) certain drugs like Inderal or cortisone must not be stopped abruptly.

Some Mysteries of Hypertension

We don't understand the mechanisms of high blood pressure in 95 percent of people who have it, so we call the disease *"essential" hypertension.* (In medical jargon, the word *essential* means "unknown cause.") In the remaining 5 percent, elevated pressure is due to some form of kidney disease or rare glandular tumors or disorders. These infrequent causes occur most often in persons under 40 and, if suspected, require a costly, time-consuming workup, which includes special blood analyses and kidney x-rays. If you are under 40 and your pressure is very high, chances are we'll have to proceed with this comprehensive diagnostic survey. But in someone over 50 years of age, we usually do only a few simple tests unless one of the rare causes is strongly suspected.

How We Evaluate High Blood Pressure

When hypertension is discovered, we always examine the urine to see if there is any disorder of kidney function. Then we measure the level of *urea nitrogen* in the blood (discussed later in the section dealing with laboratory tests). Because of the recognition of certain "risk factors" in arteriosclerosis, of which hypertension is the most important, we will also draw blood for cholesterol, sugar, and uric acid (the test for gout). Since high blood pressure affects the circulation, we will get a chest x-ray to see if your heart is enlarged and an electrocardiogram to determine whether it has been strained by having to pump its contents into the arteries against a high pressure or resistance.

Treatment—Almost as Easy as Taking Vitamins

If you have high blood pressure, I have good news and bad news for you. First, the bad news. It causes strokes, speeds up arteriosclerosis, weakens the heart, damages the kidney, can make you blind, and narrows the arteries of the legs, giving you pain when you walk. And now the good news. High blood pressure is easy to treat. What's more, if we lower the pressure, and keep it low, none of these things happen. Treatment is not difficult or painful. It involves reducing the amount of salt in your diet, achieving your ideal weight, and taking one or two tablets a day—no visits to the hospital, no fancy machines, nothing that hurts. Just a couple of pills, almost like taking vitamins.

But No Cheating

In order for your treatment to be successful, you've got to take the tablets faithfully. You're harming only yourself if you don't. Also, if you are fat, you must lose weight. If you do, you'll probably need fewer tablets. Cutting down on your salt intake is not so hard these days because of the many tolerable salt substitutes available. In most cases, you don't have to eat special, unsalted foods, but should avoid the very salty ones like pickled herring, dill pickles and bacon. You should try not to add salt to taste in the cooking, and don't use the shaker at the table. So many of us are extremely careful about the amount of salt we take, and then, unwittingly, more than make up for it in other ways. For example, did you know that one dose of such products as Alka-Seltzer, Bisodol, Bromo-Seltzer, and Sal Hepatica contain more salt than you should be taking all day if you have high blood pressure?

We've been able to relax many of the older rigid restrictions on salt intake because the mainstay of modern drug treatment of high blood pressure is the *diuretic,* which lowers blood pressure by causing your body to lose salt in the urine. So if you do take a *little* salt in the diet, it doesn't affect the pressure significantly.

Commonly Used Blood Pressure Medicines—How They Work and Their Side Effects

In addition to the diuretics, there are several other agents widely used for blood pressure control. These work in different ways—on the nerves that contract the arteries, on the brain itself, by a chemical action on the arteries, by neutralizing a hormone in the blood, or by making the heart pump less hard. Your pressure can be normalized by giving very small amounts of several of these agents in combination—if one alone doesn't work. There is so little of each drug in the mixture that troublesome side effects usually do not develop. Years ago, when we had only one or two drugs at our disposal, we had to give more and more of them until the blood pressure came down. This often produced side effects, and was responsible for the mistaken idea some people still have that blood pressure treatment has intolerable toxicity, that the "cure" is worse than the disease.

Even though treatment is successful and usually well tolerated, there may be some *undesirable individual reactions*. These can almost always be managed by changing the dose or the drug itself. Some of the side effects we may encounter are (1) with the diuretics—cramps in the legs, gout, dry mouth, frequency of urination, elevated blood sugar, and weakness due to potassium loss; (2) with Inderal—slow pulse, impotence, diarrhea, asthma, heart failure; (3) with Aldomet—tender breasts, impotence, retrograde ejaculation (the sperm, instead of coming out of the penis, goes into the bladder and there is no ejaculate); (4) reserpine—nasal congestion, depression, impotence, slow pulse, stomach ulcers; (5) Apresoline (in large doses)—arthritis. But remember, in almost every instance, these *side effects can be eliminated* by decreasing the dosage or changing the drug being used.

FEELING YOUR PULSE

I now check the pulse at the wrist to determine whether it's regular or irregular, too fast or too slow, and of good quality. Later in the physical I will check all the pulse points in the body to see how the blood is flowing to your brain, abdomen, and legs.

The normal resting pulse rate is somewhere between 60 and 90 per minute. If you are an athlete, it may be as low as 45 or 50 beats per minute, reflecting a well-conditioned heart. But medications can slow the *pulse below 50 a minute*. These include reserpine (prescribed as a tranquilizer and for lowering high blood pressure), Inderal (an agent widely used for the treatment of high blood pressure, angina pectoris, overactive thyroid and irregular pulse), and digitalis (the most widely used cardiac drug). If you're not taking any medicine and are not a well-trained athlete, a pulse below 50 per minute may be due to low thyroid function or some disorder of your heart. This slow rate then requires clarification.

Pulse Variations and What They Mean

A *rapid pulse*, faster than 90 to 100 beats per minute at rest, is most often due to nervousness, excitement, or fear. But if you're calm and not apparently upset, yet on repeated determinations your pulse rate remains elevated, you may be anemic or have a chronic illness, heart trouble, infection, or an overactive thyroid.

What about an *irregular pulse*—one that is neither too rapid nor too slow, but simply jumpy? Any such irregularity of the pulse or disturbance of the heart's rhythm is called an *arrhythmia*. Many variations in heart rhythm are harmless; most people, sometime during the day or night, have some irregularity without even being aware of it. But an arrhythmia can be a signal of heart trouble, and its precise identification is absolutely necessary.

A disturbance in heart rhythm can occur as either a single "skipped beat," a run of "extra beats," or a sudden change in the heart rate. Even when an arrhythmia is of the harmless variety, it is frightening to most people.

The commonest variety of changing heart rhythm is that caused by respiration. Try it yourself. As you take a deep breath in, the heart rate increases; when you breathe out, the heart slows. This variation associated with breathing is never a sign of disease. When you exercise, your heart goes faster and the respiratory irregularity disappears.

What about the "skipped beat"? In most cases, you are unaware of it. If you are, you feel like your heart has stopped for a moment. The terms "skipped beat" and "missed beat" are actually misnomers, because what we are in fact dealing with are neither "skipped," "missed," nor "extra" beats, but *early (premature)* beats. Let me explain.

Suppose you have a regular heart rate of 60 per minute. The

heart beats once every second, or in three seconds it contracts three times. Let's further suppose the second of the three beats comes early, say half a second after the first instead of a full second. Even though the second beat was early, the heart has no intention of overworking, and will still beat only three times in those three seconds. This means that there will be a longer interval or pause between the early second beat and the third beat, which is on time. What you feel when you think you have a "skipped" beat is, not the early beat, but the pause between it and the succeeding one. This is sometimes alarming because you may feel the heart is stopping and may not start up again. Don't worry; it always will.

Premature beats occur in a variety of circumstances, most commonly fatigue, emotional stress, cigarette smoking, alcohol use, and certain forms of heart disease. They are also observed in persons who take too much strong coffee, tea, carbonated cola beverages, or certain medications in excess (digitalis). Occasionally, foods that are very spicy, excessively hot, very cold, or to which you are allergic can induce such rhythm changes. These beats usually disappear spontaneously, but some persons are troubled by them and require treatment.

When bursts of rapid consecutive beats lasting a few seconds or longer interrupt the normal, regular cardiac rhythm, treatment is usually needed even though the cause for the abnormal rhythm does not necessarily lie in the heart. An overactive thyroid gland or too many thyroid pills can cause such paroxysms of rapid heart rate.

What Should Be Done About It?

Whatever the variation in cardiac rhythm, further testing is usually necessary to determine its cause, significance, and treatment. This is especially true in persons over 40 years of age or those with other evidence of heart disease. Additional investigation will include blood analyses for thyroid function, an electrocardiogram (ECG) before and after exercise, and a 24-hour ECG monitor. All these techniques are described in detail in the chapter dealing with special tests.

Having felt the pulse for its rhythm, I now check its *quality*. Whether it's strong or weak is not always easy to determine, even for me. For example, if you are fat, with a lot of flesh overlying the radial artery in the wrist where I feel for the pulse, it may appear to be of low volume.

More important than a small pulse is a very forceful one, which may indicate a variety of cardiac disorders—high blood pressure, an overactive thyroid, anemia, or valvular disease of the heart.

How to Take a Pulse Reading

I often ask a patient or a member of his family to count the pulse and report it back to me. This information is important when you're taking medication that can slow the pulse (Inderal, reserpine, or digitalis) or are being treated for some irregularity of rhythm and I want to assess the treatment's efficacy without bringing you back to the office too often.

You wouldn't believe how many people can't take their own, or anyone else's, pulse. And it's so simple. All you do is find the artery at the wrist (with the palm upward). It's in a straight line back from the index or middle finger. Doctors usually put the pads of their ring, index, and middle fingers over the pulsation in the wrist. Then, using the second hand of a watch to get the number of beats per minute, count for 15 seconds and multiply by 4, or count 20 seconds and multiply by 3, or count for a full minute. Note not only the pulse rate, but whether or not it's regular.

YOUR SKIN

The internist views the skin somewhat differently than does the dermatologist. The latter can distinguish one eruption from another; if he wants to identify a particular fungus, he will take a scraping of the skin, look at it under the microscope, and culture the organism on artificial media. If there is a rash or a mole or other growth, suspicious for malignancy, he will cut away a small piece of it (biopsy) and send it to the laboratory for identification. But the internist views the skin for evidence of internal disease. In addition to the obvious infections, tumors, parasites, and irritations that appear on the skin, the surface of your body may tell me if you are allergic (a rash or hives appear); are a drug addict (needle holes near veins); have internal cancer (characteristic lesions, jaundice, pallor); have disease of the liver, lungs, and heart (blue lips), kidneys (pallor), or glandular system (hair distribution). So you may shuttle between the skin doctor and the internist. If I find something local, I send you to him. If he finds something he thinks reflects an internal problem, he sends you back to me.

Skin Color and What It Reveals

We have already seen that "paleness," or *pallor,* of the skin can be very misleading. When I test the blood later, I will measure your hemoglobin and do a hematocrit, which will tell me whether you are pale because you are anemic (too few red blood cells or not enough oxygen in them) or simply because of your particular pigment endowment or lack of exposure to the elements.

Your skin may also have additional or unusual color, sometimes so subtle that neither you nor those in constant contact with you are aware of it. A yellowish hue may be due to a medication you're taking (dinitrophenol, Atabrine—quinacrine) or to excessive amounts of carotene in the diet (carrots, leafy vegetables, or oranges). Too much carotene stains the skin yellow, especially the palms and soles, and makes you look like you have jaundice, except that it never discolors the eyes, as does jaundice. Pernicious anemia and low thyroid function confer on the skin a pasty, almost yellowish hue.

Black and Blue Marks

Minor trauma such as knocking against an object gives some people, especially women at the time of their menses, "black and blue" marks. If you've been taking cortisone for a long time, you may bleed easily under the skin. Elderly persons, in whom blood vessels are more fragile because of the loss of surrounding protective fat, bruise easily too. None of these situations necessarily mean that there is similar bleeding inside the body.

Hemorrhages in the skin are important if they reflect trouble with the blood-clotting mechanism. If that's the case, you run the risk of an internal hemorrhage into vital organs like the brain, kidney, lungs, and intestinal tract. Abnormal bleeding is seen in a variety of disorders such as hemophilia, in which the blood does not clot properly, leukemia, and drug allergy when certain factors necessary for normal clotting are disturbed by the allergic process.

Pigment may be deposited in the skin and may involve the whole body or only certain areas. The most important such condition is a dark hue seen in a serious glandular disorder called *Addison's disease,* in which the glands that make cortisone are depressed.

Quality of the Skin—Is It the Kind One Loves to Touch?

Is it dry? This may be due to dehydration, vitamin A deficiency, low thyroid function, old age, kidney trouble, diuretics, skin disease, or too much exposure to the sun.

Is it moist? This may be from fever, anxiety, or an overactive thyroid.

Is it loose? I pinch the top layer of the skin to see whether it falls back into place immediately. If it doesn't, you either are dehydrated or have recently lost a great deal of weight. If I can pick skin up off the underlying fat (try it on your upper arm), that is also a sign of weight loss, although in older persons it is a common finding due to loss of elastic tissue.

Is it tense? There may be some tumor or swelling beneath it.

Rashes and What They Mean

A skin rash can be due to so many things I can't begin even to list them all here. Causes may range from insect bites to allergy, from typhoid fever to leukemia. Even if your skin appears to be free of any eruption, I will look in the folds and around your genitals for evidence of *syphilis.* Its earliest sign is a chancre—a painless, hard sore which may look like an innocent cold sore.

Patients don't always draw it to my attention, because unlike the cold sore due to a virus, it doesn't hurt, and so they think it's of no consequence. To make matters worse, if left alone, the chancre clears up completely after a few weeks, leaving no trace, and is soon forgotten. That's the reason most patients who are indiscriminately sexually active must have frequent blood testing for syphilis (Wassermann, VDRL, FTA). As in rheumatic fever, after the earliest symptoms of the disease, there is a long interval of "good health" before its deadly effects become apparent in the brain, heart, and other tissues.

I will also look for scratch marks due to chronic itching from a variety of causes. Older people, and women after the menopause, may have little brown-yellowish spots, usually slightly raised, on the face, hands or body. These are called *keratoses* and are a manifestation of aging or sun damage.

I search for warts and moles, paying particular attention to whether they have been bleeding or crusting or have changed in color or size. Such moles can be very malignant, especially those that look bluish-black (malignant melanoma).

Most "Skin Cancers" Are Not Cancers at All

Every now and then, someone will come to the office distraught and panicky. "I've just been told I have skin cancer. What do I do now?" The term skin "cancer" is most unfortunate. It should be called something else. The scientific name for the commonest skin cancer is basal-cell epithelioma. Such skin "cancers" are usually easily recognizable and for the most part completely curable. They are called "cancer" because the component cells multiply and look cancerous under the microscope, but in virtually every case they multiply only locally—that is, the tumor just gets bigger. It does not invade distant tissues. To call it "cancer" is as reasonable as calling a fly a kind of airplane.

And Can Be Safely Treated

When told they have skin cancer of the basal-cell type, some patients are suspicious of the honest reassurance we give them, and remain fearful of the implications of having a "cancer." Although there are malignancies of the skin that are life-threatening (like the blue-black malignant melanoma), the common basal-cell epithelioma should cause you no anxiety once it is removed. This is usually done surgically, although newer anticancer ointments can be applied directly to the skin (5-fluorouracil, 5-FU) in some patients.

You may have noticed that some people have soft yellowish plaques (*xanthomas*) around the eyes, the palms, the elbows, or other parts of the body. These usually coalesce. Because they are often associated with a high blood cholesterol, their presence warrants an analysis of the blood for disorders of fat metabolism.

Your Hair and Scalp

At this point I run my fingers through your hair. (You've already assured me it isn't a wig. It doesn't do me much good to evaluate someone else's hair even if it is on your scalp. Sprays also confuse my assessment of the hair texture, so please don't visit your hairdresser before your checkup.) If you have low thyroid function, your hair is apt to be coarse, brittle, dry, and fall out easily, especially on the scalp, outer third of the eyebrows, beard and sexual areas. Fine, silky hair, normal in many people, may be evidence of thyroid overactivity in others.

Graying is due to loss of pigment in the hair follicles. Although it is part of the normal aging process, it may be accelerated by emotional upset. Some people, even in their thirties, are "prematurely" gray—a trait that seems to run in families.

Baldness may affect several members of the same family. "Premature" balding, independent of aging, is a familial trait. Fever and chronic illness, as well as injury by cosmetics and chemicals, can also result in hair loss, much of which grows back after the offending agent has been removed.

Remember that for every instance of baldness in which the hair thins because of factors or causes we don't understand, there are many more due to injury—as, for example, using curlers, bleaches, and chemicals in permanent waves. Infection from bugs like nits (lice) may also result in hair loss.

After I look at and feel your hair, I will examine the scalp, where serious disease is rare. Your most likely complaint will be dandruff, and the embarrassment it causes when you wear something dark blue. The "dermatitis" causing the "snowflakes" on the shoulders can easily be cleared up with appropriate shampoos, creams or soap.

CHAPTER **8**

EXAMINING THE UPPER PART OF YOUR BODY

YOUR EYES

You Name the Disease, They Reflect It

Examination of the eyes constitutes a very important part of the checkup. Some patients are surprised when a doctor other than an eye specialist (ophthalmologist) pays a lot of attention to the eyes. We do so for very much the same reasons we look at your skin—not necessarily for evidence of local disease or to assess your vision (although we do that too) but for signs of a general disorder. Careful examination of the eyes, both inside and out, by an internist may reveal arteriosclerosis, high cholesterol, diabetes, vitamin deficiency, tuberculosis, anemia, cancer, cataracts, a brain tumor, a lung tumor, high blood pressure, stroke, viral infection, infection of a heart valve, thyroid trouble, multiple sclerosis and other neurological diseases, and even syphilis.

And that's only a partial list. Let's go through the highlights of such an exam together.

What the Eyes Tell About You

As I look at you, I immediately see whether your eyes are bloodshot from fatigue, infection, eyestrain, or drinking; bruised from fighting; swollen from crying; or yellow from jaundice—an enormous amount of information just from the first glance. If the skin around them is puffy, you may have kidney disease or low thyroid function (or simply be a candidate for plastic surgery). Most of us get dark rings under the eyes if we've been under strain, without sleep, or very tired. I'm not sure what causes this discoloration. Bulging or very prominent eyes often indicate toxic overactivity of the thyroid gland, but may simply be a normal familial or personal characteristic. One eyeball may protrude because of a tumor in the socket pushing it out from behind. The two eyelids are not always symmetrical, but if one or both really droop, we may be dealing with myasthenia gravis. On the other hand, a lung tumor may press on a nerve in the chest which controls the eyelid muscles, causing the eye on that side to droop and its pupil to become smaller. An old stroke can cause ocular asymmetry, as can Bell's palsy (a viral infection of the facial nerve with residual paralysis of the facial muscles). Feeling the eyeballs through your eyelids is also important. When they're unusually soft—not very common in healthy people—it suggests dehydration or severe vitamin A deficiency.

Do You See Spots?

If your eyeballs are unusually hard, you may have *glaucoma*. I will then ask if you see halos of light when you look straight ahead.

If I suspect that your ocular pressure is too high, I will either measure it myself with a *tonometer* or send you to an eye doctor.

When I look at the inside of your lower lid, I can see whether it's a healthy pink or is pale, indicating anemia. A white ring in the cornea (the front transparent part of the eyeball surrounding the pupil) is called *arcus senilis* (arc of aging) and is common in older persons. When present below the age of 40, it may indicate a disorder of cholesterol metabolism and a vulnerability to early arteriosclerosis. This is particularly true if it is associated with little raised yellow plaques on the eyelids (xanthelasmata). If either one is present (arcus or plaques), I will get a complete blood analysis later to check out your fat metabolism.

Testing Your Eye Muscles

When I ask you to follow my finger up, down, and sideways, I'm testing to see if any of the muscles responsible for eye movement are weak or paralyzed. If when you look up or to either side your eyes oscillate, this points to a possible visual disorder or a viral infection of the inner ear. As we sit facing each other, I have you cover your left eye, and I cover my right eye. I then stretch my arm out to the right and move it toward the midline. I want to know at what point you can see my fingers. You should see them at the same time I do, since my vision has been tested and found to be normal. This maneuver, done on each side, is a simple test to assess *peripheral vision,* which is impaired by certain brain tumors, strokes, or glaucoma.

She Wasn't Wearing Blinders

I remember one unfortunate case in which this simple test was not done. A woman in her middle fifties complained of a loss in peripheral vision. She felt as if she was wearing blinders, like a horse. She was reassured that this "tunnel vision" was related to emotional problems she was having at the time. She was sent to a psychiatrist who, assuming the referring physician had excluded a physical basis for the symptoms, formulated an interesting hypothesis to account for them. According to him, she had the feeling that her field of vision was constricted because she had put on "emotional blinders" and was shutting the rest of the world out of her life. Months of psychotherapy did not help. Then, one day the women got a cinder in her eye and went to the emergency room of a local hospital to have it removed. The intern on the eye service insisted on examining her eyes with an ophthalmoscope. There he found evidence of a great increase in pressure within the brain, due to a slowly growing tumor which had given her the "blinders" all these months.

What the Pupils of Your Eyes Tell Your Doctor, or "I'm Dilated to Meet You"

Your pupils, too, can tell me a great deal. They may be very small in older people, in those with glaucoma, or in drug addicts (morphine and its derivatives cause *constriction* of the pupil). *Dilated pupils* may be the result of fever, brain injury, eye drops, and some forms of blindness. *Irregular pupils* (they are normally round) may be a sign of late-stage syphilis of the nervous system. Although both pupils are usually the same size, one may be larger than the other. If the difference is obvious, chances are you've had a cataract operation on the dilated side.

When I shine a light into your eyes, both pupils should contract. If you first look into the distance and then abruptly at my finger in front of your nose, the pupil should become smaller, or *accommodate*. Failure to do so may indicate syphilis.

Inside Your Eye

After I've completed the external examination of the eye, I look into its interior with the ophthalmoscope. A clouding of the lens means you have a cataract, and that may prevent me from seeing in just as it interferes with your seeing out. I point at a spot on the wall opposite the examining table on which you're sitting, and ask you to fix your gaze on it. It's very hard for me to examine the eye unless you keep it perfectly still.

The inside of the eye is the only place in the body where I can actually see an artery. Everywhere else I can only listen to them or feel them. When I look at your retinal arteries I note if they are narrowed by arteriosclerosis, whether there are hemorrhages due to diabetes, or spasm resulting from high blood pressure. Even tuberculosis or other infections can be recognized by a characteristic appearance in the back of the eye.

My Ears and Your Eyes

Having looked at the inside and outside of your eyes, I now listen to them. When there is important narrowing of the large blood vessels, I will hear a "whooshing sound" or "bruit" over your eyeball.

Seeing Eye to Eye

Recently, as I was about to examine the interior of a new patient's eyes, he suddenly and with great intensity confronted me eyeball to eyeball. Every now and then doctors encounter strange and unexpected behavior in the examining room, some of it, as in this case, frightening. It's best to be prudent, so I tactfully averted his gaze, withdrew to adjust my stethoscope and returned to examine him—hoping the attack of curiosity, aggression or whatever would pass. I was wrong. He drew even closer to me, and finally broke the silence. "You're wearing my glasses," he said accusingly. "No, no," I replied, "they're mine. See? These bifocals were especially fitted to me." He was adamant. "You're wearing my glasses," and with that, he suddenly pulled them off my face. "I'm going to break them," he threatened. What to do? It was late in the afternoon. He was my last patient. Everyone in the office had left. I had the choice of a physical showdown or a psychological approach. I chose the latter—he was bigger than I. "Please give me my glasses. Don't break them," I asked. "Why not?" "Because I won't be able to see to go home this evening." He thought for a moment, and then, slowly and reluctantly, he returned the glasses to me.

"I should have broken those glasses," he murmured ruefully. "But why?" I asked. He replied, "You see, they really are mine. Look at the name printed on the frame." I did. "That's my company. I make those frames," he said, "and they should never have been sold to you. They are esthetically wrong for your face—wrong shape, wrong style, wrong color. Please don't wear them. I'll send you new ones tomorrow." And he did. I now have six pairs of glasses. What's more, he was right. The ones he almost broke were all wrong for me.

YOUR BREATH

While looking into the back of your eyes, I can get a good whiff of your breath (and you of mine). I once had a devoted secretary who for lunch insisted I eat salami and dill pickle, which I love. A candid patient commented on this one day while I was examining his eyes. I decided it was time to change my midday menu.

Even Your Doctor Won't Tell You

Bad breath—or halitosis, as it is referred to on television—like body odor and dandruff, is something your best friend and even your doctor may not tell you about. It may be due to your diet, poor oral hygiene and dental decay, or infection in the respiratory tract. In my experience, and despite the fact that so many patients insist otherwise, it is not often due to stomach upset.

Chronic sinusitis and infection of the lung both cause bad breath, usually associated with foul-smelling, greenish-yellow sputum. Alcohol on your breath is of great diagnostic significance to me. As I come close to examine you at 9:30 in the morning, and am overcome by a gust of bourbon or Scotch, your breakfast "menu" should definitely be discussed. If you complain that you're "oh so tired" in mid-afternoon, and I smell whiskey at 2:30 P.M., the cause may be too much booze at lunch. Finally, if you protest that you drink only moderately or "socially," and each time I examine you or talk to you, you have a whiskey breath, then you're either being less than candid (a characteristic of alcoholics) or we're witnessing a remarkable coincidence.

Important though it is to assess your breath, tragedies can result from overreliance on mouth odors in emergency situations. For example, when someone loses consciousness, we must consider an unwitnessed head injury, stroke, epileptic seizure, heart attack, diabetic coma or insulin overdosage, as possibilities. But if before passing out, he happens to have had a drink, a bypasser who smells the breath and detects alcohol may conclude that the victim is simply a drunk. He is then allowed to "sleep it off," losing valuable time which could be lifesaving. *Never conclude on your own, no matter how obvious the circumstantial evidence, that a comatose or stuporous patient is simply a lush.*

YOUR EARS

If you have a *hearing problem* you will probably go directly to an ear specialist, who has the equipment to measure the hearing deficit and can tell you what kind it is (bone or nerve) and what can be done about it.

In the routine physical, however, I make a gross assessment of your ears. I pull the ear lobe up in order to straighten the canal, which is normally curved. The skin of the ear canal is subject to the same eczema, infections, and irritations as is skin anywhere else on the body, especially if you are constantly probing and scratching it.

Incidentally, ear wax—though it can be a nuisance—serves a useful purpose. It protects the eardrum by trapping small particles that get into the canal. *Excessive wax* is not necessarily a sign of poor hygiene, but more likely due to actively secreting glands in your ear canal. In some persons, the angle of the canal is so sharp that the wax is inaccessible to normal cleaning and needs to be removed from time to time. There are some solutions you can buy which, when instilled, will liquefy the wax, permitting you to rinse it out gently with a syringe and warm water. Frankly, I advise you to let your doctor do it. It's a whole lot safer.

In some patients we can make the diagnosis of gout if they have hard little lumps on the tops of their ears or along the tendons in the hands and feet (tophi). These contain and sometimes discharge a chalky substance made up of uric acid crystals.

Different Kinds of Deafness

Hearing loss may be due to different causes. In order for you to hear a sound, it must first be conducted through your ear canal to the membrane (eardrum) inside. If the canal is blocked by wax or a foreign object, this will impair your hearing. Not long ago, one of my older patients cleaned his ears with a piece of cotton and simply left it there. By the time he came to see me, the canal was infected by the deeply embedded cotton and he was stone deaf. Removing the cotton restored his hearing.

Beyond the eardrum are three little bones which are connected to each other. The "sound wave" that makes the drum vibrate moves these bones. As a result, tiny hairlike structures or nerve endings in the inner ear are stimulated, sending a signal to the hearing center in the brain, which interprets the sound. When deafness is of the conductive type, these bones cannot make the drum vibrate, the nerve endings deep inside the ear are not stimulated, and no message is sent to the brain. This form of deafness can usually be corrected by surgery. Other causes of *conductive deafness* are an infection with pus or fluid in the ear, or a perforated eardrum.

By contrast, *nerve deafness* stems from damage not to the bones or the eardrum, but to the hearing nerve itself, which is then unable to transmit to the brain the message it receives from the vibrating drum and bones. Although a brain tumor is sometimes responsible, the usual cause of nerve injury is arteriosclerosis of the blood vessels supplying the nerve, or injury due to excessive noise. Nerve deafness is the type we usually find in older people. It progresses very slowly, and doesn't often cause severe deafness. More commonly, the ability to discriminate high-pitched sounds is lost. Telephones may go unanswered, and women's conversation, especially in a noisy room, is poorly understood. Unlike the conductive form of deafness, surgery cannot help such patients, and even hearing aids are of limited help.

Incidentally, noise (and it doesn't have to be too loud) not only causes deafness but also raises blood pressure and heart rate.

YOUR NOSE

No Place for Your Finger or a Jelly Bean

I look at the membranes of the nose to see if there is evidence of low-grade allergy, irritation, or polyps. Chronic "colds" and a recurrent stuffy nose are usually due to long-standing allergic reactions. Children, especially, with this problem are always pushing the nose up to help them breathe—an "allergic salute." Not infrequently, again among children, we find a jelly bean there, too. Although the bulbous red nose of the drunkard is a fact, a red nose does not always mean alcoholism. A potentially serious disease called lupus erythematosus, acne rosacea (caused by excessive flushing of blood vessels in the nose and cheeks), and certain vitamin deficiencies and infections can make the nose red.

I also look in the nose for dilated blood vessels that may bleed, for deviations of the septum that may force you to mouth-breathe, and for infections. An infection of the skin at the angle of the nose and cheek can be serious, because this area is drained by veins communicating with the brain. Before the era of anti-biotics, infections spreading from the nose to those veins were sometimes fatal.

If you have any real problems with your nose, you'll likely end up having a specialist look at it.

YOUR MOUTH AND TONGUE

Even Though I Am Not a Dentist

I will look carefully around and inside the mouth. Your lips—unless you've covered them with lipstick—tell me if there is enough oxygen in your blood. If there is not, as in patients with advanced heart trouble and in children born with abnormal shunts of blood from one part of the heart to the other (the "blue" baby), they are apt to be blue. If you have large adenoids (lymph glands in the throat) or your nose is obstructed by a con-gested lining or polyps, I'll find you breathing through your mouth. Sores at the angles of the mouth may indicate vitamin deficiency (usually B_2), while the chancre of syphilis sometimes occurs on the lips. Swollen lips may be a clue to allergy.

Say "Ah"

The usual examination of the tongue is a cursory affair. You stick it out for a moment and say, "Ah." If it comes out straight, without falling over to one side like your dog's, and if there is nothing obvious to see on it—that's the end of the examination. But if you've told me it pains you, I will look more closely. Only recently in the course of a routine examination, a man of 60 complained of pain in his tongue. Careful examination revealed a tumor behind it which was ultimately found to have spread there from his bowel.

The Morning After

The tongue is a favorite organ of self-examination, which some of us look at in the morning to help start the day right. A "furry" coating the morning after a binge is of no medical significance. But the appearance of the tongue can tip me off to some meaningful things. For example, in older people who are feeble, in alcoholics, and in those with an overactive thyroid, it quivers abnormally. If you have had a stroke and stick out your tongue, it hangs toward the paralyzed side. When you have been taking antibiotics, it may have a black coating after a few days. The antibiotic kills not only the bacteria that are making you sick but the harmless ones which are normal and useful residents in your body. As a result, fungus, which is normally held in check by the benign bacteria, takes over and gives your tongue the black color.

Cancer Warning

I touch the tongue to test its moisture and to feel for tumors. High fever, decreased water intake, or more commonly excessive loss of water from the body (severe diarrhea or uncontrolled diabetes) make it very dry. I also note whether it is smooth and beefy red, suggesting pernicious anemia, vitamin B deficiency, or lack of iron. A tongue too big for your mouth (and I don't mean this socially) may be due to underfunction of the thyroid or a tumor of the pituitary gland in the brain producing too much growth hormone. The tongue can also appear shrunken or wasted in some cases of paralysis. If you are a heavy smoker, especially a pipe smoker, I will look for little white plaques caused by irritation of the pipe and the heat of the smoke. These are precancerous and constitute a very effective and dramatic warning to stop smoking.

The *gums* are also of medical interest. Leukemia and some medications such as Dilantin (used in the treatment of epilepsy) cause them to become thick and overhang the teeth, whereas in vitamin deficiencies the opposite happens—they shrink from the teeth. Lead poisoning, still seen these days in children who eat flakes of paint containing lead, will result in a dark blue line on the gums. Though the law in most communities now requires paint to be lead-free, there are still some ghetto areas where the old lead-based paint is found—and eaten.

Your Teeth

I am not competing with your dentist when I look at your *teeth.* They provide useful information about your general condition. Are they in good repair? Multiple cavities, loose or absent teeth—all may reduce the biting surface or so impair occlusion that you can't chew properly. This is an important cause of malnutrition in older people, especially those who are poor. Bad teeth may be the source of facial pain and also of enlargement of lymph glands (or lymph nodes) in the neck. In certain diseases, the teeth assume a diagnostic shape. For example, in congenital syphilis, the incisors in front are notched, due to loss of enamel. In acromegaly (pituitary brain tumor) they are wide apart, and the lower teeth extend beyond the upper. In heavy smokers, they are yellow. And believe it or not, just looking at your teeth, as appraising your attire, gives me a good idea of your economic status (could you afford to have the teeth fixed and the bite corrected) and your personal habits.

YOUR THROAT

Now you open your mouth a little wider so I can examine the back of your throat. This is sometimes easier said than done. We all have a *gag reflex,* with which nature endowed us to prevent accidental swallowing of foreign substances. But in many people, this reflex is so sensitive that when I put a tongue depressor on the back of the tongue, they heave, burp, threaten to vomit, and occasionally do. In order to minimize this reaction, I soak the tongue depressor in hot water before using it. I've found that when the stick is warm and moist, the gag reflex is very much less active.

It's Embarrassing to Gag, But Worse If You Don't

A *hypersensitive gag reflex* is embarrassing for you and makes it difficult for me to examine your throat. But the reverse situation—the absence of this reflex—is an ominous finding because it may reflect disease of the brain or of its major nerves. We assess an unconscious person by testing the gag reflex. Its absence suggests a very serious complication, but in addition, there is no protection against inhalation of saliva or vomitus into the lungs.

When you say, "Ah," if your soft palate doesn't move or is pulled over to one side, you have a serious disorder of nerve or muscle (stroke, myasthenia gravis), which will need further study. The throat may also be the seat of many infections and ulcerations ranging from syphilis and tuberculosis to the simple irritation seen among smokers.

The *vocal cords* can be examined only with the help of a little mirror put down the back of your throat. It is warmed first in order for it not to fog up. This procedure is not done routinely except by ear, nose, and throat specialists, but it must be performed whenever you complain of persistent hoarseness.

COSMETIC FACIAL SURGERY

Beauty Is Only Skin Deep, But . . .

Before leaving the face and head, let's consider the status of *cosmetic facial surgery*. The idealized versions we have of ourselves rarely approximate what we really look like. Even the most physically beautiful among us are sometimes not happy with their natural endowment. Because such dissatisfaction is frequently based on existing cultural tastes, cosmetic surgery has become a major and rapidly growing area of medicine.

People request plastic surgery or repair for many different reasons. You may want certain deformities corrected which were present at birth (cleft palate, harelip) or are the result of injuries, accidents or burns. These may be disfiguring or interfere with your speech or breathing. You may have other physical features which you find objectionable—cauliflower ears, an unsightly nose, or perhaps a birthmark or "portwine" stain on the face. Most of us can live with these blemishes, but some would rather not have them. Before the era of cosmetic surgery, when we didn't really have this option, our culture compensated for these superficial variations. I was reminded of this one day while examining a man of fifty. He had a really unsightly dark wartlike affair near the tip of his nose. I asked him how long he had it. "Oh you mean my beauty mark?" That birthmark could not be beautiful in the eyes of any beholder, yet he was emotionally protected against its ugliness by calling it the socially acceptable "beauty mark." And finally, there are those changes that occur with age—the loosening of the skin around the face and neck, and bags under the eyes.

When It's A Good Idea

If you have any of these problems, you may well ask your own doctor whether he thinks you should see a plastic surgeon. His personal philosophy will determine the advice he gives you. While beauty is, in fact, only skin deep, often a gross deformity does interfere with one's social development and personal happiness. If surgical correction is possible and you would like to have it done, I will advise you to go ahead. But remember that most of us can cope with and compensate for debits in our appearance. Just look around at the well-adjusted couples you know, not all of whom are beauties.

Sometimes It's a Waste of Time

If a middle-aged woman finds her husband philandering and attributes this to her wrinkled skin and baggy eyes, and if she becomes convinced that a change in her appearance will make a difference, who am I to dissuade her from trying it—even if she's probably wrong and the root of the problem is something other than her appearance?

Before you rush off to the plastic surgeon, remember that some of the major cosmetic procedures can only be carried out under general anesthesia, that is, with the patient asleep. This still carries some risk, especially in persons with heart trouble or lung disease. *Whatever emotional uplift is to be derived from cosmetic surgery must be weighed against the risk of the operation.*

The most commonly performed plastic procedures done on the face include removing the bags from under the eyes, face-lifts, "nose jobs," and correction of prominent ears. Puffy bags under the eyes are removed under local anesthesia and a sedative—that is, you are not put to sleep. The surgeon will cut away excess skin and this eliminates the tired look of baggy eyes.

Plastic surgeons usually recommend a face-lift if you're having the eyes fixed anyway. Stretched-out, extra skin of the face and neck is removed, eliminating sagging cheeks and jowls. This does confer a more youthful appearance, if that's what you're after. Since the aging process is relentless, one such correction may not be enough, and additional "tucking in" is usually necessary later on.

Nose and Ear Jobs

The operation to alter the size and shape of the nose (*rhinoplasty*) is also often done under local anesthesia and sedation. When properly performed, the scars are hidden within the nose and are not visible externally. Ten or fifteen years ago, most people having such surgery looked like relatives because they all ended up with the same "bobbed-up" noses. But today, it's not so easy to detect a surgically altered proboscis.

Children born with ears that are too prominent and unsightly can have them corrected in childhood through an operation called *otoplasty*.

Plastic surgery is here to stay. Many of us who were more conservative are now coming around to the idea that if correction of a deformity will make you feel better and look better—and you can afford it—why not?

There is one exception to this generalization, and at the risk of offending the plastic surgery community, it must still be stated. The eternal search for youth and the physical self-criticism that induces some of us to change our appearance may represent an underlying emotional disorder. When this is so, the patient is never satisfied with the repair, and spends his days between the operating room, having the latest "job" fixed, and the court-room, suing the surgeon who did it.

Where Not to Look

A word of warning at this point. Ever since the usually staid and conservative medical profession was told that its own ban on advertising was unconstitutional, consumers have been flooded with directories and other circulars describing the availability and fee schedules of "specialists" in their community. Most medical societies have little or no control over what claims for expertise are made in these ads, and you may find yourself in undesirable hands. It is always best to consult your own doctor, community hospital, or local medical society for the names of qualified specialists.

THE NECK

We don't think of the neck as a critical part of the body—like the heart, kidney, or liver. It does get stiff sometimes, or you get a "crick" in it—but that's about all. As a matter of fact, we even refer to a trivial irritation as "a pain in the neck," probably because the annoyance makes you tense and puts your neck muscles into spasm.

Actually, the neck—that small area between the jaw and the upper chest—contains some very special organs and conduits. All the arteries, veins, and nerves connecting the brain and the rest of the body pass through the neck. The thyroid gland, which controls your metabolism so that you act either like a vegetable or a dynamo, is in the neck. Lymph glands, which when enlarged may indicate cancer somewhere else in the body, are felt there too. The windpipe and the foodpipe originate in the neck. And so, a thorough examination of the neck will tell me a great deal about your glands, nerves, arteries, and bones.

The Sentinel on Guard—Your Lymph Glands

I was doing a routine checkup on one of my patients not long ago. As I pushed and probed various parts of his body, he just sat there, apparently without the least curiosity. At one point I pressed a finger into the space above his left collarbone and asked him if he knew the significance of what I was doing. He hadn't "the slightest idea." "Would you like to know?" "Of course." So I explained to him that in that space there are lymph glands, collections of tissue found throughout the body, one of whose functions it is to filter fluids flowing through them, trapping infections or cancerous cells in the process. Normally these glands are so small they can't be felt. But when there is an infection or cancer somewhere within the chest, abdomen, or pelvis, one (or more) may become large enough to feel by virtue of having trapped the infectious or cancerous material passing through. Because it guards the drainage routes from other parts of the body, and signals trouble there, doctors call such a swollen gland the "sentinel" gland.

Where Are the Swollen Glands?

A swollen lymph gland anywhere tells me there is trouble in the area filtered by that particular gland either nearby or at a distance from it. But a generalized infection like mononucleosis will enlarge glands all over the body. I will move your head about so that I can relax the muscles and detect any big glands behind them. Suppose I find some swollen glands in the *back of the neck*. Since they drain the scalp and the head, I will search for infection there, like bites from head lice, ringworm, or chronic dermatitis with dandruff. But if the glands *behind the ears* are swollen, then you probably have German measles or an infection in the ear canals. Swollen glands in *front of the ears* result from disease in the face and eyes, while big glands *under the jaw* mean you have either a cold or some infection in your tongue, mouth, teeth, or lips.

Swelling of the same gland as the "sentinel," but in the right collarbone, points to trouble in the lungs or esophagus (food pipe). Finally, if the glands are enlarged along the sides of your neck, I will look for trouble in your throat, chest, or scalp; it's also possible that a process in some distant part of the body has leapfrogged and ended up there.

In addition to enmeshing traveling bacteria, viruses, and cancer cells from somewhere else in the body, lymph glands are sometimes swollen because they are diseased themselves. A form of cancer called *lymphoma* is an example of such a primary disorder of the lymph tissue. Malignancies involving the blood, such as leukemia (cancer of the white blood cells), will also cause generalized glandular enlargement, as opposed to swelling of just a few glands draining a particular area.

Other Enlarged Lymph Glands

Having searched for glands in the neck I now go looking for them elsewhere in the body, even before I finish examining the other structures in the neck.

Where are they to be found? Mainly in the armpits (axillae), above the elbows, and around the groin. An old infection of the hand can leave you with a few chronically enlarged armpit glands, and that's not anything to worry about. But the sudden appearance of swelling there is very significant, especially in women, where it may indicate cancer in the breast.

The glands behind and above the elbows swell when there is an infection of the forearm and hand. Glands around the groin are important because they drain the legs, the genital area, the lower part of the abdomen, and the rectum—common places where cancer can be detected early.

The Feel of a Swollen Gland

What does an enlarged gland feel like? It may be soft, hard, or rubbery. When I push it, you may or may not find it painful. Usually a gland with cancer in it doesn't hurt. An infected one does. A very hard gland is likely to represent a cancer, while a soft one does not. And if it has a rubbery quality, it may indicate a lymphoma, such as *Hodgkin's disease*—a malignant disorder of the lymph glands that used to be almost always fatal and today is virtually curable. For some unknown reason, patients with Hodgkin's disease have severe pain in the affected glands when they drink alcohol.

When I detect an enlarged gland, because I am an optimist by nature I first look for some simple explanation, like an infection. More often than not, there's nothing more to it than that. If you've been to the dentist or have some infection in your mouth, I expect to find some tender glands under your jaw. But if there is no apparent reason, and I come across painless, hard glands, I have to look further.

First I will do a blood count to see how many and what kind of white blood cells you have. In *leukemia,* these cells increase greatly in number and are abnormal-looking when studied under the microscope. In simple infections, there are also increased numbers of these white blood cells, but they look all right. If your blood count is normal, I will take a chest x-ray to see if any other lymph glands are swollen inside your chest. If I still don't know what the gland enlargement means, and if it's unchanged in size for three weeks or more, I will have to remove it and study it under the microscope. This will tell me definitively whether the enlarged gland represents something harmless like a local infection or is harboring a cancer.

Not all lymph glands are within the reach of my fingers. Many are deep within the chest cavity or abdomen, and their enlargement can be detected only by other special techniques, such as injecting a dye and taking x-rays of its course through the lymphatic drainage system—*lymphangiogram.*

The Thyroid Gland—Your Thermostat

Now let's get back to the neck and continue the examination there that was temporarily interrupted by our body search for lymph glands. We can start with the *thyroid gland.*

The thyroid is about two inches high—the largest compact gland in the body. It lies over the windpipe (trachea) and is shaped like a shield, with two elongated lobes on either side of the midline connected by a broad passage. (The name "thyroid" comes from the Greek word for "shield-shaped," *thyreocides.*)

If the thyroid gland is overactive (*hyperthyroidism*), you may feel nervous, with a rapid heart rate, palpitations, sweating, and diarrhea, your menstrual periods may be short, your eyes may bulge and you may lose weight despite a good appetite and adequate food intake. If your thyroid activity is below normal (*hypothyroidism*), you're apt to feel sluggish, have dry skin, coarse hair, heavy menstrual periods, and a puffy face. You go through life constipated, tired, cold, and with less sex drive than you might ordinarily have.

The Thyroid Is Not Its Own Boss

The thyroid gland does not act independently—is not its own boss, so to speak. It works in concert with the rest of the hormone system. For example, the pituitary gland in the brain produces a hormone of its own, which in turn stimulates the thyroid to make thyroid hormone. In health, this balance is perfect. But if the pituitary itself is diseased, so that it secretes too little of this thyroid-stimulating hormone, then the thyroid gland will be sluggish. Actually, a small hormone-producing tumor called an *adenoma* can form within the thyroid and sometimes make excess hormone on its own, without stimulation from the pituitary gland.

I feel your thyroid gland to see whether it is enlarged or has any lumps (nodules) in it. (But it is important to remember that a malfunctioning thyroid gland may feel normal.) If I suspect that it is making too much or too little hormone, regardless of what I find on the physical examination, I usually have to depend on other tests to confirm that suspicion. These are described in the chapters dealing with laboratory procedures.

Normally, except in very thin people, the thyroid gland cannot be felt. Also, it's the only gland in the neck that moves on swallowing (actually it's the cartilage of the thyroid that moves). So if I feel a lump or enlargement in the front of the neck, and I want to know whether it's the thyroid, I have you swallow some water. If the tissue in question moves under my fingers, it's in the thyroid.

The thyroid gland may become enlarged in various ways, in

which event it's called a *goiter*. For example, the swelling may be soft, in which case it is often associated with overactivity, or it may be hard and smooth, or lumpy, and obviously visible. Size has nothing to do with function because a goiter may make either too much, too little, or the normal amount of thyroid hormone. Regardless of its hormonal action, the goiter may on occasion be so large as to press on neighboring structures—for example, on a branch of the vagus nerve, causing hoarseness or cough. It may even push on the food pipe, making it difficult to swallow. When that happens, the goiter may have to be removed surgically.

Sometimes, even when there is no overall enlargement of the gland, I may feel a small lump in it. This may simply be an extra piece of thyroid tissue, working just like the rest of the gland and making hormone. Unless it's producing too much hormone, when it is called a "hot" nodule, it may not need to be treated. However, if the *nodule is "cold,"* that is, not making hormone, it may be malignant, and some physicians recommend its surgical removal. *Cancer of the thyroid gland,* when it does occur, is usually extremely slow growing and usually curable by surgery even after it has been present for several years.

The Big Arteries in the Neck

I can easily feel, listen to, and even see the pulsation of the major arteries (carotids) as they pass through the neck on their way from the heart to the brain. *Narrowing or blockage of these big vessels can lead to a stroke, but if detected early enough, the obstruction can sometimes be removed surgically or treated with medicines.* That's why their careful assessment in the neck is so important.

The *carotid arteries* do not usually pulsate visibly except during strenuous exercise or emotional upset. But in older people or those with high blood pressure, certain heart valve disorders, an overactive thyroid gland, or anemia, the pulsation may be very prominent.

I now feel the artery and note whether its pulsation is equal on both sides. An apparent difference indicates that the vessel is narrowed, probably by arteriosclerotic plaques. When I push on the neck to evaluate these arteries, I have to be very careful not

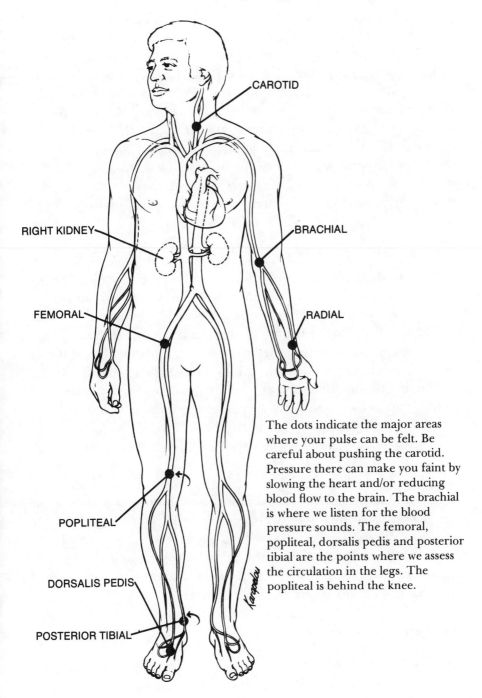

CAROTID

RIGHT KIDNEY

BRACHIAL

FEMORAL

RADIAL

POPLITEAL

DORSALIS PEDIS

POSTERIOR TIBIAL

The dots indicate the major areas where your pulse can be felt. Be careful about pushing the carotid. Pressure there can make you faint by slowing the heart and/or reducing blood flow to the brain. The brachial is where we listen for the blood pressure sounds. The femoral, popliteal, dorsalis pedis and posterior tibial are the points where we assess the circulation in the legs. The popliteal is behind the knee.

to do so too hard or for too long in someone whose blood supply to the brain is already reduced by arterial disease. Also, there is a little bit of specialized tissue within the walls of these vessels which, when stimulated, slows the heart rate dramatically. If I am too enthusiastic in hunting for the artery in the neck (or your shirt collar is too tight), you may pass out because of a slow pulse and decreased blood flow. This is the origin of the story about the man who had fainting spells for no apparent reason. A complete neurological workup was normal. The diagnosis was finally made, not by any of the specialists consulted, but by his haberdasher, who warned the patient that if he continued to wear a tight shirt collar, he would have fainting attacks.

When a Thrill Is Not a Thrill

After looking for their pulsations and then feeling the arteries, I listen to them with my stethoscope. The magnified sound of your voice and heartbeat will hurt my ears. That's why I ask you not to speak during this part of the examination. If there is an area of constriction within the vessel due to a plaque, blood flowing through it will make a whooshing noise called a *bruit* (French for "noise"). Sometimes I not only hear a bruit, but my fingers detect the tactile equivalent—a purring sensation called a *thrill*. (If you should happen to be there when I dictate the findings of your examination, and you hear me say I felt a "thrill," don't get the wrong idea.)

Just as I temporarily interrupted the examination sequence in the neck to look for glands elsewhere in the body, so I leave it now to examine other arteries that are accessible to me. These are located in the abdomen, the groin, the legs, and the feet. I already looked at the ones inside the eye, and felt both radial arteries at the wrist when I took your pulse.

CIRCULATORY SYSTEM

Looking for an Aneurysm

I now look at your abdomen for *abnormal pulsations of the aorta.* This, the largest artery in the body, leaves the heart, swings around, and comes down to the abdomen. The pulsation is very prominent if you are thin and don't have a "pot." But if you are of normal build, the pulse in the abdomen should not be bounding. If it is, you may have a dangerous widening of the aorta called an *aneurysm,* which can be felt in the midline of the abdomen. I then listen with my stethoscope for a bruit here, too, because it reflects plaques in the aorta or in the large branches going to the kidneys and down the legs.

I now feel the pulsations in the groin (*femoral artery*), which may be normal, reduced, or unequal in volume. I listen here too.

There is another pulse point behind the knees, and two more in the feet. One of these runs over the top of the foot. You can find it yourself by placing your fingers about one and a half or two inches above the cleft that separates your great toe from the one beside it. The other artery is on the inner side of the foot just below the ankle.

Arteries may vary somewhat in their location from person to person, so that I don't always feel a pulse exactly where I expect to. You mustn't be alarmed if, in testing yourself, you don't find one where I said it would be. Occasionally, we have to hunt around a little. But if after a careful search I really can't find one or more of these arteries, there are other ways of assessing the adequacy of the blood flow to the legs.

Remember that the arteries bring blood to your legs from the heart, and the veins carry it in the other direction. If your arteries are diseased, when I elevate your legs they will become pale quickly, because the veins continue to drain the blood from them while the narrowed arteries, no longer aided by gravity with the limb elevated, send in only a trickle. When I lower the leg after it has blanched, the speed with which its normal color returns is also a reflection of the patency of the arteries—the more diseased they are, the longer it takes.

Going Pale in the Legs

When your feet don't get enough blood, certain other changes take place. First, they feel cold to you and to me. I always touch both limbs because a perceptible temperature difference tells me that either blood flow is reduced in the colder one, or there is some infection or inflammation, usually of a vein (phlebitis), in the warmer one.

Cold feet do not necessarily mean poor circulation. Cold hands and feet are more often due to temporary spasm of the smaller arteries in the skin, induced by nerve signals as a result of fright or perhaps some reduction in thyroid function, rather than impaired circulation.

When the blood flow to your lower extremities is reduced, other changes take place. The legs lose their normal color, becoming violet or bluish red. Look at your toes for a moment. You should see little tufts of hair on them. When the circulation is bad, this hair is lost prematurely. (As we get older, we begin to lose hair on the toes and lower legs.) The skin begins to shrivel too, and the toenails become thick and ridged.

These are all the signs of arterial disease in the legs. What symptoms are you likely to experience? When you walk quickly, you'll get a cramp in the calf of one or both legs. When you stop (the pain is usually severe enough to make you do so), the discomfort clears in a very few minutes. One of the interesting characteristics of this disorder is that after you've been forced to stop because of pain, when you start walking again, you can usually go much farther.

When Not to Use a Heating Pad on Your Legs

As the disease of the arteries progresses, and they get narrower and narrower, the distance or pace necessary to produce the pain when you walk gets less and less. Finally, when the circulation is very bad, and unless we've fixed it surgically, you will have a burning or tingling sensation at night because there is not enough blood reaching the legs while they are horizontal in bed. These symptoms are improved by hanging the legs down so that more blood gets into them because of gravity. They are worsened by applying a heating pad. Never do this because warming the skin opens up the small blood vessels near the surface, drawing blood away from those obstructed arteries deeper down that are already short of blood and need it much more.

Surgery Can Help

Only when your symptoms become disabling will we want to find out whether surgical relief is necessary and possible. This is done by an arteriogram, discussed in another chapter. Surgery consists of either reaming out the narrowed arteries or, more commonly, bypassing the obstructed area with a Dacron tube. One end of the tube is connected to a normal portion of the artery above the area of obstruction, while the other end is attached beyond it—a *bypass graft*. Such operations usually are successful, but can only be done when there is a piece of good artery above and below the obstructed portion.

Other Blood Vessels Take Over the Job

Even when one or more of the arteries in the leg are obstructed, the circulation is not necessarily totally inadequate. Other vessels too small to be felt or seen, called *collaterals,* may take over the responsibility of nourishing the leg. Whether they succeed depends on many factors, such as the size and number of vessels that are diseased and their location. Keeping the leg active stimulates the development of these collaterals. That's why we encourage you to *walk a great deal if you have vascular disease in the legs*.

Effective Treatment of Vascular Problems

I have not found dilator drugs very useful in the treatment of arterial disease of the legs, although some doctors prescribe them. A little whiskey at bedtime, if you're not an alcoholic on the wagon or otherwise averse to taking some, and a warm pad on the abdomen (not the legs themselves) for a couple of hours are probably as effective as any medication we have.

When evaluating arterial blood flow to the legs, I also note how well it flows from the legs back to the heart—in the veins. Everyone knows what varicose veins look like. They vary in size and appearance from a profusion of small vessels to big, tortuous, dilated cords. When severe, they cause discoloration of the feet due to pooling of the blood, swelling (sometimes mistaken for heart failure), phlebitis (when they become injured or infected), pain and fatigue in the legs, and in some cases ulceration of the skin from the chronic distention by fluid.

If You Have Varicose Veins

Avoid prolonged standing. The interminable cocktail party where the guests outnumber the chairs is bad for you. Always elevate your legs on a stool or ottoman when sitting. This counteracts the effect of gravity, which retards the flow of blood back to the heart and tends to keep it down in the feet. If you're on a long airplane flight, make sure you get up at least every half hour to walk about. When you walk, the muscles contracting in your legs squeeze the veins, milking the blood back up to the heart. Many persons develop phlebitis after a long air trip because they don't move around enough. Finally, wear elastic stockings. They promote the return of blood from the veins. Such support hose now come in fairly sheer fabrics so that even women can wear them without cosmetic embarrassment.

Dangers of Varicose Veins and Phlebitis

Varicose veins make you vulnerable to pulmonary embolism. A small clot may form in the diseased vessel because blood flow within it is sluggish. This clot may break off, travel up the system of veins into the right side of the heart—and from there, to the lungs. It lodges in one of the pulmonary blood vessels and blocks it, injuring or destroying a portion of the lung tissue. This is called an *embolism,* and the death of lung tissue it sometimes produces is referred to an *pulmonary infarction* (just as blockage of a coronary artery in the heart gives a myocardial infarction). Whether you live or die after such an event depends on the size of the lung artery that was blocked by the clot and how much pulmonary tissue was destroyed as a result.

We treat phlebitis of the veins deep within the leg, but not the superficial ones, with blood thinners to prevent embolization. Veins on the surface of the leg hardly ever cause embolism when inflamed. You're at greatest risk for developing complications from your varicose veins if you injure your leg or are put to bed for any length of time (as, for example, after some operation or heart attack). Then the blood in the veins, already slowed in its flow because they are tortuous and dilated, is further retarded by inactivity, making it easier for clots to form.

Correction of Varicose Veins

When varicose veins are disfiguring and cause recurrent phlebitis, swelling or pain, they need correction. This can be done in several ways. Sometimes a material that shrivels the veins is injected, or the dilated veins (which are no good to you anyway) can be removed (stripping). When a vein is cut away, there are many others to take its place, so don't feel you've been crippled or otherwise deformed by the operation. As a matter of fact, in the aortocoronary bypass operation for coronary artery disease (discussed later), perfectly good veins are taken from the legs and grafted within the heart to improve the blood flow.

EXAMINING YOUR SHOULDERS, ARMS, AND HANDS

Continuing an orderly progression of examination, I now evaluate the upper limbs—the shoulders, arms, and hands.

Pain or stiffness of the shoulder may be due to several causes. The shoulder is a joint. As such, it consists of connecting bones, an envelope to protect the areas that hinge together, and muscles or sinews (tendons) which provide stability to the joint so that it doesn't flop around. *Chronic dislocation of the shoulder* occurs when this supporting mechanism is weakened because of repeated strain or injury. Surgery to stabilize the joint is often required and is almost always successful.

Infection, disease, or injury to any of the components of the complicated shoulder joint will make it painful or restrict its movements. For example, you may develop some form of *arthritis* in the bones. When the envelope of the joint called the *bursa* becomes irritated or inflamed from injury or overuse, you have *bursitis*. Finally, the straps or tendons that stabilize the joint may be inflamed, giving you pain, and when that happens, you have *tendinitis*. Calcium deposits have a tendency to form in these tendons, and sometimes require local injections of cortisone-type drugs, if warm, moist packs, aspirin and other antiinflammatory drugs like Indocin or Butazolidin don't work.

Even if you have a painful shoulder, the source of the trouble may be elsewhere; in other words, the pain is referred to the shoulder from another site. For example, if you have arthritis and disc trouble in your neck, the nerves that come out of the neck and go to the shoulders are either pinched by the slipped discs or compressed in the bony canals they pass through, which have been narrowed by the arthritic process. This gives pain where the nerve is distributed, which in this case is the shoulder and upper arm.

A Symptom of Heart Trouble

Perhaps the most important cause of pain in the shoulder and arms, especially on the left side—pain that doesn't originate there—is heart trouble. Angina pectoris may start in the chest and then spread to the shoulders and down the arms.

Other Shoulder Problems

There is another condition called *frozen shoulder,* associated with pain and stiffness. Its cause is unknown, but it is not the result of injury or arthritis. Occurring in the fifties or sixties, it often disappears after varying periods of time as mysteriously as it came, leaving no trace.

When I examine your bad shoulder, I first determine where the pain is greatest. I push hard with my finger to see if it is on the tendon. I rotate the arm with one hand on your shoulder, to feel for crackles due to calcium deposits. I will determine its range of motion by moving the shoulder joint in all directions. To make certain the pain isn't referred from the neck, I will rotate your head and push on your spine to see if I can reproduce discomfort in the shoulder and arm by doing so. Complete evaluation of shoulder pain requires x-rays, usually of the neck as well.

In some patients with chronic shoulder or back pain, I can feel hard, tender little lumps called *trigger points*. These are more painful when I push on them. Interestingly, they are more common in people with an underfunctioning thyroid gland. I discuss their significance and treatment in the chapter dealing with examination of the back.

Treatment of Shoulder Pain

This may range from simple heat (ice is better for bursitis), rest (or exercises), and aspirin to injections, neck collars (to minimize the pressure of discs), or rarely surgery. Acupuncture is still in vogue. Some patients swear it helps, others aren't so sure.

If one shoulder is chronically painful, so that you use it much less than the other, the muscles in the affected upper arm shrivel, and that part of the limb becomes thinner (atrophic). This indicates that your complaints of pain are not only real but significant.

The Elbow and the Unfunny Bone

I look at your elbow for any deformity due to an old injury or arthritis. If because of habit or occupation you spend a lot of time on your elbows, the irritation results in swelling ("student's elbow"). If you have chronic gout, a sac full of uric acid crystals can develop behind the elbow. This is not usually painful except during an acute attack of gout. The elbow is also the site of little lumps in rheumatoid arthritis and of deposits of fat in people with severe cholesterol disorders.

If you accidentally strike your elbow, you may feel an uncomfortable tingling there and all the way down the inner aspect of your forearm into your little finger. You say you've struck your "funny bone." In fact, you've hit a nerve (the ulnar nerve) which is cradled in that part of the elbow. Despite the pain this causes, it's still referred to as the "funny bone" because its real name is "humerus."

Your Hands—We Can Do Without a Fortune-Teller

Your hands, like the eyes, are a most revealing part of your anatomy. In my final written test at medical school, one of the questions asked was "What diagnoses can be made from examining the hands?" When I deal with some of the more important answers to that question in the next few paragraphs, you will realize why a fortune-teller uses your palms to make her predictions. So do I, and, I hope, more accurately. As you follow my descriptions, it may be interesting for you to look at your own hands and see whether you have any of the findings I describe.

I've already discussed the significance of the way you shook my hand when we first met. I observed whether you were paralyzed or weak from an old stroke. I made note of the temperature of the hand. (Hot and dry suggests fever, hot and moist may mean an overactive thyroid, cold and moist usually reflects anxiety, cold and dry may indicate hypothyroidism).

The *color of your palms* is important. There is the yellowish discoloration of carotenemia from eating too much of the pigment carotene, which is found in oranges, carrots, leafy vegetables, peaches, and squash. This staining is not limited to the palms, but occurs wherever sweat glands are present, since they excrete the pigment from the blood. Remember that it can be distinguished from jaundice (a serious sign) in that it doesn't stain the eyes. Carotene in the diet is converted to vitamin A by the liver and thyroid. When either of these glands is diseased, the pigment accumulates in the blood even if you are not taking excessive amounts of it in the diet. So if I find you discolored with *carotenemia*, I will check out your liver and thyroid function.

Are your fingers stained because of chronic cigarette smoking? No matter how much a patient protests about not smoking "much" (or admits to 60 cigarettes a day, but only a "couple of puffs" on each), yellow fingers indicate a minimum of 20 to 30 per day.

In liver disease and severe malnutrition, the palms of the hands are mottled red, the so-called *liver palms*.

The *size and shape of your hand* offer useful clues to disease. An *acromegalic*, who has too much growth hormone because of a tumor of the pituitary gland in the brain, has hands that are enlarged and wide fingers that look like paws or spades. *Marfan's syndrome* is a hereditary disorder affecting different parts of the body, especially the heart. The fingers are long and thin and are called spider fingers—*arachnodactyly* (*arachne* being the Greek word for spider and *daktylos* for finger). In *mongolism,* a congenital disorder in which there is lowered intelligence and a characteristic mongoloid appearance with slanted eyes, the hands are stubby and the little finger is always curved. Sometimes the fingers are webbed at birth or the hand may have an extra digit.

The Distorted Hand

When nerves supplying the hand are damaged or paralyzed, the fingers assume distorted positions. For example, when the *ulnar nerve* (remember the "funny bone?") is injured, the little and ring fingers, which it supplies, are bent while the thumb, forefinger, and middle finger remain straight. If you simulate this position, you can see why we call it the "preacher's" or "benediction hand." The *radial nerve* comes down the other side to the thumb and forefinger, and also controls the movement of the wrist. When it is paralyzed, as, for example, by alcoholism, polio, or lead and arsenic poisoning, the wrist droops.

There is a common disease of unknown cause affecting the tissues in the palm which become thickened and shortened, pulling in the little and/or ring finger. *Dupuytren's contracture,* as it is called, runs in families, is painless, and for some reason is seen most frequently but by no means exclusively among diabetics and patients with liver disease. Surgery is often required to release the scar tissue in the palm.

You may have noticed, especially in some athletes, a swelling of the lowest joint of the finger—*"baseball" finger.* While this characteristic enlargement may be due to repeated trauma, it also occurs in menopausal women. It is called *Heberden's node,* and represents a localized form of arthritis. Fortunately, it does not produce pain or stiffness and is not the forerunner of generalized arthritis. This is in contrast to the swelling of *rheumatoid arthritis,* which is generalized, not localized, involves many joints, and is accompanied by deformity and pain. Also, in rheumatoid arthritis, the swelling is not at the tip of the finger but in the middle joint, which is enlarged and tender, with fluid in it. Little nodules, either along the fingers or more painful ones in the pads, may indicate rheumatoid arthritis, rheumatic fever, or infection of a heart valve.

Trigger finger is a common condition involving the middle or ring finger, not at all the one you use to pull a trigger. You can bend the affected finger to make a fist, but when you try to straighten it out, it hurts. And when you do, you hear a snap. The underlying problem is not arthritis but a thickening in one of the finger tendons. Why this occurs is not known.

If your work makes it necessary to keep your hands in water for long periods, you may develop chronic infection, ulceration, and pain around the nail bed (*paronychia*). This will clear up with antibiotics, but you should wear rubber gloves to prevent recurrence.

Your Nails Are a Source of Information

Your nails may provide a wealth of diagnostic information. First I look to see if you bite them. That tells me something about your personality. The shape of your fingernails is of great importance. For example, they may be rounded or convex, like a face-down spoon, with a characteristic thickening of the nail bed (a condition called *clubbing*). If only slightly so, it is of no consequence, but when very obviously convex, it may reflect chronic lung diseases like tuberculosis, emphysema, lung cancer, bronchitis, and abscesses, as well as congenital heart disease and infections of the heart valves. The mechanism of clubbing is not understood but probably has something to do with increased blood flow to the fingers. Interestingly enough, if the responsible illness is cured—for example, if a lung abscess is removed—after a few months, the nails reassume their normal shape.

In contrast to clubbed, convex nails, spoon-shaped or concave ones (think of a spoon, face up) may be found; these are usually seen in chronic iron deficiency anemia.

When the fingernails are very thick, we sometimes find a fungus there, but there may be no apparent cause. Color of the nail beds may be significant—they are pale in anemia and blue when there is not enough oxygen in the blood, as happens in chronic lung disorders or certain kinds of heart disease.

Do Your Hands Shake?

At the beginning of our interview, I took note of whether your hands trembled. I will now evaluate this more closely. Your hands will shake if you're nervous, an alcoholic, or have an overactive thyroid. When you stretch them out in front of you and spread your fingers, a very fine tremor suggests thyroid overactivity. In Parkinson's disease, the tremor is most apparent at rest, and actually disappears with any voluntary movement such as reaching for an object. So if the patient with a parkinsonian tremor wants to eat soup, he's fine as long as he moves the spoon, but when he brings it up to his mouth and stops, the soup will spill. The thumb is involved in the shaking in a characteristic way, so that the patient looks like he is rolling pills—hence the term "pill-rolling tremor" of Parkinson's disease.

Although tremors are more common in older people, they also occur in younger persons, in which event they are usually familial or of unknown cause. Tremors in the young differ from the parkinsonian form in that they are aggravated by voluntary movement, not abolished by it.

Patients with multiple sclerosis have no tremor until they attempt to perform a voluntary movement, and then the tremor starts. Remember something that is not commonly appreciated— all tremors disappear during sleep.

CHAPTER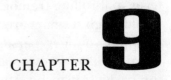

YOUR CHEST

IN EXAMINING your chest (thorax), I will be looking for evidence of disease of the chest muscles, the ribs, the diaphragm, the lungs, the heart, and the breasts (although some doctors examine the breasts when they check the lymph glands).

I use four of my five senses and the stethoscope. (The fifth sense, taste, is not ever used.) You may wonder why, as long as I'm going to take an x-ray and ECG anyway, I bother with the stethoscope or waste time tapping your chest with my finger (percussion). The fact is, these "primitive" techniques remain useful and important. Moisture in the lungs, an early sign of heart failure, can be heard with the stethoscope, but is not apparent on the chest x-ray. Neither can the x-ray hear the wheezing of asthma, the "rub" of pleurisy, or the variable noises of bronchitis. And, of course, even though the amount of radiation is very small, you don't want exposure to x-rays every time you

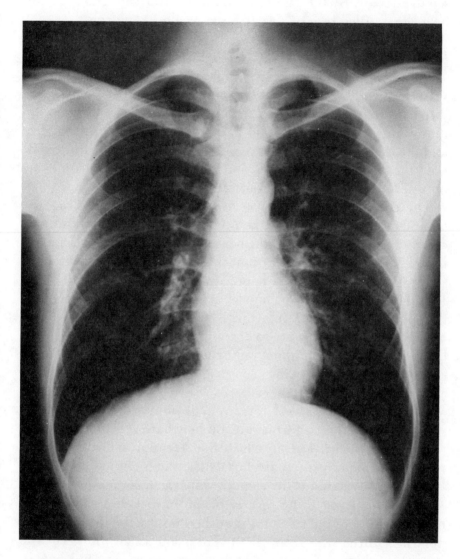

This is the chest x-ray of a healthy man. Solid tissues are white and the dark areas on either side represent air in the lungs. The white mass in the center is the heart. A chest x-ray also reveals information about the bony rib cage, the position of the diaphragm, and the great vessels entering and leaving the heart.

see the doctor. By the same token, the electrocardiogram cannot hear the muffled beat of a weak heart or a heart murmur.

The Structure of Your Chest

The chest, or thoracic cavity, contains the heart, the big blood vessels which flow in and out of it, the lungs and the air passages (bronchi) that connect it with the outside world, the nerves communicating between the brain and various organs in the body, and the esophagus which delivers food to the stomach. But really only the heart, lungs, and bronchi can be examined from the outside, and not the other internal structures.

The chest contents are protected from injury by the cage of bones and vertebrae that make up the thoracic wall. Twelve ribs connect to the spinal column behind and to the breastbone in front. The breastbone (sternum), in the midline of the chest, is shaped like a sword with a handle at the top, a blade, and a tip. If you press on the tip it moves. It is sometimes prominent in thin people and painful in arthritis. Chest pain due to heart disease is often felt as a sense of pressure in the front of the chest behind the sternum, and not on the left side as so many think.

The Shape of Your Chest

I first look at the chest for any deformities or alterations in shape. A common malformation you may have seen in the locker room is the *funnel chest,* in which the sternum or breastbone is pushed in. Some people are born that way, or years ago got it from rickets (vitamin D deficiency), which is uncommon today.

The *pigeon breast* is the reverse of the funnel chest. Instead of being depressed, the sternum is pushed out by the distorted upper ribs, so that the front of the chest looks like the keel of a ship. Again this deformity used to be due to rickets, but now is more often a congenital abnormality. As medical students, we used to learn of other deformities of the ribs caused by rickets, but I haven't seen a case in years.

The most frequent thoracic wall distortion is the *barrel chest.* The chest itself is long, wide, and deep. This may be normal, but more frequently it develops when the bronchial passages are chronically obstructed, that is, by spasm, infection or emphysema. The chest wall and its muscles are stretched as the volume of air retained in the lungs increases. The chest thus assumes a position of fixed inspiration. Try it yourself. Notice how when you inhale deeply and hold it, your chest changes in shape. When it remains in this position because of lung disease, the barrel chest develops.

Curvature of the spine (scoliosis) is a surprisingly common finding which can affect the function of the lungs by altering the size and shape of the chest wall, and even the position of the heart within the chest. A spinal deformity may be something you were born with or be the result of an old injury, arthritis, or certain bone diseases. Finally, disease and enlargement of the heart early in life, while the overlying rib cage is still soft, will also produce a bulge and deformity of the chest wall.

Your Breathing Pattern

Having observed the shape of your chest, I now watch your respirations. Sitting quietly, most of us breathe reflexly about 10–18 times a minute, without needing to be reminded to do it. Imagine having to remember to take a breath every few seconds of your life. What keeps you breathing rhythmically and without effort? There are control mechanisms in the brain called the *respiratory centers* which respond to changes in the inflation abilities of the lungs and to the chemical composition of the blood. Thus you breathe faster or slower, depending on how stiff or compliant your lungs are, and according to how much oxygen and carbon dioxide are present at any moment in your circulation. The moment you do think about your breathing, something is wrong. This awareness may be on an emotional basis or because of some disease changing the properties of your lungs or altering the level of these gases.

Is It Labored, Rapid, Irregular?

Persons with advanced arteriosclerosis of the brain have a pattern of breathing called *Cheyne-Stokes,* in which respiration is cyclical. It starts with a short breath in and out, the next one is a little deeper, the next one deeper still. This pattern works its way up to a pitch of very deep and rapid breathing. This blows out too much carbon dioxide, the chemical in the blood that stimulates the respiratory center. As a result of too little carbon dioxide, respiration stops completely for several seconds, which is a frightening sight unless you understand it. After a pause that seems like an eternity to the observer, but not at all to the patient, the carbon dioxide level builds up again, stimulating the respiratory center, and the breathing cycle commences once more. This pattern is sometimes also seen in children and in those with other disease or injury of the brain. In anxiety, in heart trouble and in fever, breathing may be rapid and/or shallow. Respirations at rest greater than 20 per minute may be abnormal.

DETAILED EXAMINATION OF YOUR CHEST

Your Lungs

Having inspected your chest for deformities and watched your breathing for a few moments, I now feel your chest with my hands (*palpation*). Then I *percuss* it: I place my left hand on the chest wall, and then tap its middle finger with the tip of my right middle finger, listening for the sound that is produced. After percussion, I listen with the stethoscope (*auscultation*).

Before describing these techniques in greater detail, let's review the anatomy of the respiratory system, which below the voice box (larynx) resembles an upside-down tree. The trunk is the windpipe (*trachea*), which has two major branches called *bronchi*, one going to each lung. They subdivide into progressively smaller bronchial limbs, which open into little air sacs called *alveoli*—the foliage of the tree.

The outside of the lung is covered by a two-layered envelope of tissue called the *pleura*. The inner layer covers the lung; the outer layer is on the inside of the rib cage. These layers are normally stuck together without any intervening air or fluid. When the lung is diseased, the pleura may become inflamed, and the inner leaf rubs against the outer. This causes pain, especially when you take a deep breath in, and that's what *pleurisy* means.

If I examine you at that time, I can actually hear the rub. After a while, fluid forms between the two irritated layers, the friction stops, the rub disappears, and the pain goes. However, this does not mean that the disease that caused the inflammation in the first place has cleared.

Palpation—Feeling Your Chest

I place my hands symmetrically on various parts of your chest and back, and ask you to breathe deeply to see whether all parts move evenly. If they do not, I am alerted to underlying disease such as pneumonia, in which the affected lung moves less, or emphysema, wherein the ballooning out of the chest results in very little overall motion with breathing. I then press various muscles in your chest wall to see if they are tender, especially if you've had any chest pain. So often, local muscle tenderness is mistaken for more serious conditions such as angina pectoris. I press on the ribs to see if this elicits pain, and it will if you have arthritis of the rib cage.

I next use my hands to test the resonance of the sounds that come through your chest wall. When you speak (I generally have you say "99" or "1, 2, 3"), the vocal cords set up vibrations which are transmitted down the air passages into the lungs. These can be felt on the surface of the chest. If the vibration does not come through to my examining hand, there may be some blockage in the air passages interfering with the transmission of sound. Damping of the vibrations may also indicate fluid or air in the pleura, on the outside of the lung. If, by contrast, you have an infection of the lungs such as pneumonia, the vibrations coming through to my hand will be enhanced, because the millions of little sacs in the lungs that are normally filled with air now contain blood and fluid. This makes the lung solid, and vibrations are conducted much more strongly to the chest wall than when just air is present.

Percussion—Thumping Your Chest

Like the stethoscope, percussion is traditional and symbolic to the medical man. Unfortunately, it is being neglected somewhat by today's medical students who rely more on technological aides and less on their senses than they should. In percussion, the sound produced differs according to the nature and thickness of the portion of the body under examination. For example, if I tap over a gas bubble in your upper stomach, I will hear a high-pitched hollow sound. Over healthy areas of the lung which contain air, there is a resonant note like a drumbeat. If I were to thump on your buttocks (which I never do), the sound would be very flat because this part of your body is solid.

The Sounds of Health

The percussion note over the lung tells me whether or not this organ is healthy. For example, in pneumonia or pleurisy, when there is fluid in the lung or between the layers surrounding it, I will elicit a flat note rather than the normal resonant one. I will also hear a dull sound if any part of your lung has collapsed and lost its air. This sometimes happens after an operation, when a plug of mucus forms in the bronchial tubes. But when there is emphysema—that is, too much air in the lung—the normal drumlike sound is exaggerated and becomes hyperresonant.

When I percuss from left to right across the front of the chest, I listen for a change in the quality of the note, to determine the outline of the heart. This tells me, without requiring an x-ray, whether there is any cardiac enlargement. Another piece of information I derive from percussing the front of the chest is the location of the top border of the liver. The liver is situated just below the right lung. As I percuss down the front of your chest on the right side, the resonant note produced over your air-filled lungs becomes flat as I reach the upper border of the solid liver.

You now see how much invaluable information I can accumulate by looking at, feeling, and thumping yur chest.

Using the Stethoscope—Auscultation

The stethoscope is the hallmark of the physician, always peeking out of his pocket when he is on duty in the hospital, or hanging around his neck as he sits and talks to you in the office. Before the stethoscope was available, the doctor used to listen to the heart and lungs by putting his ear directly on the chest wall.

Then someone invented a long wooden cone, the narrow end of which was placed in the ear and the wider end of the patient's chest. Finally, the stethoscope as we know it today was designed. Originally, it had thick rubber tubing. The old rubber tubing has been replaced by flexible plastic so that newer models are very much lighter and distort my clothes a lot less.

The modern stethoscope has a flat diaphragm on one side and a bell on the other. I switch them around depending on what kind of sound I want to hear best. The bell picks up the lower pitches, like certain heart murmurs, while the diaphragm detects higher notes. For children, we use a bell with a rubber rim on it, sparing them the shock of cold steel on a warm chest.

Breathe Through Your Mouth

The main purpose of listening to the lungs with a stethoscope is to hear how the air moves in and out of the chest. When the bronchial tubes are unobstructed and free of disease, and lead into a healthy lung, your breathing has a distinct, clean sound. There are many diseases, starting in the air pipes themselves and ending up in the lungs or the coverings of the lungs, which can change this sound.

Here are a few examples of what I listen for as I have you breathe deeply in and out, moving my stethoscope over your chest as you do so. (Incidentally, when I ask you to breathe in and out deeply, it's always to be done through the mouth. The reason is obvious: You move more air that way than through your nose.)

If you have *chronic bronchitis* or *asthma,* I hear a wheeze as you breathe out. In fact, this musical sound may be audible even without the stethoscope during an asthmatic attack. As he exhales, the asthmatic's constricted bronchial tubes become even narrower. It takes longer to get the air out of those lungs, and its flow through the constricted passages produces the high-pitched wheezing sound.

If there is fluid or air in the pleura surrounding the lungs, the breath sounds will be poorly transmitted to the outside of the chest where my stethoscope is placed, and so they are diminished in intensity or absent.

In the presence of *pneumonia,* when areas of lung are solid with infected fluid instead of air, the breath sounds are accentuated. When the lungs have water in them because of heart failure, I hear crackling sounds due to congestion in the air sacs. But crackles can also be due to the mucus of bronchitis rather than the water of heart failure, and the difference is a very important one. To distinguish between the two, I have you cough. If the crackles clear after the coughing, chances are (in conjunction with other physical findings) that they are in the air tubes— in other words, you have bronchitis. If they persist, then they are in the lung tissue and likely, in the absence of infection, indicate heart failure.

Just as I had you say "99" or "1, 2, 3" to feel any change in the vibration with the palm of my hand, I will also ask you to recite these numbers as I listen to your chest with the stethoscope. When there is solid material in the lung instead of air (pneumonia), the sound will be much louder.

One day, I was examining a patient's chest. After working all of the previous night, I was dead tired and not functioning at my best, a hazard to which doctors are vulnerable. As I inserted the earpiece of my stethoscope, I was momentarily confused and thought I was on the telephone. Instead of asking the patient to say "99" or "1, 2, 3," I said, "Hello." She looked startled. I suddenly realized what I had done, but it was too late. I didn't quite know how to explain it, so with an air of authority, I repeated, "Say 'Hello.' " Well, the rest of that examination was taken up with the patient saying "Hello" to me instead of "99" or "1, 2, 3." If your doctor asks you to say "Hello" when he's examining your chest, be tolerant. He may be overtired.

Examining the Breasts, a Critical Procedure

The "name of the game," the "bottom line," as far as evaluation of the breasts is concerned, is the detection of *cancer.* Unlike internal organs, the breast is so accessible that *careful examination by you and me is a must.*

There are many different ways to describe the magnitude of the problem of breast cancer. If you are an American woman 39 to 44 years of age, this is the disease most likely to kill you. At any age, it is the cancer you are most likely to get. What are your chances of developing it in your lifetime? About 1 in 14, or 7 percent. There are about 90,000 new cases of breast cancer detected each year, of whom 33,000 die. Put yet another way, every 5 minutes a woman is found to have it—and every 15 minutes, there is a breast cancer death. I emphasize this grim picture so starkly because *early detection* is the only way we're going to improve those figures—and that means careful examination by me and you. *You should be as adept at examining your breasts as I am.* As a matter of fact, statistics show that most women are, since more than 90 percent of lumps in the breast are discovered by them, not by their doctors.

Are Your Breasts Too Big, Too Small, or Too Many?

That is a matter of preference, both cultural and individual. Neither are they always equal in size, the left usually being slightly larger than the right. Most people have only two breasts but some have three or more. The additional ones are rarely developed, and consist of an extra nipple somewhere in a straight line with the normally located nipple, lower down on the chest or on the abdominal wall. These "accessory" nipples or breasts can be mistaken for birthmarks or moles. But if you look at them carefully, you will find they have the same general structure as a nipple, even down to the presence of a surrounding pigmented area. Although I personally have never seen a fully developed third breast (what a problem that would pose to the brassiere makers), they do occur. In fact, medical history has it that Anne Boleyn, Henry VIII's second wife, was so endowed— together with twelve fingers.

Assessing Your Risk for Cancer

The risk for developing cancer of the breast is greater than average if you (1) have a strong family history of cancer in any location, but especially in the breast; (2) have cysts in the breast; (3) have never been pregnant or had your first baby after 30; (4) are fat; (5) started menstruating at an early age (before 11); or

(6) had a late menopause. But any woman is vulnerable at any time in her life. And here's another fact that may surprise you: *One to two percent of all breast cancers are found in men.* I have seen three cases in the past twenty-five years, all malignant. Men have very little breast tissue, so the cancer spreads more rapidly because there is less to buffer its advance. I suggest that men occasionally examine their breasts and don't be surprised when I do during a routine examination.

Looking for Cancer

Since the breasts become engorged just before the monthly period and during pregnancy, they are most difficult to examine at those times. It's best not to schedule a routine visit in the premenstrual period. I examine your breast first just by looking at it. A tumor often causes a dimpling or redness of the skin overlying it or some change in the symmetry of the breast. As you sit on the examining table, I have you raise your arms to see if this pulls in the nipple or dilates the veins on the surface of the breast. I also look for some swelling or bulging and for evidence of increased heat in any part of the breast, suggesting an underlying infection (mastitis) or tumor. I then ask you to press your hands on your hips. This may expose lumps within the breast. If your breasts are very large and of the hanging variety, I can examine them more easily while you sit with your trunk bent forward. I now have you lie down, and I carefully feel every area of the breast, including the nipple. Remember that many women have depressed or inverted nipples from birth. When they have been normal in shape all along and suddenly become retracted, the possibility of underlying cancer is raised.

I now gently squeeze the nipple to see whether there is a discharge. After pregnancy, such discharge is normal, but at other times, especially if it is bloody or cloudy, a discharge may be due to infection, tumor, or a common type of cancer of the nipple called Paget's disease (usually slow growing). Several drugs may cause nipple discharge, including reserpine (an agent used as a tranquilizer and against high blood pressure), Aldomet (another blood pressure medication), Aldactone (a mild diuretic), and female hormones.

Do You Have a Lump in the Breast?

Remember that while *every breast lump is suspicious,* most are innocent. The presence of several tender lumps, especially on both sides, suggests *chronic cystic mastitis,* not tumor. These are worse just before and during the menstrual period and disappear with the menopause—evidence that they are due to a hormonal effect. Sometimes, however, benign lumps occur only in one breast, in which case a biopsy may be necessary to make sure that they are in fact harmless. Many women have lumpy, slightly tender breasts and swollen glands in their armpits. Again, if both breasts are involved, the likelihood of cancer is remote, but a biopsy is still usually required. Single cysts of the breast or breast abscesses are common, too. Neither of these is cancerous.

Drugs That Affect the Breast

Several medications and certain diseases may frequently cause painful enlargement of the breasts in both men and women. The drugs include digitalis, Aldactone, Thorazine (a commonly used tranquilizer), and isoniazid (the most important agent for the treatment of tuberculosis). Men who are treated with female hormones for cancer of the prostate always have breast enlargement. Remember that chronic alcohol abuse damages the liver, which is no longer able to break down the tiny amount of female hormone normally present in all men. This hormone, then, accumulates and female characteristics develop, including enlargement of the breast.

The Mammography Controversy

Mammography, a simple, painless x-ray of the breast, is invaluable for the detection of early breast cancers before they can be felt by the most conscientious woman or skillful examiner. Forty-five percent of the cancers picked up in a mammogram are not noted in the regular exam. It is in these small, early cancers that we obtain a 95 percent cure rate. That's why mammography is so important, and why women who are at greater risk or over 50 should have it done every year.

In 1975 after the wives of the President and Vice-President of the United States both developed breast cancer, there was a rush to mammography for early detection. We have now become more conservative and selective in its use.

Years ago, when irradiation was used to treat certain disorders of the breast, women were exposed to very high cumulative doses—some 100 to 500 times the amount of radiation used in routine mammography. When examined 15 or so years later, these patients were found to have a higher incidence of breast cancer than the general population. This has made us rethink the advisability of exposing younger women—in their thirties—to annual, routine mammography. *We now recommend a mammogram every year in women over 50, very careful yearly physical examination between the ages of 30 and 50, and monthly self-examination.* But remember, if you are "vulnerable" or have suspicious lumps or cysts, you should not hesitate to be x-rayed.

Although it is estimated that mammography every year for 15 years increases your risk of getting breast cancer from 7 percent to 8 percent, the virtues of early detection outweigh the risks. Incidentally, if you are pregnant, you should not have it done, because the radiation may be harmful to your unborn child. Also, you should try not to be x-rayed just before your period, when the breasts are engorged, since the mammogram may be more difficult to interpret at that time.

Variations on a Theme

A form of mammography currently being used in some screening centers is called *xerography.* The image is recorded on a xerographic selenium plate instead of conventional x-ray film and is then transferred to a special plastic-coated paper. This produces a clear, very detailed picture of the breast, which is available immediately.

Another diagnostic technique for evaluating breast lumps, one that involves no x-rays and can therefore be repeated as often as desired, is called *thermography.* This procedure records even slight variations in the temperature of various portions of the breast. The underlying theory behind its use is that multiplying cancer cells throw off more heat than does healthy tissue. Thermography is an ancillary tool, which may add information to that obtained from a physical examination and mammography, but should never be accepted as the only screening technique. It is not the equivalent of mammograms for that purpose.

How You Should Examine Your Breasts

You already know how important it is for you to examine your own breasts. *Do it every month.* The best time is about two weeks after your period, when they are not tender or swollen. If you no longer have periods—that is, you're menopausal or have had a hysterectomy—simply pick a regular time each month, say the 1st or the 15th, and do it then. A good place to start is in the shower, when your skin is wet and your hands can easily glide over the breasts. Keep your fingers flat and together. With your left hand examine the right breast, and with your right hand, the left, feeling for any lump, thickening, or irregularity. Every area of the breast should be examined.

Now stand in front of a mirror. With your arms at your sides, first look at your breasts. Can you see any asymmetry, dimpling, or swelling of the skin, any changes in skin color or in the shape of the nipple? If the nipple is retracted (pulled in or inverted), this is important and must be reported, especially if you've just noted it for the first time.

Next, just as you did on my examining table, press your hands on your hips and again look at the skin for dimpling. Now lie down and put a pillow under your right shoulder. Put your right hand behind your head, and using your left hand—again, as described previously, with your fingers flat—press very lightly in small circular motions around every part of your right breast. Think of your breast as a clock. Start your self-examination at 12 o'clock (on the top part of the breast) and move your fingers to 1 o'clock and so on, completing the circle back to 12. Then go down an inch or two and repeat the same process, circling every part of your breast. You should go through at least three such circles. Also examine your nipple by squeezing it gently between the thumb and index finger. Look for any discharge. Now repeat the procedure in your left breast with a pillow under your left shoulder, your left arm under your head and using your right hand. Should these examinations reveal any lumps, thickening, or discharge, whether they are painful or not, you must immediately report them.

Supposing We Find a Lump

What then? We will need other tests. First, there's the mammogram, which, when the lump is cancerous, gives a characteristic x-ray picture. If that's "positive," you'll go to surgery without delay. If it's "negative," we may still want to biopsy it to be absolutely sure it's benign. The surgeon takes a small piece of the tissue, often under local anesthesia, sends it to the laboratory and awaits the result. If prior to the biopsy we have the impression that the lump is malignant, we will wait in the operating room for the pathologist's report, so that the appropriate operation can be done then and there. Sometimes, if the lump feels like a cyst, its contents are aspirated with a needle instead of doing a full biopsy.

The Odds Are Good—and Getting Better

If the lump we find is malignant, your chances are better than 50 percent that it has not yet spread. If it was picked up by the mammogram, and is too small to feel, you have a 95 percent chance of cure. Although some doctors—a minority—believe that surgery is not necessary to remove breast cancers, and prefer radiation alone, most favor operation. The extent of the surgery will depend on the kind of cancer it is, how far it has spread, its location, and also the judgment of the surgeon. Most breast surgeons remove the entire breast when they find a lump in it, but some simply take out the cancer, leaving the rest of the tissue intact. This is called a *lumpectomy*. Naturally, it is the most appealing technique for the patient, but although it has its proponents, it is not as widely recommended as total removal of the breast.

At operation, if the surgeon believes that a radical mastectomy offers you the best chance for survival, he will remove the chain of lymph glands that leads from the breast to the armpit (axilla). This *radical mastectomy* is in contrast to the *simple mastectomy*, in which only the breast itself is excised and not the glands.

Unfortunately, cancer of the breast may recur long after surgery—sometimes fifteen to twenty years later. A second tumor may develop. Women who have had cancer of one breast are especially vulnerable to getting it in the other one. However, the new anticancer drugs now being used may reduce the incidence of such late spread. Because of an increased awareness of the importance of careful breast examinations by doctors and patients alike, together with improved diagnostic techniques and surgical procedures and the development of anticancer drugs (many of which are used in combination), the cure or remission rate for breast cancer appears to be improving.

Causes of Breast Cancer

Nobody knows for sure what causes breast cancer, although certain agents have been implicated. Estrogen is not one of them. However, we now try to avoid prescribing estrogen (female hormone), which makes many menopausal women feel better, because of the greater incidence of cancer of the uterus associated with its use.

An agent implicated in possible breast cancer formation not long ago was reserpine. This is a derivative of rauwolfia, a plant that comes from India and which several years ago was very important in the treatment of high blood pressure. Newer drugs have to some extent supplanted it for that purpose, but it is still used as a tranquilizer. Subsequent analysis of the data implicating reserpine as a cancer-causing agent has not been sufficiently incriminating, so that it is still being used when needed.

Another agent suspected in breast cancer is a drug marketed as Aldactone. It's a very useful agent with few side effects. It helps lower blood pressure and is a mild, well-tolerated diuretic used for the treatment of fluid retention. More importantly, it is a potassium-sparing agent. While most diuretics make you lose potassium, Aldactone usually helps to correct low potassium. When given to men, Aldactone often causes sensitivity and enlargement of the breasts. Whether or not it really increases the risk of breast cancer in women is not known for certain.

Finally, another recent study has shown that women who have been taking thyroid supplements over a long period of time appear to have a higher incidence of breast cancer. Again, this association is not conclusive. What to do in the meantime? Take thyroid pills only if your thyroid function is low, and not otherwise.

The Danger of New Drugs

If because of something you have heard or read you are worried about any drug you are taking, check with your doctor. Very often we prescribe a new product because it appears to have a desirable or necessary action, such as lowering cholesterol, controlling weight, or strengthening the heart. Then 10–15 or more years later, we find it has delayed side effects which are sometimes dangerous. So my advice to you with regard to any medicine is to take it if you need it, but don't experiment, don't look for miracles with unproven agents, no matter how "good" they make you feel.

Enough of the morbid with regard to breasts. Let's go on to consider the cosmetics of breast surgery.

Are You Thinking About Cosmetic Surgery for Your Breasts?

Plastic surgery of the breasts is popular and widespread—probably more so than you suspect. As in cosmetic repair of the face, corrective surgery of the breast is done because it's needed or simply wanted. Basically, it involves making them smaller, bigger, or more attractively suspended.

Why would any woman want to make her breasts smaller when big breasts are considered so sexy and, as far as I can determine, the major attributes of the centerfold in most girly magazines? In young teen-agers, rapid and "excessive" growth of the breasts may be embarrassing, but this should rarely be an indication for reduction. In some women, very large breasts are uncomfortable and a strain on the body frame, rather like carrying a heavy weight around the neck. Such women may have trouble finding clothes that fit, and they often have indentations across their shoulders where their brassiere straps have dug in because of the weight they have to support. Pain and later arthritis in the neck, middle and lower back, and shoulders may on occasion also re-

sult from such very large, heavy breasts. If you have this problem, and are considering surgery, you should know that it leaves
visible scars. Although these may become less obvious in time,
the breasts in many cases do look mutilated. So if you're thinking
about surgery because of a compelling medical reason, go ahead,
but if you're having surgical reduction purely as a cosmetic procedure, you ought to think twice about it.

What's Sexier?

In some cultures, like the Chinese, the flatter the chest, the
sexier the woman. Not so in America. There are two main
groups of women who want bigger breasts (*augmentation mammo-
plasty*): young women who have not developed a significant
amount of breast tissue in the first place (the classic "Twiggy"
type), and women in their late thirties and early forties who,
having had children and nursed them, notice that their breasts
have become looser. Although successive pregnancies sometimes
make the breasts larger, much more commonly they become
more stretched and looser. These older women feel very much
about their breasts as do others about their face. The sagging
and drooping breasts tarnish their self-image, especially at a time
in life when the husband may be maintaining an overall youthful
appearance.

The New Techniques

Modern techniques of enlarging the breast consist of putting a
shapeless gel or water-filled sac between the breast and the underlying chest wall. When properly done, this can result in a soft,
attractive, and natural-looking breast in which the prosthesis is
virtually undetectable. More often than not, however, a surgical
scar is visible.

Some years ago, *silicone injection* into the breast was all the
rage. This resulted in a very hard breast which looked attractive
under a sweater but certainly didn't bounce. What's more, it felt
akin to caressing the Statue of Liberty—hard as a rock. This
technique is illegal and no longer used in the United States.

Sagging breasts which follow pregnancy and nursing are apt to occur in women whose breasts are large to begin with. In a society where the bra is losing its popularity, some women are disturbed about their inability to go "braless" because of sagging breasts. Surgical correction to uplift them also results in scarring under the nipple and across the bottom of the breast. This operation is not very popular and the least commonly employed.

If you've had a breast removed, you should know about a recently developed reconstructive procedure. The technique is very much like the one used in breast enlargement—that is, a gel or saline-filled sac is placed on the chest wall. It is progressively enlarged, and when a suitable size is reached, a new nipple is constructed. Plastic surgeons used to be taught that patients should wait five years after radical mastectomy before engaging in such reconstructive work, since most cancer recurrences appear during that time. But more of them are recommending it be done earlier. Loss of a breast is often emotionally traumatic; in fact, some of my psychiatric colleagues equate it with deprivation of the penis in the male. Because of this conceptual loss of femininity, surgery for breast cancer is dreaded physically and emotionally. This plastic procedure, when possible, may improve morale.

YOUR HEART

By the time I get around to a clinical examination of your heart, I already have a good idea of whether or not you have cardiac disease. This judgment will have been made much earlier on the basis of the history you gave me and your answers to my questions. Symptoms like chest pressure, especially with exertion, undue shortness of breath, chest pain radiating to the shoulders, jaw, or through to the back, unexplained "indigestion," and palpitations are some of the complaints that I will already have explored in depth.

In the physical examination of the heart, I first use my eyes, then my hands, and finally my stethoscope. This is only the beginning, however, because later I will want to look at the size and shape of your heart on the chest x-ray, take an electrocardiogram, and very likely have you perform a stress test.

Structural Disorders of the Heart: You're Not "Soft-Hearted"

Heart disease doesn't mean just one "condition." The term embraces a wide spectrum of trouble. To help you understand the different kinds of disturbances, what is necessary to detect them, when they should be treated, and how (surgery or pills), I will first outline the heart's anatomy and functions. Don't be deterred if it seems complicated. It really isn't. Keep referring to the simple accompanying diagram, and even if you have to do it more than once, take the time. It's worth it, if you want to understand the function of the most important organ in your body.

We tend to forget that the heart is a very powerful muscle because of our cultural preoccupation with its "fragility." Our language is replete with expressions like "tender-hearted" and "soft-hearted." Even "hard-hearted" people die of "broken hearts." We grow up with a subconscious and unwarranted fear of the vulnerability of this really tough organ.

Just consider the work done by your heart day in, day out, year after year, without its ever stopping—except once, at the very end. What machine has man ever made that, like the heart, can go for 70 or 80 years—or more—without adjustment, oiling, refueling, or having some part replaced periodically? We take all this for granted because, like the breathing process, we are unaware of the action of the healthy heart. Even the dreaded heart attack doesn't invariably kill and often goes unnoticed, the pain or discomfort being attributed to something trivial like "heartburn" or "indigestion." Many who have unknowingly had such an attack continue to lead normal lives, attain full life expectancy, and ultimately die in old age of some other cause. When their hearts are examined after death, the muscle damage from the unrecognized attack is seen as a firmly healed scar.

The Heart of the Matter

The heart is about the size of your fist, and is situated in the chest a little to the left of the midline. A wall down the middle

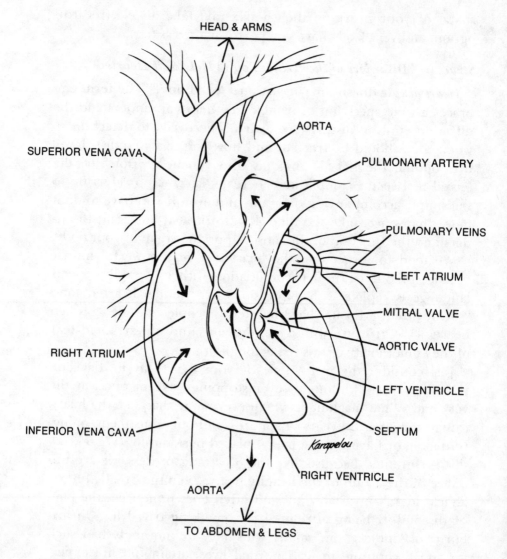

Notice the direction of blood flow entering, within, and leaving the heart. Blood enters the right atrium from the superior vena cava (the large vein from the head and upper body) as well as from the inferior vena cava, returning blood from the legs and lower body. From the right atrium, this oxygen-poor or "used" blood enters the right ventricle, which it leaves via the pulmonary artery to go to the lungs. Here it is recharged with oxygen. This fresh blood returns to the left atrium via the pulmonary veins. It then enters the thicker-walled left ventricle through the mitral valve and then out the aortic valve into the aorta.

(*septum*) separates it into left and right chambers. A set of *valves* on each side further subdivides each half into an upper portion called the *atrium* and a lower one called the *ventricle*. So there are four chambers in all. The right and left atria on top are small and thin; the ventricles below are much thicker, the left ventricle more so than the right. Thus, the chambers on the left side are separated from those on the right by the wall, while the atria above are separated from the ventricles below by the valves. If you have a "hole" in your heart, that means there is an abnormal communication, or defect, in the wall separating the left from the right side. Such openings almost never are the result of disease, but are faults in development occurring before birth. This communication, which can exist between the right and left atria at the top of the heart (*atrial septal defect*) or between the two ventricles below (*ventricular septal defect*), permits an abnormal flow of blood from the left (where the pressure is higher) to the right side of the circulation. We often have to close such defects surgically.

Normally, when the heart contracts, all the blood in the left ventricle is squeezed out directly to the body, while at the same time that from the right ventricle goes to the lungs. When there is a hole in the ventricular wall, some of the blood destined for and needed by the body is diverted to the right ventricle and into the lungs. The body therefore gets too little, and the lungs get too much. This increased flow at higher pressure from the powerful left ventricle is more than the lungs can handle and, in time, may damage them.

The valve separating the left atrium from the left ventricle is called the *mitral valve,* that between the right atrium and right ventricle, the *tricuspid valve*. If you have mitral valve disease (usually caused by rheumatic fever), that valve is deformed so that the normal flow of blood between the two chambers it separates is disturbed. This often requires surgical replacement.

There are two more valves in the heart. The *aortic valve* separates the left ventricle from the aorta, into which that ventricle ejects its blood on its way to the body. The *pulmonic valve* is situated between the right ventricle and the pulmonary artery, which is the conduit for blood flowing from the heart to the lungs.

So much for the heart's anatomy. Now for its function.

Even If You Stand on Your Head

The left ventricle has and needs the thickest muscle of all four chambers because its job is to pump the blood to the rest of the body. If you stand on your head, the left ventricle is powerful enough to defy gravity and force blood all the way up to your feet. You can remain in that position and even pedal for some time, and the heart will still supply the leg muscles with enough blood to keep them working.

When Heart Valves Must Be Replaced

When the left ventricle contracts, the aortic valve opens, allowing blood to leave the heart. When the contraction is over and the blood has been squeezed out of the ventricle, the aortic valve closes tight to prevent any of it from leaking back into the heart.

If this valve is diseased, as a result of either some congenital malformation or infection (usually rheumatic fever but sometimes syphilis), it may not open widely enough. This forces the left ventricle to squeeze extra hard to get all its blood out through the narrowed opening. In time, because of the strain, this chamber becomes thick and large. But there is a limit to how big it can become to compensate for the obstruction. When it can no longer enlarge, it weakens and fails. This narrowing or inability of the valve to open widely is called *aortic stenosis*. It is a serious and common disorder which fortunately can now be fixed quite easily when necessary. The surgeon cuts out the diseased valve and puts in an artificial one.

In contrast to an obstructed aortic valve, a bad valve may open normally but not close tightly, allowing blood to leak back from one chamber to another or from the aorta into the heart after it is expelled. Like stenosis, such regurgitation of blood also eventually causes the affected chamber to enlarge because of the extra load of blood it is forced to accommodate. Frequently, replacement of the diseased valve becomes necessary. Stenosis and leakage (*insufficiency*, regurgitation) of a valve can occur together.

The opening and shutting of the valves create sounds for which I listen with the stethoscope. I can tell if a given valve is working properly. The sound of a narrowed opening is entirely different from that of a leaky one—in loudness, in quality, and in timing.

The Course of the Blood Through Your Body

After the blood leaves the heart via the aorta, it flows into the arterial tree whose branches become progressively smaller, finally ending up as tiny *arterioles*. The function of the arterial system is to deliver oxygen-rich blood to every organ and tissue of the body. The waste products of metabolism are returned via a system of veins to the heart.

The junction between the arterial system, which brings the blood to the tissues, and the venous system, which carries it away, is not abrupt, but consists of a network of tiny blood vessels—*arterioles, capillaries,* and *venules.* As the veins return to the heart, they become larger and larger, just as the arteries get smaller and smaller as they move away from the heart. The veins finally coalesce into very large vessels which empty into the right side of the heart (right atrium). This "used" blood from the right side of the heart is squeezed into the lungs to be reoxygenated. Because the lungs are in the chest adjacent to the heart, and blood within them is at a fairly low pressure, the right ventricle doesn't have to pump very hard to move blood into the lungs. So it is normally a lot thinner than the left ventricle, which has to supply remote parts of the body, often against the force of gravity.

In the lungs there is a network of tiny vessels which brings the blood into contact with the little air sacs that make up the basic lung tissue. Here, waste products and carbon dioxide are blown off and oxygen is supplied to the blood cells. The oxygenated blood is returned from the lungs to the left side of the heart to be recirculated to the body.

Why the Feet Swell When the Lungs Are Scarred

When the lungs are diseased and scarred, as by chronic infection, heart failure, or emphysema, their circulation is distorted.

As a result, the right ventricle has to pump harder than it normally does to get the blood to circulate through the lungs. In these circumstances, it may become thickened. If the pulmonary disease is long-standing, serious and extensive enough, the right ventricle can end up being as thick as, or thicker than, the powerful left ventricle and ultimately fails. When that happens, it cannot expel all the blood brought to it by the veins. The circulation then backs up, fluid under pressure oozes through the blood vessels, the feet and abdomen become swollen, and surface veins are distended.

How High Blood Pressure Weakens the Heart

When pressure in the arterial system is high or the aortic valve is narrowed, the left side of the heart has trouble squeezing the blood out. It must work harder, and over a period of years it becomes progressively thicker and larger. When it can get no bigger, ultimately fails, and blood backs up into the lungs. The initial consequence, then, of left heart failure is not swelling of the legs but congestion in the lungs, and you become short of breath. If this continues untreated for any length of time, even the lungs can't accommodate all the blood, so it backs up into the right heart and the veins entering it. Finally, the legs and abdomen swell, the liver enlarges, becomes tender, and you are in *congestive heart failure.*

What Is Arteriosclerosis?

Arteriosclerosis, which is responsible for so much death and disability, refers to a narrowing of the arteries anywhere in the body due to fatty and cholesterol deposits in their lining. When the disease strikes the vessels in the heart (the *coronary arteries*), *angina pectoris* and a *heart attack* may result.

The Difference Between Angina Pectoris and a Heart Attack

Heart muscle, in its incessant contractions, requires a continuous supply of energy, which is provided by the blood carried in the coronary arteries. When these arteries are significantly narrowed by arteriosclerosis, and the heart muscle requires more oxygen than is available, it "cries out" for more blood. That cry is the symptom of chest pain or pressure we call *angina pectoris*. It usually occurs during some physical activity or emotional stress, when more blood is needed than when you are at rest. When a coronary artery is abruptly and completely blocked (*thrombosis*), not merely narrowed, the area of the heart muscle dependent on it dies. That's what *myocardial infarction* (or a heart attack) is. "Infarction" means death of tissue. If the area so destroyed is large, it is a big heart attack. If the obstructed artery was small, then the attack was minor. Whether you live or die depends on the size of the blocked artery and how much muscle tissue was actually lost.

Good Collateral—More Important for the Heart Than for the Bank

Before a coronary artery closes, it first usually narrows progressively as it becomes more and more arteriosclerotic. In order to provide an alternate, standby blood supply, the heart develops a network of new blood channels called *collaterals*. When the closure is very gradual, by the time the artery is completely blocked, a heart attack may not occur—that is, muscle does not die, because the collateral circulation has had time to develop and take over the function of the diseased coronary artery. That's why people with severe angina may go on for years without having a heart attack, and may even eventually lose their chest pain. You can see why we have to be so very careful in assessing the benefit of any treatment for angina pectoris (medical or surgical), since nature is constantly helping out behind the scenes.

The foregoing is a simplified view of what causes a heart attack. While narrowed coronary arteries are the most important and common prerequisite, there is more to it than that. As you will see later, sudden changes in heart rate and rhythm can hurt the heart, especially if the coronary arteries are narrowed to begin with. We are also seeing more and more patients with heart attacks whose coronary arteries are not closed or even badly diseased. Perhaps the attack is due to abrupt vessel spasm or to some sudden chemical changes within the heart muscle itself independent of its blood supply.

There is one other disorder of the heart you should know about—*pericarditis*. Remember the envelope surrounding the lungs? The same kind of tissue, called *pericardium,* also wraps around the heart. It is vulnerable to infections, mostly viral, which cause it to become inflamed and irritated. Like a heart attack, pericarditis gives pain, a little fever, and ECG abnormalities. The two conditions are not always easy to distinguish one from the other, but unlike a heart attack, pericarditis is not usually life-threatening. The commonest form often follows a simple cold, and is called *benign viral pericarditis.*

How We Examine the Heart

Now that you have an understanding of the heart's structure and function, and the major diseases to which it is vulnerable, you will better appreciate its physical examination.

First We Just Look . . .

As you sit on the examining table, I look for any deformity of the rib cage over the heart area. This may be caused by enlargement of the heart in early childhood, pushing out the ribs while they are still soft. I then identify the thrust or beat of the underlying heart on the chest wall, which should be within the left nipple line. If the heart is enlarged, however, it can extend out as far as the armpit. The presence of a strong pulsation and where it is located on the chest wall tell me whether the heart is enlarged and how much. Actually, a very forceful pulsation but one that occurs within the nipple line is often present when the heart itself is normal but the thyroid gland is overactive or when you have fever or anemia.

. . . Then Feel

After inspecting the chest wall, I will then move my hand lightly over the front of the left side of the chest, feeling for impulses which I may not have seen. I may also perceive a purring sensation under my fingers, like the "thrill" I felt over a diseased artery. If a thrill is present, I can expect to hear a very loud murmur when I listen later with my stethoscope.

I now use the same technique of *percussion* as I did when I examined the lungs. I do this to outline the shape of your heart and to determine whether it is enlarged. Providing that you are not very fat or don't have huge breasts, I can do this fairly accurately (but I know that if there is any doubt about my findings I will have the chest x-ray and ECG to fall back on later to make sure I'm right).

... And Finally Listen to the Beat of Your Heart

Finally I use the stethoscope, which can tell me so much about your heart. I assess its rhythm. Is it regular? Then I listen for murmurs. Diseases of the valves and other abnormalities that result in abnormal flow can be diagnosed with the stethoscope because they produce characteristic *murmurs*—the noises that result from a sudden interruption or change in the course of blood flow.

Murmurs That Tell a Story

As I try to interpret the significance of a heart murmur I will have you sit up, lie down, do a few knee bends, turn over on your left side, hold your breath or breathe out. These maneuvers are calculated to elicit murmurs that may not otherwise be audible. For example, one of the murmurs of mitral valve disease is rarely heard except when you lie on your left side after exercising.

Depending on where a murmur is loudest, in which direction it is transmitted (to the neck, the back, the left armpit), and what its timing is in the heart rhythm (while the heart is contracting or between beats), I am able to diagnose where within the heart it originates and what it means. Its radiation to the neck suggests a defective aortic valve. If, on the other hand, the murmur extends to the left armpit, the mitral valve is probably at fault. If it is loudest over a certain area when the heart is contracting, it means a valve is blocked. If it occurs when the heart has finished the contraction and is resting, it may mean the valve is leaking.

Not all murmurs are significant. Many are harmless, come and go, and are due to eddying of the blood around the valve before it passes through. Such *functional* or flow murmurs can usually be distinguished by the doctor from the *organic* or important ones. So if you have a heart murmur, that doesn't necessarily mean that you have heart trouble.

Aside from the murmurs, the quality of the heart sounds—the well-known "lub-dub, lub-dub"—is also revealing. Do they have the clean, firm tone of a healthy heart, or the soft mushy beat of a flabby, failing one? Sometimes I hear various clicks and extra sounds which also give me clues about the quality and strength of your heart muscle. If you've had heart surgery and have an artificial valve, the stethoscope is the best means I have of telling whether it is functioning properly.

Remember—the commonest cardiac disorder, coronary artery disease, is not usually diagnosed with the stethoscope. During the phase of angina pectoris, while the heart muscle is still intact and only the coronary arteries are narrowed, listening to the heart provides few clues. The diagnosis is suspected from the correct interpretation of the symptoms you describe to me and is confirmed by the electrocardiogram taken at rest, or if that is normal, which it often is, after exercise.

This concludes my clinical examination of your heart, except for one more observation. I look at your *neck veins* as you lie on the examining table. If you are in heart failure, they are swollen even when your head is slightly raised. If they are not, I then press for about a minute on your abdomen, over the liver area, turning your head to the side so I can see the neck veins. This is sometimes embarrassing, because patients think I'm doing this to them because they have bad breath. Pushing on your abdomen increases the return of blood from that area to the heart. The normal heart can easily handle this sudden greater volume of blood, and expels it with the next beat. But when the cardiac muscle is weak, it cannot accommodate the increased volume. Blood backs up from the right side of the heart into the veins, which then become distended in the neck.

Most of the things I look for in the clinical examination of the heart—the murmurs, the quality of the heartbeat, the neck veins—are not detectable in the electrocardiogram or chest x-ray. So when you're having a checkup, don't think that what you need is a bunch of blood tests, an x-ray, and an electrocardiogram and that the clinical examination is superfluous.

CHAPTER **10**

EXAMINING YOUR ABDOMEN

"When You Push Here, What Are You Feeling For?"

Before describing how I actually examine your abdomen, let's review the location of the organs situated within it. The abdomen is separated from the chest by the *diaphragm,* the muscle that moves with respiration. The food you swallow goes down the *esophagus,* which lies deep in the chest behind the heart and lungs. The esophagus passes through a small opening in the diaphragm and then expands to become the *stomach,* a J-shaped organ whose function it is to begin the process of digestion.

After an appropriate amount of time in the stomach, the food continues its transit through the gut. The stomach narrows into some 23 feet of *small intestine,* which winds back and forth within the abdominal cavity until it widens out to become the *large intestine,* or large bowel. The first part of the small intestine beyond

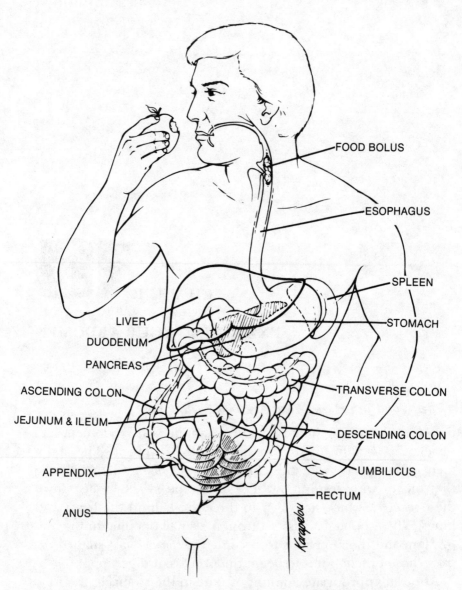

FOOD BOLUS

ESOPHAGUS

SPLEEN

LIVER

STOMACH

DUODENUM

PANCREAS

TRANSVERSE COLON

ASCENDING COLON

JEJUNUM & ILEUM

DESCENDING COLON

APPENDIX

UMBILICUS

RECTUM

ANUS

Karapelou

This "busy" drawing shows only some of the many organs there are in the abdominal cavity. The pancreas (above) and urinary bladder (below) are shaded. The ascending, transverse and descending colon make up the large bowel, which ends in the rectum and anus. The stomach leads into the duodenum, which is the first part of the small intestine. The kidneys are not shown here.

the stomach is called the *duodenum*—a common site of ulcers. The large bowel, about 4–5 feet long, begins with the *cecum* (to which your *appendix* is attached) in the lower right-hand portion of your abdomen, and then it assumes almost a rectangular course. It goes straight up to your rib margin on the right (that first part is called the *ascending colon*) and directly across to the rib margin under the left side of the chest (the *transverse colon*). It then descends toward the left lower part of the abdomen, the *descending colon,* whence it prepares to exit from the body in the segments called the *sigmoid,* the *rectum,* and the *anus.*

What's Inside the Abdomen—and Where?

Apart from the gut—made up of the stomach, small bowel, large bowel, sigmoid, rectum, and anus—the abdomen contains several other organs. The *liver* is situated in the right upper part of the abdominal cavity. When enlarged, it is easily felt. The *gall-bladder,* which can be detected from the outside only if it is swollen or distended by a cancer blocking its outflow of bile, also lies in the right upper portion of the abdominal cavity, peeking out from under the liver. The *pancreas,* which is very deep inside the abdomen, can never be identified by the examiner's hand (or even by the ordinary x-ray)—even when enlarged. It is the site of important diseases such as diabetes and cancer. The tip of the *spleen,* which is situated in the left upper portion of the abdomen, is often detectable. The spleen itself is enlarged in many diseases, especially of the blood. The *kidneys,* one on either side, lie deep within the body behind the abdominal cavity and are therefore not easily felt under normal circumstances.

All of the abdominal organs are supplied with blood from branches of the aorta, which, after it leaves the left ventricle, passes down the chest and through an opening in the diaphragm into the abdomen. Lower down, it divides, one major branch going to each leg.

DISEASES OF THE ABDOMEN

When the Trouble Is High Up in the Gut

In order for you to understand what I am looking for when I examine your abdomen, you must know the major disorders that can affect the various organs within it. Let's start at the top of the intestinal tract. A common problem in this area, especially in middle-aged and older people, is *hiatus hernia.* This is caused by a weakening of the usually tight ring in the diaphragm which keeps the stomach in the abdomen where it belongs. As a result of this weakening, a portion of the stomach actually slides up into the chest cavity. The stomach acid coming in contact with the food pipe causes *heartburn,* especially immediately after eating. If you have a hiatus hernia, eat small quantities at any one sitting so as not to allow regurgitation of food into the esophagus. Sleep with the head of the bed elevated on blocks so that gravity can pull the stomach down and out of your chest. Finally, antacids (Gelusil, Rolaids, Maalox) will neutralize the stomach acid which causes the heartburn.

Hiatus hernia is diagnosed clinically from the characteristic symptoms and is confirmed by x-ray examination. The hernia cannot be detected by physical examination. I cannot see it or feel it.

Many people over 50 years of age have a hiatus hernia. It may be large or small, but is nothing to panic about. Unlike other hernias, it hardly ever needs surgical correction. It is almost never dangerous except when it ulcerates and bleeds, just as any other part of the gut, owing to some irritation like excessive alcohol, or too much aspirin.

Why You Get Stomach Trouble

The *stomach* itself is vulnerable to several disorders, the most frequent of which is ulcer, and the most important *cancer.* The x-ray is the best way to make the diagnosis of gastric cancer.

Gastritis is an inflammation of the lining of the stomach. It may result from dietary abuse, heavy drinking, and chronic use of some medications, especially aspirin.

Ulcers of the stomach, too, can only be diagnosed with certainty by x-ray, but when I examine you, applying pressure on the abdomen will often give you pain.

What Is an Ulcer?

An ulcer is a hole, erosion, or break in the integrity of the lining of an organ. There are ulcers of the skin, eye, mouth, rectum, and so on. They also occur in the stomach or duodenum (the first part of the small intestine) and, when they do, often cause pain and sometimes bleeding. *A duodenal ulcer is never malignant, but ulcers of the stomach can be. So, any stomach ulcer that has not healed (as seen on x-ray) after several weeks is suspect* and may have to be biopsied. The term *"peptic" ulcer* means it is somewhere in the stomach or the duodenum.

What Kind of People Get Ulcers?

Ulcers are thought to occur in nervous, frustrated persons. This has given rise to part of our social vocabulary: "This job is giving me ulcers," or "Unless I get a divorce, I'm going to end up with an ulcer." Aside from the *ulcer-prone personality,* which I personally find hard to identify because so many of us are nervous and so few have ulcers, there are other causes. If you take cortisone in high doses for any length of time, you may develop an ulcer. Patients who are severely burned may also get one by some poorly understood mechanism (*burn ulcer*). Persons who undergo very prolonged operative procedures occasionally get ulcers (*stress ulcers*), and I have seen them develop after prolonged use of aspirin and other antirheumatic drugs.

The ulcer patient usually has a lot more acid in the stomach than you or I, and this is one of the reasons for the pain and break in the lining. There are other mechanisms too. After all, many of us have hyperacidity yet our stomach lining is not eaten away. What makes some of us resistant and others not is a mystery.

New Drugs for Ulcers

If you have an ulcer, you will be treated with three main agents—*antacids, antispasmodics,* and a new drug called Cimetidine. Antispasmodics reduce the irritability and acid secretion of the gut, while antacids neutralize acid. Cimetidine is one of a new group of medications called *histamine-2 blockers,* which represent an important advance in ulcer management. They do not merely neutralize acid that has been formed, as do Tums, Rolaids, and other antacids, but work in the following way. Histamine-2 is a chemical produced by one of the cell types in the stomach, and it stimulates another kind of cell to make the actual acid. Cimetidine and related drugs block the formation of hista-mine-2, so that no gastric acid is produced in the first place.

We used to place a great deal of emphasis on diet in the man-agement of ulcers. We don't anymore. Eat what you will, except for frankly hot, spicy foods and strong coffee. *But you must stop drinking.*

Small Bowel—It's Actually 23 Feet Long

The most important disease to which the 23 feet of small bowel are vulnerable is not ulcer or cancer but some disturbance of absorption and reabsorption or an inflammation called *"regional enteritis"* (Crohn's disease). The food we eat is prepared in the stomach for its subsequent digestion in the small intestine, where most of the major nutrients are actually absorbed. When the lining of the intestine is diseased, it doesn't properly absorb them, so that diarrhea, dehydration, abnormal foul-smelling stools, and malnutrition result. The ability of the small bowel to absorb the food passing through it depends not only on the in-tegrity of its lining but on how well the pancreas is working, since many of the digestive enzymes are produced in that gland.

Large Bowel—Short, Wide, and Prone to Cancer

The small bowel ends and the large bowel begins in the right lower portion of the abdomen where the appendix is tacked on. We used to think the only function of the appendix was to be-come inflamed (*appendicitis*) and help send the children of sur-geons through college. Recent work, however, has shown that it may play a role in protecting the abdominal cavity against can-cer. That doesn't surprise me, really. Why should so compli-cated, fantastic, and incredible a creation as the human body have a "useless" appendage? And maybe the routine removal of the appendix during an operation for something else (gallblad-der, ovary) should be discontinued.

Unlike the small intestine, the large bowel is frequently the site of malignant tumors, which may be found anywhere along its five-foot course. It is characteristic of such cancers that for months they may not produce any symptoms—no pain or obvious bleeding. (Later you will see how a simple chemical test of the stool can detect bleeding not visible to the naked eye.) That's why *routine x-rays* and direct inspection with a sigmoidoscope of this part of the body are so important. *While still early enough to be cured, bowel cancers cannot be felt by an examining hand,* but may be seen on x-ray or with the scope. Later, as they enlarge, they can be so detected, but by then it's often too late. Fortunately, tumors of the bowel can be benign as well as malignant.

Polyps, little fingerlike growths, can form anywhere along the large bowel. These are almost always benign but should be removed, because after a time some of the larger ones can become cancerous.

In addition to growths of one kind or another, your large bowel can get you into other troubles, the most important of which are infections and irritations (*colitis*). Most of these occur low down, that is, around the sigmoid and rectum. The hallmark symptoms of colitis are crampy pain and diarrhea with mucus and blood in the stool. Colitis is suspected when your abdomen is tender and painful. This finding requires examination of the stool and direct inspection with the sigmoidoscope, described later.

Your Liver—the French Blame It for Everything

The *liver,* being one of the major body organs, is the seat of a great deal of potential trouble. If you're French, you probably blame it for everything from bad temperament to bad investments. Tumors do not frequently originate in the liver, except in alcoholics, but spread to it very quickly from many other organs—the bowel, stomach, prostate, and pancreas. If these growths (*metastases*) are large enough, I can feel them when I examine the liver.

The liver is also vulnerable to infection. Viruses contracted from contaminated food and infected blood cause *hepatitis,* or inflammation of the liver. In addition, infections within the abdominal cavity can spread by way of the bloodstream into the liver, where they form abscesses. Worms and other parasites in the intestinal tract find their way to the liver, where they settle down to form cysts and abscesses. The liver can be damaged by toxic substances and drugs, including alcohol, various anesthetics, and tranquilizers.

The commonest causes of an enlarged liver are obesity and *heart failure.* Fat infiltrates the liver just as it does the pot belly. As the heart weakens, so that the right ventricle cannot expel all the blood returned to it from the body, the blood backs up into the liver, which then becomes swollen and tender. When the liver can no longer accommodate this excess fluid, blood serum seeps out of the circulation and accumulates in the abdominal cavity itself. This makes the belly round and swollen.

So within the abdominal cavity, a sick liver is a common and important complication. Depending on the nature of the process affecting it, liver trouble shows up as jaundice or results in a deterioration of its important functions. Infection of the liver or chronic alcoholism may leave it scarred (*cirrhosis*), so that blood cannot flow through it from the abdomen and backs up in the veins. This distends the belly with fluid, and the normally small veins of the abdomen stand out on its surface. The legs become swollen, and later, as the veins in the esophagus, bowel, and rectum also become engorged, the cirrhotic patient bleeds massively and often fatally.

Your Gallbladder—Why We Sometimes Have to Remove It

The function of the gallbladder is to store *bile,* a yellowish-brown or green fluid made by the liver. It is carried through a small duct (*common duct*) into the small intestine, where it breaks down any fats you have eaten so that the body can absorb them. If you were to eat fat all day long, the liver would keep producing the bile and pass it directly into the gut. However, when there's no fat in the small intestine, bile is not needed there. Since the liver is always making some, the surplus is diverted via another duct (*cystic duct*) into the gallbladder for storage. The next time you eat fat, the small intestine signals its presence there to the gallbladder, which then contracts and squeezes the stored bile out into the gut.

Your gallbladder won't give you any trouble unless it starts forming *stones*. It does so when there is low-grade infection within it or because of some chemical disturbance of the bile. Whatever the mechanism, instead of remaining in the liquid state, the bile crystallizes to form stones. A gallbladder that has stones in it usually doesn't work as well as it should. So now, when you eat fat and need more bile, the gallbladder may not contract sufficiently vigorously to squirt enough into the small intestine. Some of the fat remains undigested. What's more, as it contracts to deliver whatever bile it can, the gallbladder may expel a stone or two (especially if they are small) into the cystic duct. This gives you pain in the right upper part of the abdomen. Should the stone get past the cystic duct and block the main duct coming down from the liver (common duct), you will become jaundiced. This happens because the liver continues to secrete bile which now cannot get through either to the gallbladder or to the intestine. It backs up into the liver and the bloodstream, making you yellow. When the stone eventually passes of its own accord, or is removed surgically, the jaundice and pain disappear.

Your Pancreas—So Important Yet So Hard to Find

This organ cannot be examined from the outside, no matter what goes wrong with it, since it lies deep in the abdomen. Its main function is to produce various enzymes, which aid in the digestive process, as well as insulin, which converts sugar to energy. Occasionally, those cells of the pancreas that make insulin develop a tumor (insulinoma), as a result of which there is too much insulin around (instead of not enough as in diabetes) and patients become weak and faint due to *low blood sugar*.

Cancer of the pancreas is one of the most deadly, miserable, painful, and lethal diseases of mankind. It is not curable. Its pain is typically gnawing, felt deep inside the belly and eventually in the back. It is difficult to diagnose, even with x-rays and other specialized tests because the pancreas is located so deeply inside the abdomen. For this reason, this malignancy is almost always found very late, and has a mortality rate of virtually 100 percent.

On the brighter side, the recently developed CAT or body scanner and the use of ultrasound, described later, may permit earlier diagnosis of these tumors and possibly improve the outlook somewhat.

The Spleen—Graveyard of Your Red Blood Cells

The *spleen* is a blood filter and a storage place for your red blood corpuscles. Every thirty days, old blood cells are destroyed as they pass through it. Early in life, it is also a blood-forming organ. When it is not enlarged, it usually cannot be felt, but in the presence of most diseases of the blood, such as leukemia, it becomes big enough to be felt. The spleen cannot be examined by x-rays, but radioactive scanning and echo techniques described later can tell us something about its structure and function.

Sometimes the spleen takes its job too seriously, and will go about destroying blood components with excessive enthusiasm. When that happens, we have to remove it. Also, it may rupture, for example, in an automobile accident, and has to be taken out to prevent hemorrhage. You can lead a normal life without the spleen. Other parts of the body—the liver and bone marrow—take over its function with no trouble whatsoever.

Your Aorta—Looking Out for Aneurysms

The portion of the aorta within the abdomen from which large arteries branch off to supply the gut, the kidneys, and all the other organs in the area is frequently clogged up by arteriosclerosis. If severe enough, this process weakens the aortic wall, which balloons out like a defective tire, forming an *aneurysm*. This gets larger and larger and ultimately ruptures the aorta, like a blowout in a tire. The aneurysm, a large, pulsating mass, is usually easy to feel in the abdomen except in fat persons. However, the aorta often seems prominent in thin or older persons. It's not the apparent beating that's important, but the size and nature of the pulsation. When an aneurysm is suspected, special x-rays are required to confirm the diagnosis.

Long before an aneurysm ruptures, it may give some signs

and symptoms. You may see or feel the pulsations yourself or have abdominal pain. Because of interference with blood flow to the leg, you may experience cramps in the calves when walking, and the pulses in your groin and feet may be reduced.

One of my friends and patients, a portly 70-year-old man, complained of pain in his right testicle for months. A very careful medical and urological examination failed to reveal any cause. All his pulses were normal, and he had no trouble walking. One evening, after a heavy meal with wine, he suddenly felt faint, started sweating, and complained of abdominal pain. We examined him shortly thereafter, and found nothing unusual—a typical case of indigestion. While under observation in the next few hours, the abdominal pain became worse, and now spread into his right testicle. His blood pressure dropped precipitously, and he was found to have a ruptured aorta. His disease had gone unrecognized for months, until the moment of catastrophe. In retrospect, his only symptom was the testicular pain.

Pushing, Percussing, and Listening

Now that you know the contents of the abdomen and something about the basic functions of its organs, you will understand what I am looking for as I push, percuss, and listen to it.

For purposes of reference and so that you know what area of the abdomen I'm talking about, let's divide it into four quadrants. Using the navel as the central point, we draw an imaginary line through it from left to right, and a second line up and down. The gallbladder and liver are in the right upper quadrant; the spleen and stomach are in the left upper quadrant; the right lower quadrant is the site of the beginning of the large bowel and the appendix; the left lower quadrant houses the descending colon. (The pelvic cavity, which contains the ovaries and uterus of the female and the bladder in both sexes, is not considered part of the abdominal examination and will be discussed separately, even though its organs, when enlarged, can be felt there too.)

To examine the abdomen, I first look, then listen with the stethoscope, feel, then percuss one finger with the other.

For a satisfactory examination of the abdomen, you and I have to cooperate. You should be lying flat on a firm surface, relaxed, with your hands by your side, small pillows under your head and knees, your feet extended, breathing quietly through your mouth. I do my part by having warm hands. The biggest impediments to successful examination of the abdomen are, in my experience, severe pain in the belly, cold hands of the examiner, and a ticklish patient.

What Your Abdomen Looks Like

As you lie there, what might I see that's important? First, is your belly symmetrical? Is it swollen—filled with fluid, pregnant, or just fat? From time to time patients tell me they've inexplicably gained so much weight they can't close their trousers or skirt. But nowhere else is there any evidence of weight gain. I subsequently find they have a belly full of water due, usually, to liver disease or heart trouble.

Even the Belly Button Talks

Are there any abnormal pulsations due to an aneurysm? Are the superficial veins prominent, reflecting possible liver disease? What about surgical scars? Even the belly button can be revealing. Take a look at your own. You will see that it is indented. If it bulges out, the cause may be a weakness or hernia of the abdominal wall or an increase in pressure within the abdominal cavity due to a tumor or fluid. Patients sometimes complain of "stone" formation in the belly button. This usually reflects poor hygiene, with dirt and old skin building up within it, but may represent the first evidence of a malignant tumor. If the area around the belly button is blue, there is bleeding somewhere inside the abdominal cavity.

What Feeling and Percussing Your Abdomen Tell Me

I now proceed to feel various portions of the abdomen, the sequence depending on whether or not you complain of pain anywhere. If you do, I will examine that part last for obvious reasons. If your belly is distended, I want to know if it's due to gas, fluid, or a tumor. That's where percussion comes in. Gas will give a resonant, hollow percussion note. Fluid sounds dull, and a mass (tumor or growth) is flat. I will feel for muscle spasm, for weakness of the abdominal wall through which the tissues may sometimes herniate, and for tenderness or enlargement of any of the organs in the abdomen.

In the *right upper quadrant,* an abnormal mass may represent enlargement of the liver, the gallbladder, the ascending colon, part of the transverse colon, or the right kidney. The liver normally weighs about three pounds in the adult. In certain diseases it can be as much as thirteen pounds. I feel for the liver edge by having you take a deep breath. Even in normal people, pushing up against the liver can produce tenderness, so you mustn't worry if when you are examined there it is slightly sensitive. If the liver is enlarged, but not tender, it may mean early cirrhosis or a tumor. If it is smooth but overly tender, the most likely cause is hepatitis or early heart failure. An irregular liver edge suggests the late stage of cirrhosis, cysts, or cancer, the latter especially if it is very hard to the touch. If the gallbladder is enlarged and not painful, cancer of that organ or the pancreas is suspected. When it is painful, infection is present.

A mass in the *right lower quadrant* may represent a swelling of the cecum (remember that's the first part of the ascending colon) due to infection or tumor, an abscess, or more rarely a tumor of the appendix. Such a lump can also be due to a tumor of the right ovary which, if it is sufficiently big, can be felt in the belly.

A mass in the *left upper quadrant* may mean an enlarged spleen or a tumor in the transverse colon, in the upper portion of the descending colon, in the left kidney, or in the stomach. Finally, a mass in the *left lower quadrant* represents something in the descending colon, the sigmoid, the left ovary, or an enlarged left kidney.

Two harmless conditions can mimic a tumor in the belly. One is a bowel full of stool in a constipated person, and the other is a full bladder in someone who is either unconscious and can't tell anyone that he has to void or is awake and too shy to say so.

Listening to the Abdomen

When I listen to your abdomen with my stethoscope, I can normally hear the bubbling and gurgling noises caused by fluid and air in the digestive process. When there is some obstruction in the bowel, these sounds become high-pitched and tinkling. If the intestines are paralyzed temporarily, such as after an operation or when there is rupture of one of the abdominal organs with widespread infection (*peritonitis*), the sounds of the gut can either become faint or disappear. I will also listen for a murmur or bruit over the arteries of the abdomen, which, if present, indicates narrowing due to arteriosclerotic plaques. In younger persons it may merely reflect a thin body build.

What Is Abdominal Angina?

Before leaving the abdomen, let me tell you about one not so rare type of abdominal pain which patients and even physicians don't think about enough. This is called *abdominal* or *mesenteric angina*. Angina pectoris is pain in the chest caused by inadequate blood supply to the muscle of the heart. The bowel, like the heart, is an active structure. It propels the food and is almost constantly involved in digesting and absorbing the food we eat—all of which requires energy. This is provided by the blood carried to all parts of the bowel via the branches coming off the aorta. Arteriosclerosis, which we normally think of only in terms of the heart, brain, or legs, can also involve the arteries supplying the gut. If after a heavy meal, when additional blood is required to aid the process of digestion, the narrowed arteries can't deliver enough, you will have pain. This is abdominal angina. Every x-ray we take will be "negative," and you may go home with a diagnosis of "gas" or a "nervous stomach."

The treatment of abdominal angina is not very satisfactory. Nitroglycerine, so useful in relieving cardiac pain, is not effective for abdominal angina. There are no really good drugs for it, and surgery is difficult and not often feasible. The best way to manage the symptoms is to eat lightly (and more frequently, if necessary) so as not to burden the bowel and its meager blood supply.

THE RECTAL EXAMINATION

"If I Don't Put My Finger In, I Put My Foot In"

Whether you like it or not, the rectal examination is here to stay. It must be done routinely because a tumor detected here is often completely curable, in contrast to those of the lung or pancreas, where by the time a cancer is found, it is often too late.

The entire lower portion of the gastrointestinal tract—that is, the anus, the rectum, and the sigmoid—should be evaluated routinely in adults once a year. That tract can be examined up to a length of some twelve inches, about five of which can be reached by the finger. The proctoscope, a rigid tube which feels many times its actual diameter, allows me to see seven inches' worth of lower bowel, while with the sigmoidoscope the range is extended to twelve inches.

Regardless of whether or not you have blood or mucus in the stool, chronic constipation, diarrhea, or pain, this lower portion of the gut must be looked at routinely. No examination is complete without it. Rectal examination detects hemorrhoids, polyps, and cancer. In women, it provides additional information about the ovaries and the uterus. It is particularly valuable in examining young women who are still virgins, since it does away with the necessity to perforate the hymen, as might be necessary in a vaginal examination.

A Position to Take When Your Rectum Is Being Examined (Bottoms Up)

There are several positions you can assume. Some doctors have the patient on the back with the knees flexed; others have you lying on your left side. Some prefer the knee, chest, and elbow position on the table, while others will have you stand and lean over the table with your body and shoulders resting on it.

Before inserting my gloved and lubricated finger, I will look at the outside of your anus to see if it is irritated due to chronic scratching. This is especially common in children who have *worms*. The most frequent cause of rectal itching in adults is *hemorrhoids*, either external, which can be seen as tags on the outside of the skin, or internal. Venereal sores, especially common in homosexuals, are also apparent. But if you've complained of itching, and I find none of these abnormalities when I examine your anus, then your symptoms are probably due to poor hygiene, irritation from too much coffee, tea, and beer, or allergy to foods like shellfish and tomatoes.

What We Feel For

I now feel inside your anus, the outermost portion of the rectal canal. This is about two inches long, and in it I can detect internal hemorrhoids, tumors and abscesses. I can also assess the tone of the muscles that open and close the anal canal, an important piece of information in older people or those who've had strokes and who may have problems of continence. Also, rectal exam is the only way to find cancers of the anal canal. Next I push my finger beyond the anus into the rectum itself, where I can assess its walls and the lower part of the abdomen. In men, I feel for the prostate, searching for nodules, hardness, and size. In women I can feel the cervix and portions of the uterus.

When a woman is in labor, and the obstetrician wants to know how soon the baby will come, he examines the cervix through the rectum. As the time of delivery approaches, the cervix dilates more and more to allow the baby out. The more direct vaginal route is not used in these examinations in order to avoid introducing infection into the pregnant uterus.

After examining you with the finger, I will perform an examination with the sigmoidoscope. The sigmoidoscope is a long tube with a light at the end of it. It permits a view of the interior of the bowel, where we can see evidence of inflammation or tumors. *Rectal polyps,* if they are seen with the sigmoidoscope, can be snipped right off at the time of the examination.

Sigmoidoscopic examination is uncomfortable, but don't let that scare you. It's worth it. A positive finding can be lifesaving. We estimate that silent cancer is detected in 1 of every 700 such procedures. After two negative examinations one year apart, most doctors will recommend a sigmoidoscopy every five years; others still insist that it be done every year after the age of 40.

CHAPTER **11**

EXAMINATION OF YOUR
GENITAL ORGANS

BETWEEN THE UROLOGIST, who is interested in the urinary tract in men and women (the kidneys, the ducts leading out of the kidney into the bladder, the bladder, the penis, and testicles), and the gynecologist, who deals with the vagina, uterus, and ovaries—what is there left in the pelvis for the internist? He functions as a screen, detecting any underlying disease which requires referral to those specialists.

Gentlemen First

The organs of reproduction or more appropriately pleasure (in this age of contraception and small families) are surrounded by an aura of ignorance, superstition, and fear. As a result, many significant symptoms are overlooked and some important diseases can be missed.

As we did for the other organ systems, we will review the component parts, where they are located and their function.

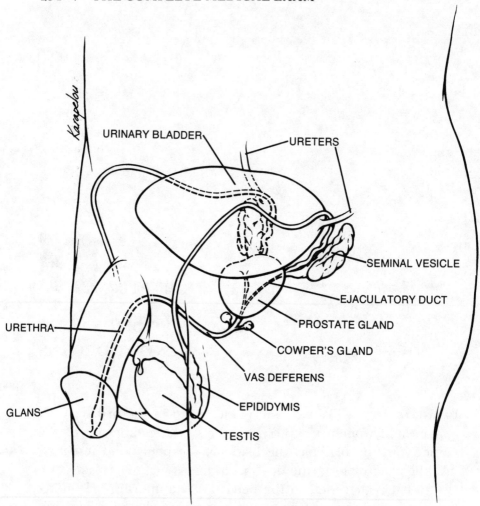

Note the pathway of the sperm from the testis out through the urethra. You can see how cutting the vas interrupts the exit of the sperm. The dotted line behind the prostate is the urethra, which can be compressed by enlargement of the prostate gland.

The Penis—Size, Shape, and Functions

First and most obviously, there is the penis, which is normally cylindrical. I say "normally" because there is a disorder called Peyronie's disease which makes it curved, a source of some pain and embarrassment.

The penis varies in size, but is about six inches long when erect. Since it is usually limp when I examine it, I can't bear personal witness to stories of exaggerated size, although some of these emanate from usually reliable sources. When uncircumsized, the head of the penis (glans) is covered by the foreskin.

By what mechanism does the penis become stiff and erect? There are two columns of tissue within it which are engorged with blood. This flow of blood into the penis is controlled by a complicated network of nerve impulses, some of which originate in the brain (reflecting sexual excitement) or tactilely (due to physical stimulation of any of the erotic zones—penis, mouth, and for some, the rectal area). The spinal cord receives impulses from these sensitive areas and sends back messages which trigger the opening of arteries and the flow of blood into the penis. Different reflexes, some of which are partially under voluntary control, are responsible for ejaculation.

Running through the center of the penis is the tube (urethra) that carries urine from the bladder to the outside and into which the various ducts from the organs that produce the sperm and seminal fluid empty. So the penis serves to perform the male sex act, as a conduit to emit semen, and to void urine.

Disorders and Treatment

What disorders can affect the penis? It's the only body organ we worry about when it *doesn't* enlarge—and that's the most common complaint I hear about. Then there are infections, the most important of which are venereal. These are contracted during sexual activity—vaginal intercourse, oral sex, and, among homosexuals, by the anal route. (One of the first things I learned in medical school is that you don't get VD from lifting pianos.) *Syphilis* is the most important and, if untreated, the most life-threatening venereal disease, while *gonorrhea* is the most common and obvious. There are other venereal infections, most of them viral, which can produce all manner of warts and ulcers at contact sites.

In the case of syphilis, a painless, weeping "cold sore" called *"chancre"* usually appears (on the tongue, lips, mouth, penis, anus, or wherever) some twelve to thirty days after sexual contact. It only lasts two weeks and then disappears. But the syphilitic infection it represents remains in the body and, if untreated, spreads everywhere, but most importantly to the heart, liver, and brain. The disease then makes itself apparent in a much more serious form later in life. And remember that with regard to possible infection, *the organism that causes syphilis, the spirochete, can be transmitted through the unbroken skin.*

Gonorrhea, unlike syphilis, does not produce sores. Instead, the bacteria that cause the disease infect the interior of the penis, the urethra, or the anus, which then release pus. But all such discharges are not necessarily due to gonorrhea. Nor are the evidences of this infection limited to the penis or anus, since it can spread via the bloodstream to a large joint, causing severe arthritis. Gonorrhea used to be more easily cured with penicillin than it is now, because the causative bacteria have, in many cases, developed some resistance to this antibiotic. If gonorrhea goes untreated, it can scar the urethra, interfering with the passage of urine and semen later on in men. In women, it results in chronic disease of the other organs in the pelvis.

Treat It As If It Did—But It Didn't

At this point, I'd like to share an amusing true story. Some years ago, a distinguished gentleman, patriarch in his family and the community, visited the clinic complaining of a discharge from his penis. It looked to me very much like gonorrhea. However, he insisted it came about when, in a moment of extreme urgency, he had found it necessary to urinate in an alleyway. At that very moment, he confided, a strong gust of wind blew on his unprotected organ—from which time on he noted the greenish-yellow discharge. Disputes of this kind are easily resolved. I analyzed the discharge—and found the gonorrhea organism looking up at me from the microscope. What to do? I had no inclination to have him think he was putting one over on me, so I said, very seriously, "I believe you. I'm going to treat this discharge with specific measures we use when it comes from a draft. I promise you it will be cured. However, I must warn you. If it didn't come from the wind, but by some stretch of the imagination you acquired it during intercourse, it will not be cured, and you will be very sick." He blanched, visibly embarrassed, but would not concede entirely. "I see," he said. "Well, in that case, treat it as if it came from sex, but between you and me, I got it from the wind." I left it at that and cured him with penicillin.

The Meaning of Blood in Your Ejaculate or Urine

Apart from looking for various sores on and discharges from the penis, I will want to know whether you have burning, increased frequency of urination, difficulty in starting the stream, and cloudy or bloody urine. *Blood in the urine must always be explained.* It can come from an infected or cancerous kidney, from a stone in the kidney or one of the ducts that lead from it into the bladder (ureter), or from the bladder itself, signifying cancer, a benign tumor, or some infection there. Prostate trouble may give similar symptoms.

Sometimes an alarmed patient will call about blood in the semen. This is often more frightening than blood in the urine, because it combines the mystery of sex with the panic most people have at seeing blood. In almost every case, however, a bloody ejaculate is a harmless sign of congestion of the veins of the seminal vesicles; these are the glands above the prostate that produce most of the fluid in the ejaculate.

If you are taking Aldomet, a drug widely used in the treatment of high blood pressure, you may be concerned about the fact that during intercourse the semen fails to come out. Instead, it is ejaculated in the wrong direction into the bladder. This is called *retrograde ejaculation*—a bizarre but harmless side effect, unless, of course, you want to have a child.

While sustained erection of the penis is a goal that most males may strive to achieve, it is not so gratifying to suffer from *priapism*—persistent or prolonged erection without sexual feelings. This can be a manifestation of some serious underlying disease, most commonly leukemia or some neurological disorder.

Sometimes the large vein that runs along the top of the penis can become varicosed just like veins in the legs. If severe enough, it may require the same kind of treatment. It most often occurs as a result of infection of or injury to the penis.

Incidentally, before leaving the penis to examine the scrotum, I will look carefully at your pubic hair to make sure that there are no lice there, a common cause of itching, notably among the unhygienic and the indiscreet.

Your Scrotum—A Bag with Valuable Contents

The scrotum is a bag of skin hanging loosely under the penis and containing the sperm-producing *testes*. Each testis is made up of coiled, winding tubules, which if stretched out would be about 800 feet long. From the testis, the sperm passes into another tube called the *epididymis* (about 20 feet long), and then into a long conduit called the *vas deferens*. *Vasectomy*, currently popular as a form of birth control, involves making a tiny nick in the scrotal sac and simply tying off or cutting the duct (vas) which carries the sperm formed in the testes to the urethra, and thence to the outside. This procedure is so simple it's usually done in the urologist's office. It prevents the sperm from reaching the outside, but in no way affects the testis itself, where the hormone *testosterone* is produced. Testosterone, unlike sperm, is not carried in the ducts, but diffuses into the bloodstream from the testis. Therefore, masculinity and sex drive are not interfered with when a man has a vasectomy in order to become sterile. Remember that you may still be fertile several weeks or for 15 to 20 ejaculations after a vasectomy. Even though no more sperm come from the testes, there are enough beyond the severed portion of the vas to give you a nice bouncing baby.

Vasectomy—You Can Change Your Mind

Unlike a hysterectomy, the vasectomy operation is often reversible should you change your mind about wanting to have children. But even when continuity of the vas is restored so that it can once more carry the sperm to the penis, fertility does not always return. The reason for this is not clear. It seems that after the vas is cut, antibodies are formed to one's own sperm. It's almost as if the body is saying to the sperm, "as long as you're not needed or wanted anymore, let's get rid of you."

Semen, the fluid in which the sperm are suspended, is a mixture of the secretions of the various structures along the pathway from the testis to the penis. It contains enzymes and proteins to ensure the survival of the sperm; it enables the sperm to be mobile in its search for an egg to fertilize and provides a favorable environment for the ultimate fusion with that egg after intercourse.

The *prostate* makes some of the fluid in the semen, but it does not produce either hormones or sperm. So if you are about to undergo a simple prostatectomy—that is, an operation to relieve obstruction due to an enlarged prostate—and you are worried that your potency will be affected, have no fear. So long as your testes, brain, and other glands in the body are intact, simple removal of the prostate will not usually have a physical effect on your ability to make love.

Sperm will live more than a month in a man's body but only about three days after ejaculation. The effect of heat on sperm is very interesting: the higher the temperature, the shorter the lifespan, because higher temperatures increase the metabolism of the sperm and burn them out faster. It is probably for this reason that the testes move down into the cooler scrotal sac from the interior of the abdomen, where they originally were situated in the development of the fetus. As you may know, sperm for artificial insemination can be stored at very low temperatures for years.

The male hormone testosterone is responsible for enlarging the penis after puberty, for determining the male distribution of body hair and muscles, and for lowering the voice. One interesting characteristic of testosterone is that it reduces the growth of hair on the head. So while baldness in a young man may be a genetic characteristic, it may also be due to an overabundance of the male hormone testosterone and is considered by some as evidence of virility.

Sometimes, women develop tumors that produce male hormone. As a result, they grow a beard like a man, they sound like a man, and they lose the hair on their head. That's also the reason why some forms of the "pill" which contain a little male hormone can cause loss of head hair in the women taking them.

The reason I have described, in some detail, how sperm is formed, how the penis becomes erect, where testosterone is made and what its actions are is that if you understand these mechanisms, many aspects of sexual function will lose their mystery, and some of the things you may have wondered about become clear. For example, *impotence* is so often a psychological state because mental stimuli from the higher nervous centers in the brain ultimately control the nervous reflexes which occur lower down to make the sex act possible. A mental or emotional block can interfere with this process. Hypnosis will sometimes restore impotent men to normal function by removing these inhibitions.

The "Morning Erection"

This phenomenon suggests that impotence can and does occur in the setting of an intact physical mechanism. Except in instances of nerve involvement, such as sometimes happens in severe diabetes mellitus, many impotent men, to their delight and encouragement, do experience an erection early in the morning. This is not the result of any sexual stimulation but a reflex from a full bladder. They run to empty it and rush back to bed, "rarin' to go," only to find the erection gone—victim of an empty bladder. However, even if you do enjoy such morning erections, their presence is not, as we used to think, proof that your problem is necessarily psychological. The isolated bladder reflex can occur even when other physical mechanisms responsible for normal sexual activity are impaired.

A Potpourri of Hernias, Tumors, and Varicose Veins

When I examine the scrotum, I first look to see that both testes are present. Then I feel gingerly but thoroughly to make sure they are not harboring a cancer (seminoma), which, when detected early, can be cured.

Tumors are not the only cause of a swollen scrotum. The generalized fluid retention seen in heart failure may also distend the scrotal sac. Also, when the veins that return blood to the heart are obstructed, blood backs up in them, and this too causes swelling of the scrotum.

I feel for hernias by putting a finger into the sac, pushing upward and having you cough. A little pulse against my finger tells me the wall there is weak.

The testes may also become infected with such diseases as gonorrhea, mumps, typhoid fever, scarlet fever, and influenza. Mumps is a serious and not infrequent cause of sterility in adult life if it happens to involve the testes. It's much better to contract mumps when you're very young, because these glands are not yet fully developed and can't be permanently damaged by the infection.

And Now for the Ladies

Every woman should have a gynecological examination at least once a year, preferably twice. It can be done either by your gynecologist (some women and many doctors prefer this arrangement) or by your internist. This examination is important because tumors of the cervix (the neck of the uterus), of the uterus itself, or of the ovaries may all be silent and detected only during a routine physical examination, which includes the Pap Test. However, not all gynecological disorders are symptomless. You may have vaginal itching (a possible sign of diabetes mellitus or of local infection); a vaginal discharge (representing anything from too much antibiotic treatment and fungal overgrowth to venereal disease); bleeding either with intercourse or spontaneously and at any point in the menstrual cycle (possibly representing a hormonal disorder, a polyp, or a cancer somewhere in the female genital tract); or menstrual pain. Again, you may have noticed changes in your menstrual cycle—in its duration and the amount of flow. These may be due to glandular disorders, such as an overactive or underactive thyroid, but also to growths within the ovary or uterus.

The gynecologist who examines the pelvis, abdomen, breasts

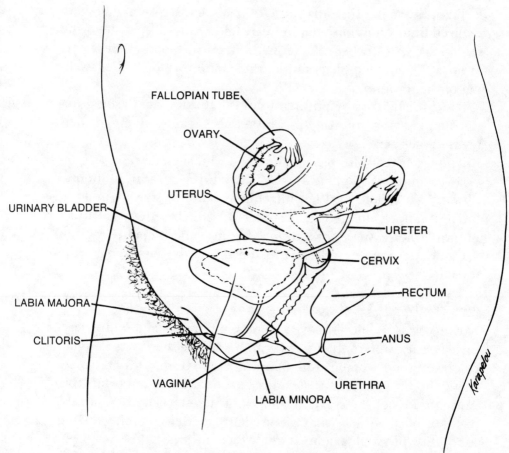

FALLOPIAN TUBE

OVARY

UTERUS

URINARY BLADDER

URETER

CERVIX

RECTUM

LABIA MAJORA

CLITORIS

ANUS

VAGINA

URETHRA

LABIA MINORA

Karapelou

This is a three-quarter view of the female genital anatomy. You can see how doing a rectal examination makes it possible to feel the cervix. The urethra (from the bladder) emerges in front of the vagina. So "vaginal" bleeding may be from either the urinary tract or the genital organs. The egg from the uterus passes down the fallopian tubes (whose top portion fits like a glove around the ovary) and into the uterus. Sperm travels up the vagina into the uterus, where it meets the egg and fertilizes it.

and rectum can probably detect about 70 percent of the cancers that afflict women, and most of these can be cured.

The Pelvic Technique

The pelvic examination consists of looking and feeling. I look at the opening of the urethra, from which urine is passed, to see if there is any discharge. The presence of pus suggests gonorrhea. I then examine the lips of the vagina for "warts" or "sores" which may indicate herpes virus or various forms of venereal disease. Just as obstruction of the veins within the abdomen causes enlargement of the testicles in man, so the vaginal lips may become greatly swollen under similar circumstances in women.

I then look for a discharge from the vagina itself and, when present, send it for analysis. If it is yellowish and frothy and accompanied by vaginal itching, it most probably indicates infection with a tiny organism called *Trichomonas*. Passed between sexual partners, it is harbored in the female and the male, but some men contract it without any symptoms. Whenever the diagnosis is made in a woman, her male partner should also be examined and both of them treated at the same time. Unless this is done, the female is constantly reinfected.

Gonorrhea (gonococcal infection) is another common cause of vaginal discharge. Unlike *Trichomonas*, which is limited to the vaginal interior, the gonococcus involves the urethra as well.

Some women who have been taking antibiotics for too long experience a persistent discharge due to the growth of a fungus. Other discharges come from infections of the cervix, the lower part of the uterus, and the neck of the uterus.

Many older ladies, especially those who have had many children, complain of losing urine on coughing or sneezing. This symptom is called *stress incontinence*. It results from the fact that the tissues supporting the vaginal walls are torn or weakened. This condition often requires surgical correction.

The "Pap Smear"

At this point in the examination, I will introduce a speculum into the vagina. This is a duckbill-shaped instrument which opens and closes, and through which I can look into the interior of the vaginal vault. I can then see whether the walls are as moist as they should be, or dry as in some older women because of insufficient female hormone, and whether there are any bleeding spots or areas of infection. It also permits me to look at the opening of the uterus (cervix), from which polyps (bulging masses of tissue) sometimes protrude. The cervix is also where I take the "Pap smear." I gently rotate a small cotton-tipped applicator around the opening of the cervix, painlessly removing some of the superficial tissue. This is then looked at under a microscope. The value of the test is that the very earliest stages of cancer of the uterus can be detected before a tumor has actually developed. Surgery at this stage will usually effect a cure.

The Pap test probably saves the lives of some 75,000 women every year with this early detection of malignancy. Why Dr. Papanicolau, the modest, brilliant doctor who devised this simple test was never given the Nobel Prize in medicine has always been a mystery to me.

Next, I do a bimanual examination—the fingers of one hand inside the vagina, the other hand feeling from the outside and pushing the organs down toward the fingers inside. This tells me the size of the uterus and whether or not there are any tumors in it. I can usually also feel the ovaries on either side for cysts or growths. If your hymen is intact I examine the pelvic organs through the rectum.

Infertility and Miscarriages—If You've Tried and Tried

It is unfortunate that the medical term for miscarriage is *abortion,* because socially this word implies the deliberate removal of an unwanted pregnancy. In medical usage, if you lose your baby, that counts as an "abortion."

If you have tried and tried, and been unable to become pregnant, you may very well have some glandular imbalance. Although this may involve the pituitary, the adrenal, the thyroid gland, or the ovaries, a common cause, in my experience, is underfunctioning of the thyroid. If that's the case, some thyroid tablets will restore your fertility. But supposing the cause is not obvious, how do we go about finding out why you can't become pregnant, or if you do, why you keep losing the baby before it is born?

Why Not Check the Sperm First?

Whenever a couple is barren, the woman is first put "through the works" of a fertility investigation—for no reason but chauvinism. As a matter of fact, about one third of sterile marriages are the fault of the man, in whom it is quite simple to do an analysis of the number and quality of the sperm. So if you're a woman, before launching on an intensive glandular and gynecological evaluation because you're supposedly infertile (a complicated and expensive affair), it is a good idea to *have your mate's sperm checked first.*

If the sperm are adequate in number and motility, and the routine gynecological examination is normal, we will go on to assess the function of your glands. This is usually done by analyzing your blood. If your hormones are normal, we must then examine the fallopian tubes, which carry the egg from the ovary down to the uterus where it meets the sperm. In women who have had chronic infections of the genital tract, these tubes may become scarred, preventing the egg from passing through it. The techniques we use to determine whether the tubes are open are the hysterosalpingogram (an x-ray technique described later) and, less commonly now, blowing carbon dioxide into the tubes to see if they are patent.

CHAPTER **12**

BENDING EVERY WHICH WAY—
EXAMINATION OF THE BACK

EVERYBODY IS AN AUTHORITY on back pain—your internist, chiropractor, osteopath, barber, best friend, and orthopedist. Those entitled to collect a fee for their opinions, however, are those licensed to do it—orthopedists, physiatrists (MD's specializing in physical medicine), osteopaths, and chiropractors.

Diagnosis of back pain is one thing; treatment is quite another. Diagnosis involves examination by looking, by touching, by assessment of muscle movement and, in order to make sure that there are no underlying bony problems, by x-ray.

What the Spine Consists Of

In order to understand how and why you develop back pain, you should know something about the makeup and function of the spine. It's a flexible structure consisting of 33 bones called *vertebrae,* separated from one another by soft structures (*discs*)

Note the spinal cord emerging from the brain, sheathed by the bony spine. On the right is a magnification of the lumbar area. You can see how a "slipped" disc pushes on the nerve, causing pain.

which prevent the bones from grating and rubbing against each other. The entire back is surrounded by muscles which keep the spine straight. The top 7 bones form the *cervical spine,* the next 12 in the chest area make up the *thoracic spine,* the 5 in the low back are the *lumbar spine,* while the 2 bottom ones—the *sacrum* and *coccyx*—consist of 5 and 4 fused bones, respectively. The coccyx is the structure that protrudes in very thin or emaciated people. If it sticks out too much, it becomes irritated or inflamed by constant pressure due to lack of supporting fat, tissue, and muscle. If that happens, try sitting or lying on a rubber tire.

Running through the spinal column are the delicate nerves (spinal cord) that pass between the brain and every organ and part of the body. They leave the skull through a large hole (foramen magnum) and branch out to all the organs through small holes in the vertebrae. The spinal column, then, in addition to giving you physical support, also serves the critical function of protecting the cables (nerves) from the central switchboard (brain) to each telephone (organ).

Your Aching Back

What can go wrong in the back to produce "backache," "back trouble," or a "bad back"? One or more of the bones in the spine may be injured or fractured. The site of the pain, its severity, and how dangerous it is will depend on which bone is hurt. Obviously, if it's the one you sit on, the coccyx, it may hurt, but it's not serious. On the other hand, an injury to the *atlas* at the very top of the cervical spine can be fatal, because all the nerves which pass from the brain into the spinal cord may be severed or damaged.

If you have some disease that makes your skeleton soft or brittle, you may fracture a bone without even knowing how you did it. Rickets in infants and young children (caused by insufficient calcium for developing bones), Paget's disease in adults (a metabolic disorder affecting the quality of bone), and the menopause (in which the bones become thin due to lack of calcium) can all result in fracture, either spontaneous or after some trivial blow. In routine x-rays of the spine, we sometimes see evidence of an old fracture without any history of injury, and only a "backache" that lasted a few days.

Cancer of the bone eats away at it, causing severe pain and spontaneous fractures. Such cancer may originate in the bone itself or spread to it from other organs, such as the breast, prostate, and lung. And any infection in the body, such as tuberculosis and syphilis, may involve the bones anywhere, including those in the spine.

You can injure a bone without necessarily breaking it. It can be bruised or is dislocated by a sudden wrench from its normal alignment. This may cause severe pain which for all practical purposes is indistinguishable from that of fracture, so that an x-ray is required to differentiate the two.

The back is vulnerable to most forms of *arthritis,* but the commonest is the kind caused over the years by wear and tear—*osteoarthritis.* Where you feel the pain will depend on what part of the spine is involved.

It's the Spasm That Hurts

The spinal column is surrounded by bands of muscles which protect it from injury and make sure that its alignment does not go "out of whack." When a bone is injured or diseased, these muscles go into spasm in order to protect it from excessive motion, and it's the spasm rather than the hurt bone that gives you most of the pain. Even a trivial bone disorder may trigger a crippling spasm, accounting for the fact that many painful backs have normal x-rays. (X-rays do not show up muscle, only bone.)

The garden variety of *muscle spasm* is not due to injury or disease but to nervous tension or bad posture. One young man telephoned from his honeymoon hotel complaining of a crippling back pain which had developed the night before—a classic example of how nervous tension and bad posture can be responsible for backache at the same time.

Where You Feel the Pain

Pain originating in the back can be transmitted to other parts of the body and mimic disease elsewhere. For example, a headache, is probably more likely to be due to spasm in the muscles at the back of the neck than to a brain tumor; spasms in the small of the back resemble the pain of kidney disease.

Back trouble is often due to disease and dislocation of the *discs* between the bones. These discs are normally of a gelatinous consistency. When they become dislocated or hardened, the bones they ordinarily separate ride on each other, and the nerves that go in and out of the spinal column are pressed upon. The result is not only back pain but numbness, tingling, pain, and weakness of the arms and legs supplied by these nerves.

The arthritic process also thickens and deforms bones. When this happens, the holes through which nerves pass out of the bony spinal column become smaller, pressing on and irritating the nerves. This produces pain, not only in the diseased bone, but wherever the involved nerve happens to be going—to an arm or leg. This explains the pain of sciatica, for example, which you feel in your buttock and down the back of the leg, even though the pressure is being exerted on the sciatic nerve in the low back.

While pain due to a back disorder can travel elsewhere, by the same token many diseases originating in other parts of the body give symptoms in the back. For example, the pain of a heart attack may be felt in the left shoulder or the midback; acute gall-bladder pain radiates to the right shoulder and the small of the back; and the pain of cancer of the pancreas or an ulcer may be referred to the spine.

EXAMINATION OF THE BACK

The first step in examining the back is to look at it for evidence of deformity and loss of its normal curvature. Is there a "hunchback"? Is the spine twisted to the left or right? I will tap each bone to detect any unusual sensitivity, and feel the muscles for spasm. I will then put you through a series of movements to see if there is any rigidity or reduction in the flexibility of the spine. In some forms of arthritis, the bones and joints actually fuse, so the spine becomes stiff and rigid—the "stiff man's syndrome."

Examining Your Neck Area

Starting with the *cervical spine,* I look to see how supple your neck is. The nerves that come out of the spine at this level supply the upper chest wall, the arms and hands. Pressure on them due to disc disease or arthritis causes pain that may be mistaken for angina pectoris. As in heart disease, such pain involves the fingers, wrists, or elbows. To make sure, then, that the symptoms are due to the spine and not the heart, I have you put your chin on your chest for a few moments. If that reproduces any of your chest pain, tightness in the back of the neck, or numbness and tingling in the arms and hands, chances are the trouble is in the neck, not the heart. Hyperextension, that is, tilting your head way back, will make you feel better. I will also have you put your chin and then each ear on your right and left shoulders. If you have arthritis of the neck, this will pinch the nerves and reproduce your complaints too. When I place my hand over various portions of your neck and have you move it, I may also feel the crackling or crepitation of the joints underneath.

"Trigger Points"

I now examine the muscles of your neck for "trigger points," tender areas about the size of a dime or smaller, due to muscle spasm. When I press on them with my thumb, it hurts. Trigger points are managed in different ways. Some doctors inject them with Novocain and mash up the concentrated spastic tissue with the needle. No fun, I'll tell you. Others use a local anesthetic spray like ethyl chloride, and then break them up by deep massage. Some physicians prescribe muscle relaxants while yet others recommend heat and rest—or exercises.

Neck Pain

If x-rays confirm that you have worn or dislocated discs, traction of the neck muscles will often give relief. We put your neck into a halter for various periods when you're at home, or have you wear a neck collar. You may even have to be hospitalized if you're uncomfortable enough.

One important and common mechanism of neck pain that has been the subject of much disability and humor is *whiplash* injury. If you are in an automobile struck from behind, your neck and head are forcefully jerked backward (hyperextending them), then forward (flexing them). You may then develop neck pain, headache, and even blurred vision hours or days later. These symptoms are exaggerated when litigation has begun, but whiplash is nevertheless a real phenomenon. In the majority of cases, we are unable to find objective changes, even though you have pain. But usually when the injury is severe enough, clinical examination does reveal absent reflexes, changes in the way your pupils react to light, muscle spasm, and distortion of your posture. The pain may be mild at the beginning and then clear up. Months and years later you may end up with some form of arthritis.

Examining Your Trunk

Moving from the neck to the trunk, I again check for mobility. How far can you bend forward to touch your toes? Does raising your legs cause pain in the back? These and other maneuvers reveal the presence and degree of any arthritis of the spine, the existence and severity of muscle spasm, and whether or not there is disc disease. Slipped discs are most common in the low back, producing pain in the sciatic area down the back of the leg. They can be detected by testing reflexes and sensation (Do you feel the pinprick?) to see whether they are reduced or absent in the ankle and at the knee.

TREATMENT OF THE "BAD BACK"

The millions of people with chronic "bad backs" who lose countless man-hours of work each year are witness to the inadequacy of treatment. The trouble started, I suppose, when in his evolution man got up off all fours to assume the upright position.

A few basic rules of treatment are generally accepted. If pain is due to bone injury, then rest and immobilization—as, for example, with a cast—may be required. If you have a slipped disc, with pain and weakness of an arm or leg, before submitting to surgery try a good long period of bed rest, aspirin, and moist heat. As you improve, a program of planned progressive exercise may help, too. But remember, there's nothing worse than the wrong exercise, so make sure it's prescribed by a specialist in the field, someone who understands the dynamics of the muscle groups involved. Recently, injection of papain into herniated discs to remove them by dissolution has been tried. However, this therapy is still in the experimental stage and not generally applicable.

Watch Your Posture

Many cases of chronic backache are due to physical inactivity, poor posture, obesity, or bad mattresses which permit excessive curvature of the spine. Occupational stresses which require unnatural repetitive movements may also give you a sore back. For example, when I use my telephone too often, cradling it on my left shoulder, I get pain in the left side of my neck. The writer or secretary sitting at the typewriter with neck bent often develops neck pain. So does the executive sitting at his desk, neck constantly flexed, looking down at papers. The television viewer, lying in bed, body flat, and neck bent forward looking at the screen hour after hour, may also develop neck pain. And if you like to read lying in bed with your neck brought forward, you may be vulnerable to backache.

So, if you get recurrent aches in any part of your body, think about your posture and the positions you assume during the day and at night. When you consult your doctor, be sure you tell him all about it, so that he can have a better understanding of the possible mechanisms that are giving you the symptoms.

CHAPTER **13**

DO YOU HAVE ARTHRITIS
OR RHEUMATISM?

WHENEVER ANY TWO BONES in the body meet, a joint is formed whose function it is to allow smooth, pain-free movement between them. Like the bones they unite, these joints are vulnerable to a variety of disorders which come under the general heading of arthritis (*itis* means inflammation, *arthron* is the Greek word for joint). So *arthritis is an inflammation of a joint.* It is not one disease, but anything that injures a joint. Arthritis may result from *infection* (for example, tuberculosis, gonorrhea, or syphilis); *injury* (traumatic arthritis) to the bone or bleeding into the joint; or some upset in the body chemistry causing irritation of a joint. Gouty arthritis is the classic example of a *chemical arthritis;* in gout, uric acid crystals form in the joint making it hot, painful, red, and swollen. Arthritis may also be due to chronic *irritation and inflammation*—the wear and tear caused by the surfaces of the joints rubbing against each other over the years. This condition causes pain and some deformity, and is known as *osteoarthritis* or *degenerative arthritis.* Then there is *rheumatoid arthritis,* whose basic cause is unknown and which deforms and cripples.

Certain diseases which appear to have nothing to do with the joints are accompanied by arthritis. Psoriasis, a skin disorder, is one such example. Rheumatic fever, which starts as a sore throat, later causes acute arthritis by virtue of some sensitivity mechanism in the joints. As a matter of fact, aches and pains in the muscles, bones, and joints are so "nonspecific" that years ago people used to have their teeth pulled when no other cause for their symptoms could be found. When the muscles, tendons, and ligaments also hurt you, and the pain is not limited to the joints, then we call it *rheumatism.*

Throughout these chapters, I have referred to joint involvement when discussing certain specific diseases or areas of the body. In the preceding chapter, you read about "your aching back." I have referred to acute rheumatic fever, gout, gonorrhea, bursitis, "student's" or "tennis elbow," and several other situations in which "arthritis" is the main complaint.

The Big Two in Arthritis

There are, however, two very common and troublesome disorders that constitute the bulk of the "arthritis problem" and should be discussed separately. These are *osteoarthritis* and *rheumatoid arthritis.* They remain important causes of disability and suffering, if not death. Their management is largely symptomatic—that is, we treat the aches and pains, but can do very little to prevent or arrest the underlying factors that cause them. Because our attention is focused on the great killers of mankind—cancer and arteriosclerosis—joint cripplers like arthritis have gone, if not unchallenged, then unconquered.

Osteoarthritis—It Hurts But Doesn't Often Cripple

If you are over 40 years of age, chances are nine out of ten that you already have some osteoarthritis. It's probably not severe enough to bother you very much (a couple of aspirin and some heat make you feel better in a few minutes). You may have some joint stiffness during the day. You "loosen up" after a while. Your hip may ache a little, and if you're among the unlucky few, it may eventually cripple you. (Fortunately, if your symptoms are bad enough, the hip joint can now be replaced with spectacular success.) You may notice swelling of the knee from time to time, which usually responds to heat, rest, and aspirin. We've already discussed how your back may be affected. Attacks of pain, wherever they occur, may come and go without reason, but if you've "strained" or used a joint too much, you're more likely to suffer.

Osteoarthritis is the result of "wear and tear" on the joints, primarily the weight-bearing ones and those that are constantly in motion. Treatment consists of exercises which strengthen the muscles around the affected joint, showing you how to protect the diseased parts from further damage, giving you splints and other supports where necessary, and operation, even replacing worn-out joints like the hip or knee. But for most of us; arthritis is a mild disorder, and all we need is occasional rest and aspirin.

Rheumatoid Arthritis—the Villain of the Piece

Unlike osteoarthritis, which is a local disorder of one or more specific joints, *rheumatoid arthritis* (RA) is an internal disease of the body, which strikes the joints in a dramatic, crippling, and painful way. Occasionally, other organs like the heart, lungs, skin, and eyes are also affected. Patients with rheumatoid arthritis are apt to have what we call "systemic" signs—a little fever, weakness, loss of appetite, as well as changes in the blood count and certain abnormal chemical tests described later. Instead of just having a "bad joint," they look and feel sick. Also, more than one joint is usually involved, and these are often symmetrically affected at the same time—both knees, both hands, or both feet. The inflamed joints are not necessarily the ones that do the work or bear the weight of the body. The hand is more frequently involved than the knees.

As much as 3 percent of the population has rheumatoid arthritis, so it is one of our most important crippling diseases. Its cause remains unknown, although everything has been implicated—stress, food, viruses, and allergy. Women suffer from it two or three times more than do men. It can begin any time in life (there is even a childhood form) but it is basically a disease of adults starting in the forties and fifties. You will be happy to know it does not run in families.

Rheumatoid arthritis may come on insidiously, with some stiffness of the fingers, and just stay that way. Or it may progress gradually, leaving you in pain, crippled and deformed. In some patients, it strikes suddenly and without warning. However it starts, it usually disappears for a while from time to time (the phenomenon of "remission"). Perhaps one in ten patients eventually becomes completely disabled. The majority continue to function, but in pain.

We Can't Cure, But We Can Help

We try to emphasize to you that rheumatoid arthritis is something you can live with. If our record with other diseases is any indication, help is on its way. If we can get you to believe this, depression, a common and understandable accompaniment of RA, is minimized. Actual treatment consists first of resting the inflamed joint. Persuading you to do that is not difficult. Then there is a long and growing list of "antiinflammatory" drugs, the key one being aspirin, which afford relief. They not only control the pain, but also exert some as yet poorly understood soothing effect on the process of inflammation. But taking one or two aspirin, as you would for a headache, is not enough. Massive doses, 8 to 16 or more tablets a day, may be necessary. In these amounts, we recommend you take some "buffer," like antacid, or use the coated aspirin preparation. But even so, you run a constant risk of stomach irritation, bleeding, and ulceration. This is true for most of the other medications used as well, including Indocin, Butazolidin, Motrin, and other newer preparations.

It is most important to avoid the use of addicting pain-killers. Remember, RA is probably going to be with you for the rest of your life. If you resort to codeine, Demerol, morphine, or similar narcotics, it won't be long before you're hooked. And then you'll have two diseases to deal with, rheumatoid arthritis and drug addiction.

Another drug, which should be used only when other measures have failed, is cortisone. Never take it without close medical supervision. I have already described its hazards—ranging from reactivating old TB to stomach ulcers, high blood pressure, bones that break easily, a big round moonface, and making your own adrenal glands sluggish.

There is one form of therapy worth a try at some point—gold. It is given by injection once a week for several weeks, and may cause a prolonged "remission" of the disease.

CHAPTER **14**

WHAT MAKES YOU TICK—
THE NERVOUS SYSTEM

No PART OF YOU is independent of the nervous system. In fact, it's the real you. The ability to think, to walk, to make love, to see, to hear, to control your bladder and your bowels, to perceive pain and interpret the meaning of that pain, to taste, to smell, to enjoy, to cry, to fear—everything, all of life, depends on the integrity of your brain and its connections to every part of your body.

When I examine each organ and system in your body—your heart and the automaticity with which it beats, your lungs and the rate and regularity with which you breathe, your stomach and its ability to transmit hunger pains—I am indirectly evaluating your nervous system at the same time. When I specifically perform a neurological examination, I am looking for direct evidence of disease within the brain, determining the integrity of the nerves that go to and from it. In addition, I may detect some problem at the nerve-muscle junction where the messages the nerves carry from the brain are translated into action.

Its Different Parts

Think of the nervous system as being made up of two different components. There is the *voluntary* part over which we all have some control. For example, if you want to raise your right arm, the thought or wish to do so originates in a portion of the gray matter of the brain and is then transmitted by the appropriate nerves via the spinal cord to the muscles that create this movement. The second kind of nervous activity is basically automatic or reflex and is called *autonomic*. Sweating, blushing, the rate at which the heart beats, the speed of digestion, and the regularity of breathing are all examples of how the autonomic nervous system works. Erection and orgasm, too, are basically reflex actions, although they can also be voluntarily modified by sexual thoughts or emotion and, so, controlled to some extent.

What Can Go Wrong

The brain and the various nerve tracts going to and from it are affected by the same disorders or diseases as the rest of the body. For example, they can be *injured,* and the consequences of the trauma depend on what part of the brain or nerve tract is involved and to what extent. The nervous system can be *infected* by bacteria and viruses. *Cancers* can either originate in or spread to the brain. *Chemical* or *hormonal disorders* disturb it. For example, diabetes out of control, liver failure, and end-stage kidney disease may cause coma because of the accumulation of toxic substances which literally poison the brain. *Drugs,* tranquilizers, narcotics, and *alcohol,* affect the brain, producing anything from drowsiness or excitability to coma, depending on the drug, its dose and for how long you were taking it. *But the most common mechanism of brain injury is some interruption in its blood supply.*

Stroke Is the Big Threat

Impaired blood supply to the brain, if severe and prolonged enough, ends up in some kind of *stroke*. The brain, like the heart, is very dependent on getting enough blood. Unlike the heart, which needs less when you're resting and much more when you're exercising vigorously, blood requirements of the brain are fairly constant. The cerebral circulation can be reduced or stopped by three major mechanisms. In *thrombosis,* a clot forms within an artery inside or outside the brain, depriving it of its blood supply. If the artery is a big one, like the carotid in the neck, the stroke is massive, with paralysis, inability to speak, coma, or death. If only a small vessel is involved, the damage is more limited; the symptoms may be mild and clear up in a matter of minutes or hours. Such strokes due to obstruction of blood flow by a clot originating in a diseased artery usually develop gradually over a period of days or hours, and may be preceded by what we call *transient ischemic attacks.* These are recognized by brief episodes of dizziness, disturbances in vision (you may see double), light-headedness, numbness and tingling of an arm or leg, or temporary slurring of speech. It is important to recognize such attacks because treatment (with anticoagulants and possibly with aspirin, Persantine, or surgery) may avert or delay the final closure.

The second mechanism that causes stroke and brain damage is the *rupture* of a blood vessel within the brain. The burst artery hemorrhages into the brain tissue, producing the same symptoms of stroke as a closure. In such cases, the attack is more likely to be instantaneous, without the warning of the transient ischemic episodes, and the outlook for recovery is not as good as when the artery is blocked. *Untreated high blood pressure is the major cause of brain hemorrhage (and the commonest contributing factor to strokes of any kind).* For example, in Japan where the high-salt diet is presumed to be largely responsible for the increased incidence of hypertension, stroke is the leading cause of death and far more common than it is in the United States.

The third way in which a stroke can occur is when a clot or *embolus* arising in another part of the body, usually the heart, travels within the circulation and lodges in one of the vessels in the brain, occluding it. Such emboli may originate in artificial heart valves around which the blood eddies and on which clots may form. These then break off and are carried to the brain.

Most patients who have prosthetic valves are kept on anticoagulants indefinitely to prevent such particles from forming. Emboli also develop (a) after major heart attacks, at the site of injured muscle inside the heart; (b) in patients with valvular disease before operation, because of sluggish blood flow within the heart; or (c) when the cardiac chambers are so weak that the blood within them isn't squeezed out properly. In this last circumstance, little clots form within the stagnant blood in the heart and may be released into the arterial system to lodge in the brain or other organs when the heart is treated. This happens because when the weakness is improved, the heart once more contracts forcefully, expelling the clots.

HOW IS THE NERVOUS SYSTEM ACTUALLY EXAMINED?

I examine the nervous system in a step-by-step evaluation of its component parts—the brain and the various nerves coming to and from it.

The Brain—a Very Complicated Switchboard

We usually associate brain injury or disease with weakness, paralysis, blindness, or other obvious, striking motor symptoms. But remember that changes in personality—sudden bizarre behavior—may also reflect brain damage. There is so much emphasis on the psychiatric and emotional basis of mental illness these days that we sometimes forget that structural disorders within the brain can also cause peculiar or abnormal behavior. Whenever I see a patient, no matter how old or how young, who recently has become "strange" or "different" in his ways, I perform an especially careful neurological examination. *Psychiatric disorders in the elderly may be the result of unrecognized small strokes.* Also, I've seen more than one brain tumor masquerading as mental illness at any age. Remember the man who died in a mental hospital with unrecognized, treatable bleeding in the skull, and the woman who lost her peripheral vision because of a brain tumor.

He Loved School—and His Baby Brother

Here's another example of why you should see your doctor before you consult a psychiatrist when behavioral problems develop. One evening, a waiter in my favorite restaurant asked me to recommend a child psychiatrist for his 7-year-old son. The boy had always been a good student, liked school, and enjoyed his work. Now, suddenly, he was no longer well adjusted. He was making all kinds of excuses to avoid going to school in the morning, his favorite one being "I have a headache." After a cursory examination, it was concluded that this behavior was due to emotional problems resulting from the birth of a new baby. The parents were advised by the pediatrician to take the "troubled" boy to a child psychiatrist as soon as possible.

When I was told about the problem, the headache part of the story worried me. Since the child was only 7, I advised that he be examined by a neurologist before making a commitment to psychotherapy. Forty-eight hours later, before such an appointment could be arranged, the child suddenly lapsed into coma. He was rushed to the hospital, where he was found to have a brain tumor the size of a plum. Fortunately, the surgeons were able to remove all of it without any permanent brain damage.

The boy now likes his school again, his behavior is normal, he even plays with the new baby—and the headaches have gone. That tumor was so large it must have been growing there for months, maybe even years. A thorough examination may well have revealed its presence, possibly even before the onset of symptoms. So it is of critical importance to separate "pure" mental illness from physical brain damage.

Headache—and What It Can Mean

An important complaint that is too often relegated to the "tension" wastebasket is headache. *Every patient who has persistent headache deserves a careful neurological examination to make sure there is no underlying physical cause.* This involves testing various reflexes and looking into the eyes with the ophthalmoscope. Tumors cause increased pressure within the brain, and this can be recognized by a characteristic appearance of the nerves and blood vessels inside the eye. Looking into your eyes is my job, as well as that of your eye doctor and boyfriend.

Fits and Starts

If you complain of *seizures*—anything from dreamlike states of only a few seconds from which you can't be roused, to abrupt loss of consciousness with convulsions or a "fit," waking up and finding you've wet your pants or moved your bowels involuntarily—then you probably have a form of *epilepsy*. Epilepsy, like migraine, may not be detectable on physical examination, and you will need other tests described later if we suspect that diagnosis.

The neurological exam really begins when you first walk into the office. At that time, I look at how you walk and for facial asymmetry or deformity. I listen to the way you talk and make a note of any slurring of speech, of appropriateness of language and behavior, as well as of your mental status. By that time I have a pretty good idea as to whether or not you have any obvious neurological disease.

The Twelve Major Nerves—What They Do and How We Test Them

To help me determine more accurately the status of various portions of the brain, I next carry out a test of the 12 major or *cranial nerves* which leave the brain. These are numbered (1–12), named, and tested separately. For example, when I ask you to show your teeth, I'm checking the 7th nerve. Shrugging your shoulders against resistance is a test of the 11th nerve. You stick your tongue out for me to check the 12th nerve.

The 1st nerve (olfactory) is responsible for smell. The commonest cause of inability to appreciate odors and aromas (anosmia) is, of course, a stuffy nose. Sometimes a viral illness, especially in older patients, can produce a loss of smell for varying periods of time, occasionally permanently. Finally, a brain tumor in a certain predictable location will also destroy the sense of smell.

The 2nd nerve (optic) permits us to see. Brain tumors that press on the optic nerve cause blindness, which is either complete or partial, affecting specific parts of the visual field. For example, you might be able to see straight ahead, but have no peripheral vision (like our lady with blinders), or you may see the bottom half of an object but not the top. In other cases, the central portion of the vision may be wiped out but the periphery is visible. Each of the several possible patterns of visual loss tells me where the tumor lies within the brain. Then, when I look into the eye itself with the ophthalmoscope, I can see whether the nerve is shriveled, swollen, or blanched, owing to pressure by the tumor on the arteries supplying it.

Three more nerves (numbers 3, 4, and 6) move the eye muscles up, down, sideways, and across. If you see double as you follow my finger with your eyes, one or more of these muscles is weak, perhaps due to nerve damage within or outside the brain. The remaining seven nerves are responsible for facial sensations, muscle movement (I ask you to whistle, show me your teeth, wrinkle your forehead), hearing, taste, the mechanism of swallowing, movement of the shoulder muscles, and tongue motion ("show me your tongue").

Testing Your Reflexes

In the remainder of the neurological examination, I will test your coordination, to give me some idea of how certain portions of the brain are functioning and cooperating with each other. I also look at your muscles generally to see whether any are wasted (atrophied), which may happen from disuse following nerve injury. I will then test muscle strength to detect any weakness of which you may be unaware. A muscle is weak because the nerve supplying it is damaged or because there is something intrinsically wrong with the muscle itself.

When I test your reflexes with a special hammer, the response may be abnormally brisk, diminished, or absent.

The intensity of a reflex varies a great deal from person to person, even in the absence of disease. So I judge overactivity or underactivity by comparing the reflexes on either side of the body. They should be equal in intensity. When a reflex on one side is either more brisk or more sluggish than that on the other side, this may indicate disease in the brain or somewhere in the nerve tracts in the spinal cord, or damage to the nerve itself within the organ being tested. The reflexes we usually test are the jaw reflex, the triceps reflex behind your elbow, the biceps, the reflex above your thumb, the knee jerk, and the ankle jerk. A reflex with an exotic response is the abdominal. When I stroke the belly lightly, the superficial muscles twitch and in normal men the testicle is drawn up within the scrotum. Also when I scratch the bottom of your foot from heel to toe, your big toe should bend down. If it goes up, there may be a significant disorder of the nervous system, most commonly a stroke.

Other tests of the nervous system involve evaluating how well you perceive pain and touch, temperature, vibration, and position sense. ("Am I moving your toe up or down?") These tests are done to identify disease within the nerve tracts going to the brain, such as spinal cord tumors or pernicious anemia.

If in the course of my questioning, observation, and clinical testing I find suspicious or definite evidence of disease, there is a whole array of special tests at my disposal to hone down on the diagnosis. These range from the lumbar puncture to the sophisticated computerized brain scanner, and are described in the following chapters.

"Pregnancy" Without a Baby

There is a fascinating disorder, *hysteria* or hysterical reaction, which will occasionally fool even the most experienced physician. In nonmedical terms, "hysteria" means frantic, wild, unreasonable behavior which generally requires a slap in the face or dousing with cold water (especially when it occurs in a movie scene). But medically it refers to symptoms that have no physical basis. For example, there is a hysterical symptom called pseudopsiesis or *false pregnancy*. Even though the patient is not pregnant, she stops menstruating and her abdomen swells so that she looks to all intents and purposes as though she is in her sixth month, or more.

Other manifestations of hysterical behavior may be paralysis of an arm or leg, blindness, amnesia, numbness, or pain. When you are examined carefully, these symptoms cannot be explained on the basis of any physical findings. For example, when a leg is paralyzed because of brain disease, the reflexes we test with a little hammer (the most popular one is the knee jerk) are either absent or very much increased. In hysterical paralysis they're normal. In hysteria, patterns of pain or numbness do not follow nerve pathways or distribution. Such hysteria, by the way, is not on a conscious level. The patient is not deliberately trying to "con" the doctor. He has no idea that his symptoms are without physical foundation and due to some emotional crisis. Treatment of hysteria is psychiatric.

When I was a medical student, anyone who wanted to become a neurologist was viewed with some suspicion. After all, why enter a field where all you can do is sit back and watch people die. That's not the case anymore. With improved surgical techniques, antibiotics and other drugs, and a better understanding of how the nervous system works, there is a great deal to be done—and that depends basically on making an accurate diagnosis.

CHAPTER **15**

AFTER THE HISTORY AND PHYSICAL—
WHAT NEXT?

WE'VE NOW SPENT about an hour together in the office. First you talked and I listened, then I asked my questions. Later I performed that part of the examination in which I used my senses of touch, sight, smell, and hearing—as well as my intuition and judgment. All of that, however, is not enough. There remain two final aspects of the examination—analysis of the various fluids and substances of the body, plus the electrical and x-ray study of its interior.

Chemical analysis of some of your specimens is easy enough. You can usually provide the urine, feces (not always when I want it), and sputum (if you are bringing any up). I will also remove a small amount of blood.

The rest of your checkup—the chest film, sigmoidoscopy, x-rays of the bowel, electrocardiograms, and stress tests—will be performed routinely at regular intervals whether or not you have any symptoms. This is so because diseases of the heart, chest, and bowel may be present without causing any symptoms or signs that I can detect early in a clinical examination; they can be recognized only by these special procedures.

Fill This Bottle, Please—the Urinalysis

My nurse will now present you with a small, clean bottle, which I hope you'll be able to fill before you leave the office. It's the one test you'll have to pass before getting insurance, joining the army, or getting a clean bill of health from your doctor. In order for you to appreciate the importance of the urinalysis, you must understand how and why urine is formed.

Making Urine

The big job of the kidney is to maintain the chemical equilibrium of the body, to filter the blood that circulates through it—and to convert it to urine. The process of life within the body produces waste products. These are excreted in the breath as carbon dioxide, by the skin as sweat, from the bowel as stool, and in the urine. To give you some idea of how efficient the kidney is with respect to this one filtering function, consider this: About 2000 liters of blood pass through it every 24 hours, yet only about 1½ or 2 liters end up as urine, which contains all the wastes that have to be eliminated. The healthy kidney does not allow anything the body needs to leak out into the urine, despite the massive volume of blood that circulates through it. So in healthy people sugar, certain minerals, proteins, the red and white cells of the blood, and other vital elements are all meticulously reabsorbed.

The amount of urine you pass is also determined by what the body needs. For example, if you drink a lot of water, you will be voiding a large volume, so that you don't drown in your own fluid. On the other hand, if you're dehydrated or lost in the desert, the kidney will form only the smallest amount of urine—that needed to dissolve the waste products—and will reabsorb the rest.

What Is an Abnormal Urine?

A specimen containing substances that shouldn't be there, or too much of what should, is abnormal. This can happen as a result of several possible mechanisms. If the kidneys themselves are damaged, they may allow needed constituents to slip through the otherwise efficient filtering system and be lost to the body. So when we find the urine to contain things that shouldn't be there, like red or white blood cells, sugar, proteins, and other elements, we report it as abnormal. By the same token, if the kidney is sick, material that should be excreted is not, but then the retained substances are detected in the blood analysis, not in the urine.

What Does the Urine Reveal?

Urine may be abnormal even if the kidneys are healthy. For example, if you have too much of a certain substance in the blood, the kidney will try to get rid of the excess by excreting it in the urine. The classic example is diabetes mellitus, with its high blood sugar concentration. Some of this excess is eliminated by the kidney and then appears in the urine. So sugar in the urine usually represents a problem of insulin deficiency, not kidney disease. Also, if there is trouble anywhere in the genital or urinary system other than in the kidney (bladder, prostate, urethra), then the urine may also be abnormal.

What You Ate

Suppose your history doesn't suggest any trouble in your urinary tract—you don't void too frequently, there is no burning sensation when you do, you haven't noticed any blood, you don't have to get up at night more than once—what routine tests will I still do on the urine? Well, first I look at it. If your urine is murky or cloudy and has a strong odor, it may have been obtained soon after eating meat or other foods containing phosphates. Vaginal secretions contaminate the urine in women and also give it a cloudy appearance. Certain foods like asparagus cause urine odors.

If you have fever or are dehydrated because of diarrhea, vomiting, or poor intake of fluid, the urine, especially the first morning specimen, is "concentrated" because the kidney is doing its job to retain scarce water, and this concentrated urine also has a strong odor. On the other hand, most abnormal substances except blood are not visible to the naked eye. For example, *perfectly clear-looking urine may be found to have large amounts of albumin,* the most common protein in urine.

It's Not Always Yellow

The *color* of the urine depends on how much water you've been drinking. Dilute urine is pale yellow or colorless, a gold-colored specimen is concentrated. Tea- or mahogany-colored urine usually means there's bile in it and is found in jaundiced patients. Deep brown, frankly red, or pink urine indicates blood or its components, but don't be alarmed if after you eat beet soup (borscht) or fresh beets, your urine becomes red. Dyes found in candy, food, and drugs also may alter the color of the urine. For example, several popular laxatives will turn it red, and a widely used pain-killer (phenacetin) may make it gray, brown, or even black. Tranquilizers like Thorazine and Compazine taken frequently may turn the urine red or brown. Vitamin pills, especially those rich in the B group, not only will give it a characteristic odor but will make the urine orange. If you've had some bladder irritation and the doctor gives you a pill called Pyridium to relieve the pain, don't be alarmed when you find your urine bright orange. Urised, a commonly used bladder sedative, turns urine green. You should know all this because there's nothing more frightening than unexpectedly passing bright orange or red or green urine, and not being forewarned about it.

Is It Strong or Dilute?

I now determine the *concentration* of the urine. Is it strong or dilute? This tells me whether the kidney is properly maintaining the body balance of water. By "concentrating" the urine, I mean is the kidney able to retain enough of the needed water brought to it in the blood? If you've been eating a normal diet and drinking at least the equivalent of 4–6 glasses of fluid a day, and your morning urine is very dilute, the kidneys are permitting too much water to leave the body. This may mean that there is not enough of a certain hormone produced in the brain which helps the kidney reabsorb water, or it may indicate that the organ itself is damaged.

How Acid Is Your Urine?

Normal urine is *acid*. But if you have lung disease or severe diabetes, the body retains too much acid. To help correct this situation, the kidneys will excrete urine that is more acid than normal. A very *alkaline* (the opposite of acid) specimen may mean infection, or simply not enough meat protein in your diet. Meat tends to make urine acid, so vegetarians who eat only fruits and vegetables have an alkaline urine.

I now screen the urine to see whether it contains any abnormal substances like sugar, proteins, bile, ketones, and blood. This is very simple and takes only a minute.

Strip Testing

Only a few years ago, urinalysis was much more involved and time-consuming. Each determination had to be done separately. Today we use a small strip of paper with several little patches on it, each of which is treated with a different chemical. The strip is dipped into the urine; we wait about a minute and look for the color changes on each patch. We can then determine at a glance the presence of bile, blood, sugar, protein, and most of the other abnormalities routinely looked for in the urine.

The Meaning of Protein (Albumin) in the Urine

Protein is an important constituent of the blood, and the healthy kidney does not permit any of it to escape. So its presence in the urine usually indicates some disorder. Normal young men may leak albumin, especially if they have been standing for long periods of time. This *postural* phenomenon is not associated with any disease. Also, some widely used drugs result in the appearance of albumin in the urine. These include oral medicines used in treatment of diabetes, various antibiotics including penicillin, dyes injected for certain x-ray procedures, sedatives, and large amounts of vitamin B.

Insurance Companies Won't Like You

Insurance companies place a great deal of emphasis on the presence of albumin in the urine. When you apply for a policy, they look for three things in the urine—blood, sugar, and albumin. If any of these is present, up goes your premium. (But should they find sperm, you're not penalized.)

Although many different kidney disorders may give you albumin in the urine, if your insurance policy is declined or rated because of it, check with your doctor to make sure you don't have the postural kind. Also be sure you tell the company if you're taking any of the aforementioned medication, which may be causing it. Very few insurance firms will go to the trouble of finding out why you have the albumin. They simply increase your premium or decline your application.

The test strip also indicates *sugar*. When the circulation is filtered by the kidney, the sugar it contains is reabsorbed into the body. However, if sugar levels are high, the kidney eliminates some of the excess, which then shows up in the urine.

What Did You See?

Years ago, physicians didn't have the technical means of detecting sugar in the urine. So they actually tasted it. The term *diabetes mellitus* means "flow of sweet urine." I am reminded of that special freshman class in medical school whom the dean was welcoming. As part of his introductory remarks, he emphasized the need for doctors to develop acuity in their powers of observation. "None of your senses may be ignored, not even the sense of taste," he said. "I have here a container of urine. Now watch closely." With this, he dipped a finger into the urine and licked it—to the horror of the budding young medicos. He then had each student fill a paper cup with his own urine and instructed them to do exactly what they had seen him do. Every student dutifully put his finger into the urine and licked it. After they had finished, the dean looked at the grimacing faces and said,

"You have learned your first lesson about the importance of your senses. It was not the sense of taste I wanted you to use, but your sense of sight and observation. I put my index finger into the urine container, but licked my ring finger. You put your ring finger in and licked it."

How Important Is Sugar in the Urine?

Just as albumin is occasionally found in the urine of normal persons, so does one find a little sugar now and then in the absence of disease. The healthy kidney reabsorbs all the sugar presented to it when the sugar concentration in the blood is normal. The level above which the kidney begins to allow sugar into the urine is called the *sugar threshold*. Some people, especially the elderly, have such a low threshold that even in the presence of normal blood sugar, a little gets into the urine. This does not mean disease, and is the reason why the diagnosis of diabetes should never be made on the presence of sugar in the urine alone without a blood test.

Aside from the low-threshold cases, the screening test for sugar in the urine may indicate its presence if you have some rare kidney disorder or are taking various medications. The list of drugs is large and includes high doses of vitamin C (which so many people now take in the hope that it will prevent or abort the common cold), various antibiotics including penicillin and tetracycline, aspirin, sulfa pills, some diuretics, and even certain vaginal powders.

The commonest cause of sugar in the urine is diabetes, so whenever sugar appears, regardless of all the harmless possibilities I've mentioned, the next step is to check the blood sugar level.

The Pregnant Male

You may enjoy a true experience I had several years ago. In my first year of medical school, we learned that sugar in the urine might mean glucose, fructose, lactose, sucrose—and so on. The simple paper strips we now use were not then available. We had to boil the urine and add a different chemical to identify each of the different sugars that might be found in human urine.

One day we were at a laboratory session devoted to this subject. Each student provided his own specimen, to which we added various sugars one at a time for analysis. One of these was lactose, a sugar excreted by the pregnant woman. The experiment was designed to show that routine urinalysis on a pregnant woman may falsely indicate diabetes because of this lactose. My bench partner was a very serious chemistry student who was taking this particular laboratory course with the first-year medical class. He was firmly convinced that a freshman medical student was practically a doctor. I was fascinated by the prank potential of lactose in the urine. I had his attention diverted at a critical moment, and while he was gone, I added some laboratory lactose to his urine specimen.

When he performed the prescribed analysis on his own fresh urine, he was amazed to find that it contained sugar. He was due for an even greater surprise, because as he went through the procedures to identify it, he found this sugar was lactose. I was paying no apparent attention to his work. As he stared in puzzlement at the brown color of his lactose-filled urine, he turned to me and asked, "Why would I have lactose in my urine?" I matter-of-factly indicated to him that it must be because he's pregnant. We laughed together at this joke, he decanted the urine and provided a fresh specimen to be retested. At this point, I had him distracted again, and once more surreptitiously added some lactose to his specimen. A repeat test, this time very meticulously done, again revealed the presence of lactose. This was no longer a laughing matter. He asked for help from the instructor, who went through the various testing procedures with him to make sure that they'd been done accurately. He too confirmed the presence of lactose.

Several of us, including the instructor, were now in on the caper. This serious young chemistry major was keenly interested in knowing the diagnostic possibilities, which, by prearrangement, were narrowed down to the fact that he was pregnant. But how could he possibly be pregnant? We explained to him that in the process of their development, both male and female embryos actually have a small uterus, but that as the fetus grows, the male uterus shrivels. In the female, it develops further. I explained to him, with the concurrence of all the "experts" in the first-year medical class, that occasionally in a male this uterus fails to disappear, and that some grown men actually have a functioning uterus. In the course of some of his sexual activity, I postulated, one of his sperm must have gotten into his own uterus and impregnated him.

This sounded so plausible to my bench partner (who incidentally is now a distinguished biochemist with children born in someone else's uterus) that he actually consulted the professor of obstetrics at our university. The latter had not been forewarned about the ruse and didn't quite know how to deal with this obviously disturbed "pregnant" young man. The professor of psychiatry was about to be called in when we came clean.

Ketones Mean Diabetes—or a Starvation Diet

The presence of *ketones* on the paper stick is especially important if there is any sugar in the urine. Ketones are the end product of the breakdown, or metabolism, of fat. If you have any in the urine, it means you are burning fat. Normally, energy is provided by glucose (sugar). When there is not enough *available* sugar as in *diabetes mellitus* (there is plenty of sugar in the blood but not enough insulin necessary to convert it to energy) or in *starvation* states (self-imposed or forced), or it is being lost or energy needs are increased (diarrhea, vomiting, high fever), the body calls on its fat reserves to provide extra fuel. As this fat is burned, you lose weight and ketones appear in the urine. Their presence is important in monitoring the status of diabetics. If such a patient is getting enough insulin by injection, he burns his sugar, does not have to use his fat reserves for energy, and no ketones appear in the urine. Urine loaded with sugar and ketones means the diabetes is out of control.

Is There Bile in Your Urine?

When blood levels of bile are high, as occurs in jaundice and certain liver diseases, it will make the urine tea- or mahogany-colored. A quick way of telling whether there's any *bile in the urine* is to shake it vigorously in a test tube. Bile makes it foam. In any event, the chemical dip strip will tell us if there is any bile present, and does so before the patient with liver disease has obvious jaundice.

There is one more patch on the strip to be looked at—perhaps the most important one—the test for *blood*. If it is positive, I examine the specimen under the microscope to see how many red cells are actually there.

Why We Need the Microscope

The urine is spun rapidly for a few minutes in a high-speed centrifuge. This moves any sediment to the bottom of the tube. I take a drop of this sediment and look at it under the microscope for red blood cells (indicating bleeding), white cells (infection), and various crystals. If you're menstruating, blood will usually appear in the urine—a false alarm.

Blood in the urine must always be explained. It can come from a cancer of the kidney, bladder or prostate, from some simple infection or one like tuberculosis, from stones, or from injury. Blood disorders unrelated to urinary-tract disease can also cause blood in the urine—for example, some abnormality of the bleeding and clotting mechanism. Also, if you are receiving anticoagulation therapy, you may suddenly and spontaneously bleed in the urine (and also the stool, mouth, or nose). This indicates that the dosage of the drug is too high and your blood is too "thin." *An insidious danger in these circumstances is to assume that such bleeding is always due to the anticoagulants.* A patient can coincidentally develop other diseases that cause blood in the urine, and these may then be overlooked.

If there is blood in the urine, I will send it out for a "Pap" test, just as we do in the routine examination of the cervix in females—again looking for cancer cells.

Is Your Urine Infected?

If I see *white blood cells* and *bacteria* under the microscope, especially if you have a low-grade fever, frequency of urination, urgency (you've got to get there fast), and burning, I will send the urine to the laboratory for "culture." The specimen will be incubated so that any bacteria in it will grow and can be identified. Different antibiotics are then added to each of a group of test tubes containing the bacteria to see which one kills most of them. Unless you're allergic to it, that's the antibiotic I'll prescribe for you. Of course, in addition to identifying and treating the infecting organism, I want to know how and why you got the infection in the first place so we can prevent future trouble.

Crystals of various shape and refraction seen under the microscope may provide a clue to possible kidney stone formation later on. *Sperm* are also normally present, even in elderly men.

No More Rabbits

Now you know how I examine urine routinely. But there are several other tests performed on the specimen when there is a special reason to do so. For example, if I suspect that you have *lead poisoning,* urinalysis for lead is a very sensitive test, becoming positive before you even develop symptoms. If you complain of severe abdominal pain and I think it may be due to inflammation of the pancreas (*acute pancreatitis*), I look for the enzymes from that organ in the urine. If you are *pregnant,* your urine will reveal it. Incidentally, frogs, rats, and rabbits will be happy to know we no longer need them to diagnose pregnancy. There is now available an immunologic procedure, the *radioreceptor assay,* which requires just a little blood and takes a few minutes to read. This test is very accurate and can be used as early as one week after fertilization. You needn't wait for a missed period to be suspicious.

Various tumors can be detected by special cellular analysis of the urine. In one, a blood malignancy involving bone called *multiple myeloma,* abnormal proteins other than albumin appear in the urine. Another rare tumor, which causes *high blood pressure,* excretes specific hormones that can be measured in the urine. The *appendix* may very rarely develop a tumor which characteristically also involves the lung and produces a measurable chemical in the urine. We use the urine also to assess your *hormone function.* I ask you to save all of it passed in a 24-hour period and then measure various hormone concentrations. Many toxic substances that cause poisoning and coma can be identified in the urine. This is especially useful in unconscious patients when we need to know what they took in order to give them the proper antidote.

In short, in addition to kidney disease, the urine mirrors a great number of normal and abnormal states in the body, ranging from pregnancy to cancer, and its analysis is often vital to accurate diagnosis and treatment. If you have a completely normal urine, that's a big plus for you in your checkup.

The Stool—Esthetic? No. Important? Yes.

The same people who are preoccupied with moving their bowels every single day without fail, whose life revolves around whether they "did" or "didn't" that morning, often consider bringing a stool to me for examination unpleasant, embarrassing, and undignified. No matter how you react to it esthetically, *stool analysis is a necessary part of your routine physical examination.* Even if you have no bowel symptoms, your stool may reveal evidence of *bleeding* somewhere in the gastrointestinal tract (due to ulcer, hemorrhoids or cancer), *infection* (by various parasites or bacteria—ameba, pinworm, dysentery), or *inflammation* (colitis—a chronic inflammation of the lower bowel which causes mucus and blood to appear in the stool). Also any disturbance in the way the bowel handles, transports, and utilizes the food you eat is reflected in the kind of stool you pass.

The "Hemoccult" Test

A stool specimen cannot usually be produced on demand in the office, and so I try to get enough on the glove during the digital rectal examination, at least to test for blood. There is now in widespread use a very convenient way for you to get a specimen back to me. It eliminates the problem of collection and delivery of the stool from your home to my office. I give you a small card with a paper portion in its center on which, with a small wooden spatula, you smear a thin film of stool. In a few minutes, when it's dry, you seal the card and mail it back to me.

We add a couple of drops of a special chemical to the area on the card with the stool on it. If it turns blue, the test is positive for blood. This "Hemoccult" test is so sensitive it will pick up even traces of blood. So if your gums ooze, or you've had a nosebleed recently, you may have a positive test for blood in the stool, If you're a big meat-eater, you may also show traces of blood. When this occurs, we put you on a meat-free diet for two or three days and then repeat the test.

A common cause of blood in the stool these days is *aspirin,* which can cause chronic, insidious blood loss due to irritation of the stomach. The stools are not black because the amount of blood lost is small—but the anemia is cumulative. If you take two or more aspirin every day, be especially conscientious about looking at your stool for evidence of bleeding. To double-check, send your doctor a stool specimen on one of the cards three or four times a year. *Whenever there is blood in the stool, a complete x-ray study of the gastrointestinal tract together with sigmoidoscopy must be done, regardless of how obvious the cause may seem to be.*

Sometimes I need more than just a film of stool. If I want to examine it for *bacteria* or *parasites,* or do chemical testing, you will have to bring a larger portion. So many people have a hang-up about getting such a specimen to the lab. They loathe doing it, they have trouble collecting it, they never know what to put it in, and no matter how securely the container is sealed, they worry about the odor. It's best to use a glass jar, close it tightly—and avoid a fancy wrapper.

All That Glitters Is Not Gold

I remember one lady who simply refused to bring a specimen despite my repeated requests. I finally told her that unless she came with a stool at her next visit, I would refuse to see her. A few days later, there she was again without the specimen. Before I could berate her, she explained what had happened. She had finally overcome her revulsion to this "debasing" procedure. She did collect the stool, put it in an empty Tiffany box—and to assuage her sensibilities, gift-wrapped it. She boarded a bus to come to the office and put the package on the seat next to her.

She was distracted for a moment or two, and when next she looked, it was gone—stolen. Can you imagine the expression on the face of the thief when he opened that box and found it was not a pot of gold?

Most of It Is Water

About 75 percent of the normal stool is made up of *water*. The rest consists mainly of *bacteria*, small amounts of the residue of the food we've eaten, vegetable fibers, fat, and other debris. Digested *protein* gives the stool its odor. If your stools are frothy and foul-smelling, they contain a great deal of fat, the result of poor digestive function or disease of the pancreas. The normal brown color is derived from the breakdown of *bile pigments* in the bowel, but its intensity largely depends on the kind of food you eat. If you are a vegetarian and take no meat, your stool will be light-colored, and because there is less protein, it will have less odor. If you're taking iron in any of your vitamin preparations, or Pepto-Bismol, your stool is likely to be black. If there is some obstruction to the normal flow of bile from your liver to your intestine, you will be yellow but your stool will be clay-colored due to lack of bile pigments. Bleeding piles or hemorrhoids give you bright-red blood, usually on the outside of the stool or on the toilet tissue. Bleeding low down in the large bowel will also give such red blood. Bleeding higher up, as in the stomach, makes the stool black, like tar. Beets not only color the urine red but simulate blood in the stool too.

You're the Best Judge

While I can assess the color and constituents of the stool, including any bacteria and parasites in it, I depend on you to describe the *size and shape* of the movement itself. *You should look at every stool you pass.* You may consider it indelicate to do so, but missing a cancer is a lot more gross. The caliber of the stool depends on the size of the tract of bowel down which it came. If you tell me that your stools have become consistently narrower and are now almost ribbonlike, you may have an otherwise silent growth in the large bowel which is reducing the width of the bowel and therefore of the stool. Occasional narrowing of stool is due to spasm and constipation.

If you've had *unexplained diarrhea* for several days or weeks, we will send the stool to the bacteriology lab, looking for any unusual bacteria in it. We then test it for sensitivity to various antibiotics just as we did the urine. Looking for parasites in the stool usually requires a fresh specimen, which means that you have to go to a lab and sit there until you're able to deliver the goods. And one session may not be enough. If the stool is especially foul-smelling and frothy, we will do special tests for fat and protein content.

How and Why the Blood Is Examined

Until a few years ago, before the development of automated techniques, all blood tests were done by hand. This was time-consuming and expensive. Under those circumstances, the more tests ordered, the greater the cost to you. So doctors tried to do as few tests as possible, and only those that were really necessary. To do a lot of expensive tests without apparent reason—in other words, to "screen" for disease—was not considered justified. "Put all your information together, and then hone in on only those blood tests that are likely to yield pay dirt," we were taught as students. "Any jackass can make a diagnosis if he takes every test under the sun." All that has changed. A tiny quantity of blood, sometimes only a few drops, fed into an automated device will in minutes perform an array of twenty or more important tests. This has resulted in the *biochemical screening* concept, by means of which most of us are delighted to make an "accidental" diagnosis. For what it used to cost to do only two or three tests, we can now run a complete blood chemistry survey. While this has reduced the challenge to my diagnostic acumen, because I find so many unsuspected disorders in this routine testing, it represents a major advance for you. After all, the practice of medicine is not a game played for the intellectual gratification of the doctor.

Automation for blood analysis is now used virtually everywhere. Smaller units which can be operated by office personnel are also to be found in doctor's offices where a checkup includes this spectrum of blood tests.

In addition to the automatic analyses, there are several others that we routinely do which require special equipment. For example, I almost always draw blood for thyroid function and serology (the test for syphilis) in new patients.

For Future or Special Reference

Let's review the analyses done on your blood, and what information they yield. You may not want to read through the following pages at one sitting. Some of it may seem a little dull, but I have neither shortened nor removed any important material concerning all the blood tests we do, because it should be there if you want it. After your checkup, whoever gets the bill or the results will see a list of tests that were charged for. You should understand what they are, why they were done, and the significance of their results, especially if abnormal. So have a little patience. At least thumb through the following pages now. You will surely have occasion to refer to them in the future.

Do You Have Venereal Disease? (Or "You Don't Have to Study for Your Wassermann Test")

Many years ago, a very astute researcher by the name of Wassermann observed that when the syphilis organism infects the body, it stimulates a defense, or antibody, mechanism. He devised a test to identify it. The old Wassermann has been modified. More sophisticated procedures are now widely used, but they are all based on the identification of the material that reflects the body's reaction to syphilis. Dr. Wassermann made one error in his brilliant discovery, and it took us many years to realize it. *The abnormal protein that is the hallmark of syphilis can result from other infections as well.* Nonvenereal diseases like infectious mononucleosis, inflammation of the thyroid gland, a whole group of poorly understood disorders in the arthritis family, even smallpox immunization, can give a positive Wassermann. Before we realized that such *false-positive* reactions could occur with the Wassermann test, we had many embarrassing experiences, including the virgin I referred to early in the book who asked how she could possibly have a positive test for syphilis. In fact she had a much more serious disease called lupus erythematosus.

Maybe Your Doctor Never Told You

Today's tests for syphilis are specific and reliable, so that no longer is anyone labeled syphilitic because he has a positive Wassermann. *But remember that any of the blood analyses for syphilis may be negative in the very early stages of the disease, and positive even after cure.* This can present a problem in treatment. Suppose that in the course of a routine exam I find your test for syphilis positive. It may have been successfully treated years ago. But if your old records are not available, and you were never told you had the disease, I have to determine if the infection is active. There is a special test for that purpose. If it is positive, I must treat you. *In a significant number of people cured with penicillin, the test for syphilis remains positive.*

Most physicians almost always perform a screening test for syphilis in new patients because this disease may be very difficult to diagnose any other way. Remember that the *first or earliest stage* of syphilis consists simply of a chancre, which is essentially painless and which disappears in a short period of time without leaving a scar. In the *second stage* of syphilis, the organism spreads throughout the body, producing a generalized rash. This is easy to overlook. Who among us hasn't had a rash at one time or another? The *third stage* follows a long period during which the organisms burrow deep inside the body and don't make their presence known for fifteen or twenty years. Ultimately, symptoms of mental deterioration due to involvement of the brain, severe heart or joint trouble, or malfunction of some other organ appear. *If syphilis is diagnosed early enough, its late dreadful stages can be prevented by penicillin therapy.* But it's too late to treat in the last stage, after the damage is done.

What a Routine "Battery" of Blood Tests Consists Of

Let's now go on to the blood tests that are "routine" and are done regardless of what history you give and what symptoms I find. This biochemical screen goes by various names like SMA

12, SMA 20, or Chem Screen, depending on which laboratory does them and what equipment it uses.

Following is the list of these tests, whose significance and results are described in the following pages. Refer to any that are of special interest to you.

1. Complete blood count (CBC)
2. Sugar
3. Uric acid
4. Potassium
5. Calcium
6. Phosphorus
7. Alkaline phosphatase
8. Urea nitrogen
9. Albumin
10. Globulin
11. Bilirubin
12. Cholesterol
13. SGOT
14. SGPT

The Complete Blood Count (CBC)

Blood is made up of fluid called *plasma,* which contains water, innumerable hormones, minerals, proteins—the very stuff of life—and *formed elements* called the *red cells, white cells,* and *platelets.* The hemoglobin within the red cells carries oxygen. The white blood cells may be considered the body's front-line troops in its fight against infection, and the platelets are involved in the clotting mechanism.

The complete blood count does not refer to the plasma, but rather to the red and white blood cells—how many there are, what types, and how they look under the microscope. A drop of blood is put into an automated machine which counts the number of these cells. I then prepare a thin smear of the blood, stain it, and look at it under the microscope to see whether in addition to having too many or too few of the cells, they are also unusual in their appearance. A decrease in the number of red cells means too little hemoglobin and therefore not enough oxygen circulating in the blood—in other words, you are *anemic.*

How You Become Anemic

Anemia, like fever, weight loss, or pain, is not a disease. It is a laboratory finding. So just discovering you are anemic, and treating it, is not enough. We must discover the cause, which may be any of the following: (1) You may not be getting enough iron, vitamin B12, or folic acid in your diet or can't absorb what you've eaten because of trouble in your intestinal tract. (2) You're losing blood somewhere. (3) You have a disease interfering with the way your body, or more specifically your bone marrow, makes hemoglobin. (4) Some process is destroying your red blood cells.

You may not be getting enough iron in your diet if you are *malnourished*, the major cause of anemia. Since iron is the most important constituent of hemoglobin, and hemoglobin is what carries the oxygen in your blood, an inadequate amount in the diet means you will have what on television would be called "tired blood." *Dietary anemias* are found in food faddists, the poor, or the elderly who live alone and can't prepare their meals satisfactorily or don't have the budget to do so or the teeth with which to chew.

Suspected or unsuspected, blood loss will make you anemic. Insidious bleeding from piles, too much aspirin, heavy menstrual flow, an ulcer, or a cancer somewhere can all produce anemia.

Since the blood cells are made in the bone marrow, and the marrow itself is vulnerable to many diseases and infections, any disorder that *depresses the bone marrow* will cause anemia. This includes infections, tumors spreading to the marrow, sensitivity reactions to drugs, and the leukemias, which prevent the production of normal blood constituents.

There are certain conditions that cause the *destruction of the red blood cells* within the body. Parasites can invade and destroy individual blood cells (malaria), and sensitivity reactions to certain drugs will break them up, as will various infections, blood disorders, and mismatched transfusions (if you get the wrong blood by mistake).

There are special tests that help me determine which of these four major categories are causing your anemia.

Too Much May Be Worse Than Too Little

Instead of being anemic, you may have *too many red cells*. Your blood then becomes thick, viscous, and doesn't flow as freely in your arteries. This occurs under two sets of circumstances. The bone marrow may make too many red cells because it is diseased, a condition called *polycythemia vera.* It is treated by frequent bloodletting or administering radioactive chemicals which depress the overly enthusiastic marrow. Polycythemia vera is dangerous because the thick blood clots more easily in arteries that supply vital organs like the brain and the heart.

Or It May Really Be Necessary

Another mechanism by which the number of red blood cells increases is essentially compensatory, that is, the marrow is responding to some real need for more oxygen. For example, at high altitudes, there is less oxygen than at sea level. In order for the blood to carry enough of it, the body simply makes more red blood cells to make up for the decreased amount of oxygen in each cell. So those living in La Paz, Denver, the Alps, Teheran, Mexico City, or wherever the altitude is high have such a secondary or *compensatory polycythemia.* Also, in patients with chronic lung disease, where the amount of functioning lung tissue available to transport oxygen between the air and the blood is reduced, there is a compensatory increase in the number of red cells. Laboratory techniques distinguish easily between these two types of red cell proliferation.

The Different Kinds of White Blood Cells

There are several different kinds of *white blood cells.* The largest number are concerned with handling infections. We call them *polys* (short for *polymorphonuclear leukocytes*). When bacteria invade the blood or settle in a specific location in the body, these white cells are chemically attracted, then surround and engulf the attacking organisms. These cells are truly white and are responsible for the color of *pus,* the material you see in an abscess or other infected area. They keep the infection localized if they can. A significant increase of polys in the blood means you have an infection somewhere and I look for it.

The second kind of white blood cell is called a *lymphocyte.* It is also involved with the body's defense mechanisms, but in a different way. It does not directly attack the bacteria, but releases substances that neutralize them; in other words, this cell gives us our *immunity*. A third type of white cell (eosinophile) is also present, but its function is not clear. It increases in number whenever there is an allergy of some kind, as may result from parasites, worms, and other infestations, or from food, inhalants, and pets. So if you have some puzzling or unusual symptoms, too many eosinophiles means it's due to an allergic reaction.

What Is Leukemia?

This is a form of *blood cancer* in which certain of the white cells previously described increase tremendously in number. They not only proliferate but also assume bizarre shapes. It's one of the few cancers where treatment has been gratifying.

Since white blood corpuscles, like their red counterparts, are formed in the bone marrow, anything that depresses the marrow will also reduce white blood cell formation, and the white blood cell count drops. This is dangerous because the body's resistance is now compromised, and the patient becomes vulnerable to even the most trivial infections. Fortunately, antibiotics can help tide one over such a crisis.

Platelets—the Key to Blood Clotting

In addition to red and white blood corpuscles there is a formed element in the blood called a *platelet*, whose function it is to make sure the blood clots properly. If you were to cut yourself, and there were too few or no platelets around, you might well bleed to death. Unlike red and white blood cells, we rarely have to worry about an increase in platelets. But they can drop in number when the bone marrow is sick—as, for example, in leukemia, viral infections, or sensitivity to a drug. A telltale sign in children that platelets may be low, and one that parents often overlook, is easy and inappropriate bruising, especially on the legs.

"Sick as Hell" Anemia

In addition to disturbances of the formed elements of the blood just described, there are several other important disorders.

One of these is the way the hemoglobin molecule within the red cell is put together genetically. In blacks, for example, a very important disease called *sickle-cell anemia* results from such an alteration in the structure of hemoglobin. The molecule breaks up abnormally under certain circumstances, with life-threatening results. So in black patients, we always screen for this particular genetic anomaly.

Sedimentation Rate—It Tells Us Nothing Specific But It's Important

A test of great importance you should know about is the *sedimentation rate*. A few drops of blood are put into a long, thin tube with numbers on it. We then see how far the red blood cells have settled at the bottom in one hour. In the presence of disease, the sedimentation rate is high—the red cells sink down the column much faster than they do when you are healthy. This is not a reaction specific to any one disease. It simply tells us that something is wrong somewhere. If you have no symptoms and your sedimentation rate is high, the ball is now in my court. I'll have to find out what's causing it—a hidden infection, arthritis, a cancer somewhere—or just a common cold. When you come to me with vague complaints that I can't make heads or tails of, a sedimentation rate may help me decide whether you are "nervous" or some disease process is actually going on. If I can find nothing on clinical examination, and in addition the sedimentation rate is normal, I can reassure you with some confidence that whatever is troubling you is not serious. But if the "sed" rate is high, I'll keep looking for something to show up sooner or later to explain your symptoms.

Measuring Your Blood Sugar Level—and What It Means

Even before laboratory testing became automated, blood sugar determinations were virtually always done in the course of a checkup. Why not screen for diabetes using the urine alone? For two reasons. First, sugar may appear in the urine and reflect, not an elevated level in the blood, but a low threshold in the kidney, as discussed earlier. Second, the kidney tries to accommodate slight or moderate increases in blood sugar before excreting the excess. As a result, you can be mildly diabetic and not spill any sugar in the urine. *The diagnosis of excessively high or low sugar must be made with the blood.*

At What Time Was It Drawn?

Blood sugar values are interpreted depending on when the specimen was obtained with respect to food intake. Was it drawn in the *fasting* state, when you had nothing to eat for eight or ten hours? This is generally done first thing in the morning, and is called a *fasting blood sugar* (FBS). Or the blood sugar is measured without any special preparation, just when you happen to be in the office. That's called a *random sugar.* Finally, we can take the blood *two hours after a meal* and see how well the body handled the food load. These are basically screening tests. If the value obtained in any of them is normal, and if you do not have any symptoms suggestive of diabetes (increased thirst, increased frequency of voiding, weight loss) and no family history of it, then we leave it at that. But there are certain circumstances under which I will want to perform a glucose tolerance test.

The Glucose Tolerance Test (GTT)—Why You?

This is how we challenge the ability of your body to handle a sugar load. If your routine sugar was borderline or slightly high, a GTT should be done. It is only when the body is presented with a sudden large amount of sugar, either by mouth (the usual route) or by vein (when there is some trouble of absorption in the intestinal tract), that abnormalities will be unmasked.

How It's Done

The glucose tolerance test is performed in the following manner: You come to the laboratory fasting from midnight. A blood sugar level is then determined, after which you are given a measured amount of sugar, usually a prepared sweet cola drink. Blood is drawn for sugar content in one half hour, in an hour, again in two hours and in three hours. When each blood specimen is taken, urine is collected to see how much if any sugar you spill at that particular time, thus correlating the blood sugar level with the amount in the urine.

If you have diabetes it's because you are deficient in insulin, the hormone made by the pancreas (a large gland deep inside the abdomen) or your body doesn't use it properly. Blood sugar levels will be high and fail to return to normal by the end of the second hour. A word of caution, however. A reliable glucose tolerance test depends on your having had a normally balanced diet for several days prior to the test. As I mentioned earlier, if you have been avoiding sweets in order to "pass" the test or to lose weight quickly, you may have a falsely positive result. It happens this way: The more sugar you eat, the more insulin the pancreas produces. If you have been taking no sugar for any length of time, the pancreas has less to do and becomes sluggish. When that happens, it cannot make insulin fast enough when challenged to do so, and your blood sugar will be high. Unless I knew about your starvation diet, I might very well label you a diabetic.

Hypoglycemia (Low Blood Sugar)—You Probably Don't Have It

There are some doctors and more patients who believe that the phenomenon of "low blood sugar" (hypoglycemia) is very prevalent and accounts for many of the complaints we are otherwise unable to explain. It must be a relief to a patient who, after going to several doctors and not getting a specific diagnosis, finally finds a doctor who can give the patient's complaint a name and prescribe something to relieve or cure it. But I do not believe hypoglycemia is as common as some proponents claim.

If we are specifically looking for hypoglycemia, we extend the glucose tolerance test from three to some six or seven hours. The symptoms of low blood sugar are nervousness, weakness, faintness, sweating, and palpitations. Sometimes, after a sugar challenge, the blood level rises briefly to a high level, and then drops sharply. The low concentration after eating sugar reflects a sudden, excessive release of insulin in the body's attempt to lower the sugar. When this happens, even if the level does not fall too low, some patients still have evidence of hypoglycemia. Presumably they are sensitive to the change in levels and not the absolute amount of sugar present. Such persons, despite the fact that they are really hypoglycemics as far as their own bodies are concerned, are not, according to the tables and charts, so no one believes them. If you have been told by your doctor that you are "prone to low blood sugar" and should adhere to a low-sugar, high-protein diet, try it. If you feel better, follow that diet no matter what the blood sugar numbers are.

Low blood sugar may occur as a result of a tumor in the pancreas which produces excessive amounts of insulin. Such an "insulinoma" is quite rare, has nothing to do with diabetes and is cured by surgical removal.

No Sugar for Low Sugar

The usual *treatment for low blood sugar is to avoid sugar, reduce carbohydrates, and eat lots of protein.* You would think that if your blood sugar was low, you could improve it by eating more sugar. This is not so. The blood sugar is decreased in the first place because of an overreaction of the insulin-producing cells in the pancreas to the presence of normal amounts of sugar. When you eat more, the pancreas continues to produce too much insulin, dropping the sugar level even farther. So the way to prevent these attacks is to eat foods that are low in sugar so as not to provoke the insulin-making cells of the pancreas.

First Low, Then High

High and low blood sugar levels are interrelated. If you are found to have an abnormally low blood sugar, chances are good that sometime in the future you will probably find yourself at the other end of the spectrum, with diabetes mellitus and high blood sugar. Why do people with low blood sugar later develop high levels—that is, diabetes? Presumably because having produced unnecessarily excessive amounts of insulin over the years, the pancreas becomes exhausted, and finally doesn't make enough, so you wind up with diabetes.

What About Diabetes Mellitus?

Diabetes in children is a serious matter. It requires insulin and very careful control of the diet. The outlook for long-term survival is not good, because juvenile diabetes is associated with premature hardening of the arteries and early loss of vision. This kind of diabetes differs in its behavior from that which has its onset in adult life and, in fact, may not be the same disease at all.

No Cause for Panic

An elevated blood sugar appearing in adult life is called *maturity-onset diabetes* or *chemical diabetes* and is not usually associated with the same dire outlook as in children. Management of adult-onset diabetes depends on how abnormal the sugar is. In most cases, if you have no symptoms, a diet low in sugar and calories (especially if you are overweight), is enough. No one has ever proven that a high blood sugar in itself is harmful in persons who have no symptoms from it, although it is suspected of contributing to arteriosclerosis. Even if your blood sugar is elevated, and you are spilling some sugar in the urine, as long as you are not excessively thirsty or losing weight other than what you want to lose, and if there are no ketones in your urine, there is no cause for panic. But you should still aim for reasonable blood sugar levels.

But Treatment May Be Necessary

In some adults, despite faithful adherence to a diet, or more often because of an unwillingness or inability to follow one, the sugar does become too high, and symptoms do develop. We then have to consider treatment alternatives. These include pills to lower the blood sugar (*oral hypoglycemic agents* like Orinase and Diabinese) and *insulin*.

A few years ago, when the oral antidiabetic agents were introduced, they were widely and enthusiastically used. (Incidentally, these drugs are related to the sulfas and it was by accident that their sugar-lowering properties were noted.) Diets were de-emphasized. Why not eat what you want to when simply taking a pill or two in the morning will keep your blood sugar normal? But then a group of diabetes specialists decided to evaluate how diabetics had benefited over the years from these agents. They stunned us all with the results. It was found that survival rates were highest among those adult diabetics who were treated with diet alone. Those taking insulin also did well. The greatest number of deaths occurred in persons using the oral drugs, and the cause of death in those cases was usually cardiac.

The Diabetes Pill—Yes or No?

Many diabetes experts insist that this statistical study is invalid for one reason or another, and continue to use oral agents. Others, including official government bodies who have reviewed the data, are equally fervent in their warnings that these agents are to be avoided—that if diet alone is not effective, then insulin should be given. And there the controversy stands.

There isn't a day goes by but that some concerned patient with diabetes asks whether he should try the diet alone, take the pill, or go on insulin. My own opinion is that you should really work at the diet first. I am not concerned if your blood sugar is a little high, so long as you feel well and are not spilling ketones in the urine. If, however, your fasting sugar is more than 250 milligrams percent, then I prescribe insulin. The adverse data concerning the pills are such that I would rather not give them to my patients. Insulin is something you adjust to very easily. You soon become skilled at injecting yourself, and as for many thousands the world over, it becomes just another routine in your life.

The *diabetic diet* is one in which you avoid concentrated sweets—sugar in any form, candy, chocolate desserts, canned fruits with sugar syrup, and so on. There are many dietetic and diabetic preparations—canned fruits, even ice cream, cookies, and candy. Some of them are so skillfully prepared it's hard to tell them from the real thing. *Cyclamates,* which were very acceptable sugar substitutes, have been banned in the United States because of their alleged tumorigenic (cancer-producing) qualities in certain experimental animals in massive doses. There is some pressure to have this decision reviewed, but thus far there is no indication that it will be. The Food and Drug Administration has also recommended a ban on the use of *saccharin* because of experiments showing it can also cause cancer in rats. This substance is still available to diabetics, and at the time of writing, the matter remains in abeyance.

If you are diabetic and are managing your sugar by diet, oral medication, or injectable insulin, you should follow the urine sugar levels daily. This is done very easily, using commercially available tablets or chemically treated strips of paper which, when put into a urine specimen, indicate how much if any sugar is being spilled.

Danger Signals

Your diabetes is out of control if you have increasing thirst, frequency of urination, ketones in the urine, rapid weight loss, and in women, vaginal itching. Whether you are taking the pill or insulin, remember the *symptoms of low blood sugar are nervousness, weakness, sweating, light-headedness, palpitations and dizziness.*

Diabetics, no matter what age, must beware of infections and fever. Even trivial ones can upset sugar levels and make you very sick. I have seen elderly patients who were doing very well on dietary regimens alone lapse rapidly into diabetic coma because of untreated pneumonia or other infection.

Alcohol is another source of trouble, because of its ability to raise and lower the blood sugar unpredictably. Diabetics may develop severe attacks of low blood sugar causing coma. In others, especially after too much beer or wine, the blood sugar rises, making insulin and pill dosages very difficult to stabilize. So if you drink, do so in moderation, and let your doctor know about it.

High and Low Blood Sugar Without Diabetes

There are circumstances other than diabetes in which the blood sugar may be elevated—for example, with the use of certain "water pills" (diuretics) or oral contraceptives or with an overactive thyroid gland. If your liver is diseased, blood sugar levels may be high because that organ is responsible for the storing of sugar. On the other hand, if you have some disorder of absorption or trouble with the lining of your stomach or intestines, so that the sugar you eat is not properly absorbed into the blood, your levels will be low. Patients who have had a portion of the stomach removed (perhaps because of an ulcer) are often left with a very rapid transit time, the food they eat going right through the gastrointestinal tract without the usual delay in the stomach. As a result, their blood sugar levels are altered.

Uric Acid Level—the Test for Gout

The determination of how much uric acid is circulating in the blood is an important one for several reasons. If you have the classic joint pains in the big toe, elbow, or elsewhere, and your uric acid level is high, you probably have gout. If you have no pain yet, such a high level suggests you are vulnerable to suffering from gout in the future.

Uric acid is derived mostly from the interior portion, or nucleus, of body cells. Why it is increased in gout is not known, but levels are also high in conditions where blood cells are excessively destroyed, notably leukemia. As it does with sugar, the kidney gets rid of some of the uric acid excess in the urine. So if the kidneys are damaged for one reason or another, this function is impaired and uric acid levels rise in the blood.

Not Necessarily Gout

What should you do if you do not have any aches or pains, and in the course of a routine examination you are found to have a high uric acid? Should you go on a diet, take medication, or just worry? The first thing to do is to make sure you're not taking pills that raise the uric acid level. Some of these are very commonly used and include diuretics, aspirin, and vitamin C.

How and When to Lower Uric Acid

There are several drugs that can reduce a high uric acid level or control the symptoms of gout. These are usually well tolerated and are always prescribed for persons whose readings are very high and who have passed urate kidney stones or who have had one or more attacks of gout in the past. These medications, Benemid and allopurinol (trade name Zyloprim in the U.S., Zylopric and Amplivix in Europe), have revolutionized the management of gout. Persons who formerly had to be on severe dietary restriction with total abstention from alcohol, red meat, and animal organs may now eat a relatively unrestricted diet so long as they continue to take the medication. Whether or not you should take these pills prophylactically, before you have the first attack of gout, depends on the level of the uric acid. This is something you should discuss with your doctor. I believe that if the elevation is only modest, these medicines should not be taken. However, if it is high enough, I may prescribe them even if you have no symptoms.

Suddenly Everyone's Interested in Potassium

I'm being asked questions I never heard before. "Are you checking my potassium too?" "Is my level too low?" "Is that why I'm tired and have leg cramps?" Why the current interest? Because of diuretics ("water pills"), among our most widely used drugs. "If I could only knock off these five pounds, I'd look great. I think I'll take a water pill for a few days." "I have some puffiness under the eyes, and my rings are tight. It's time for my diuretic."

There are also legitimate uses of these pills—in hypertension, glaucoma, heart failure, and fluid retention associated with menstruation. Most *diuretics cause potassium loss* (Lasix, Diuril, Esidrix, Hydrodiuril, Hygroton, and others)—although not nearly as much as most of us believe.

Potassium is a mineral found in high concentration in every cell of the body, as well as in the bloodstream, where it can be measured. Its two major functions involve muscle contraction and the cardiac rhythm. So too much or too little potassium can give you fatigue and serious heart problems as well.

The determination of the potassium concentration in blood is not a test I would normally order if you have no complaints, unless you are taking diuretics or have high blood pressure. But its content in the blood is especially important if you are taking any form of digitalis (Lanoxin, Digoxin, Digitoxin) and diuretics at the same time, because *low potassium sensitizes the heart to digitalis.* This can cause serious disorders of cardiac rhythm.

When the Level Is High

In my experience, the commonest cause of a *high potassium* reading is an accidental or technical one—usually resulting from the analysis not being done right away. If your blood specimen is kept overnight in the refrigerator, or shaken up as it is being transported to a laboratory, the red blood cells in the test tube break up and release their potassium. This adds to the amount already in the serum, giving a falsely high level. But if the test is freshly done, then a high potassium level may mean kidney disease or deficiency of the naturally produced corticosteroid hormones in the body (Addison's disease). Your potassium content may also be too high when sometimes in our enthusiasm to correct low levels we give more supplement than you need, especially when your kidneys aren't in good working order. *Too much potassium is more dangerous than too little, especially to the rhythm of the heartbeat.*

Or Low

Low potassium results from the body losing it. This may be due to chronic diarrhea, certain kinds of kidney disease, overproduction of corticosteroid hormones in the body (Cushing's syndrome, the opposite of Addison's disease), and the use of diuretics. The last make you lose not only water and sodium, which is their purpose, but also potassium.

If you have too little potassium, you may feel weak, have palpitations due to disturbances in heart rhythm (especially if you happen to be taking digitalis as well), and get cramps in your legs.

How to Raise Your Potassium Level

Potassium loss or deficiency can be supplemented by diet, drugs, or pure potassium (ugh!). Foods rich in potassium include citrus fruits, bananas, tea, apricots, and figs. Tomato juice also has a high potassium content, but contains a great deal of salt (sodium) as well. Salt is bad for high blood pressure and heart failure with fluid retention, so if you're taking diuretics for either of these conditions, tomato juice is not a good way to supplement your potassium. You can also take potassium directly in liquid or tablet form. The syrups are not usually great delicacies and may irritate the stomach, so always take them after meals. Newer preparations are said to be more palatable. The enteric-coated tablets which were supposed to protect the stomach from irritation may cause ulceration of the bowel lower down. Avoid them. There are other medications, like Aldactone and Dyrenium, which help prevent potassium loss by diuretics. These drugs act on the kidney, making it reabsorb the potassium it would otherwise excrete.

Your doctor may not always give you potassium supplements with your diuretic. Why wouldn't he—routinely? Some diuretics come with built-in potassium sparers (Dyazide, Aldactazide), or your kidneys may not be working perfectly, so that you have too much potassium to begin with, and any more either is unnecessary or might hurt you.

Do You Have a Potassium Problem?

One's potassium level is now a favorite cocktail party topic, as witnessed by this true account. One of my friends recently attended a dinner party at which the food was superb and plentiful, and the wine outstanding. Dessert in the form of a huge cream pie was simply beyond his ability to manage. When offered a substantial piece of it, he quietly demurred. His hostess asked, "Won't you have any of this delicious dessert?" He replied, "No thank you, really." She pressed him further, "A little taste? I made it myself, you know." "No thank you, I simply can't." Not to be so easily rejected, she asked, "What's the matter, are you on a diet?" To this he replied, leaning over and whispering very confidentially, "No, I have a potassium problem." "Oh," she said, "I understand," and there the matter was dropped.

I Hope Your Acid Phosphatase Level Is Normal

Acid phosphatase is an enzyme normally found in the prostate gland. A small amount of it circulates in the bloodstream of men where it can be measured. When cancer of the prostate spreads out of the gland, the acid phosphatase level in the blood rises significantly. Such spread may occur from a tumor too small to feel on rectal examination. To make sure that I am not missing such a prostatic cancer, I routinely measure the acid phosphatase level in the blood of all men over 50 years of age. But the blood for this test must be drawn before examining the rectum, since a vigorous digital examination there may cause the normal gland to release enough acid phosphatase to elevate the values in the blood. Prostate infections and some blood diseases will also increase the test levels.

Calcium and Phosphorus—Organizing the Skeleton

Calcium and phosphorus levels are measured routinely in the automated processing of the blood. This is a good example of how "screening" in apparently healthy persons can pay dividends.

Calcium is a substance that is vital in the metabolism, formation, and strength of bones, in maintaining normal blood clotting, in the transmission of nerve impulses, and in the contraction of muscles, including the heart. *Phosphorus* acts with calcium in many of these same functions, but in addition is involved with energy use by the body. These two minerals have a reciprocal relationship in the blood. In other words, when the serum calcium is high, the phosphorus is low, and vice versa.

Detecting a Hidden Tumor

Both calcium and phosphorus are the matrix of bone, moving in and out between the skeleton and the blood in response to different stimuli. The most important regulator of normal calcium and phosphorus levels is a hormone produced by the four *parathyroid glands*. The parathyroids are tiny glands in the neck behind the thyroid. Sometimes a tumor develops in one of them, but even then the gland cannot be felt during an examination, because of its small size. This tumor secretes an excess of the *parathyroid hormone*, which in turn sucks too much calcium out of the bone and into the blood. We *diagnose a parathyroid tumor by a high calcium reading in the blood.*

You May Not Be Neurotic After All

An elevated calcium level is responsible for many symptoms which are so common that we never think they may be due to a parathyroid tumor—until we do the blood test and find the calcium level abnormal. These symptoms include something for everyone—a little deafness, numbness and tingling of the hands and feet, muscle cramps, constipation, decreased appetite, nausea, weakness, stomach pain, and ulcers. Think of all the people you know who complain of these things from time to time. Soon, we stop listening to them. They're just "chronic complainers" or have a "personality problem." Then, one day, they go for a routine physical examination, a few drops of blood are sent through an automated machine, a test that wasn't even specifically asked for is performed, and a "high serum calcium" comes back in the report.

Parathyroid tumors most commonly occur in middle-aged women, who are simply told they are menopausal when they offer all these complaints. If the parathyroid tumor remains undetected, it eventually leads to deposits of calcium in the kidney and its ultimate failure, spontaneous bone fractures because the parathyroid hormone is removing calcium from the bone, deformity of the skeleton, and finally death due to irritability of the heart.

When to Operate for a High Calcium Level

Suppose in the course of a routine examination I find your calcium high. What then? Too much vitamin D in the diet, bone cancers, chronic confinement to bed without movement (as, for example, being put in a body cast) and certain diseases can all elevate the amount of calcium in the blood. Calcium leaves the bone, causing its demineralization as it enters the bloodstream. If you are over 50, female, *and have no symptoms,* we'd probably just observe you. Above 50 years, women may have some elevation in serum calcium due to increased activity of the parathyroid gland, rather than tumor. *In women under 50, in whom other causes of elevated calcium have been ruled out, by x-rays and blood tests, a consistently high serum calcium with or without symptoms is usually an indication to operate and explore the area of the neck where the parathyroid glands are situated.*

Low serum calcium is usually the aftermath of an operation for a parathyroid tumor in which too much normal tissue has been removed. Now, instead of an overproduction of hormone with too much calcium, there is a deficiency. Too little vitamin D will also result in a low calcium, as will certain kinds of kidney disease.

The most important symptom of low blood calcium is *tetany*—muscle twitching and sustained contraction with very little provocation.

When calcium levels are low, they can be elevated by supplemental calcium and vitamin D preparations.

Your Urea Nitrogen Level (BUN)—a Sensitive Kidney Test

The concentration of urea nitrogen in the blood is a key test of kidney function. Protein is constantly being used and broken down in the body. The end product of that process is urea, which is formed in the liver. Urea is carried in the blood from the liver to the kidneys, where it is excreted in the urine. So there is always a certain amount of urea circulating in the blood. An increase in the normal reading may indicate, among other things, that the kidneys are not getting rid of this waste product. Many kidney disorders may result in a high blood urea level. These include chronic infections, injury, and obstruction to the outflow of urine from both kidneys so that it backs up, causing a ballooning out of and damage to the kidneys.

Since urea is the end stage of protein metabolism, any process that suddenly causes a great deal of protein to be broken down quickly and challenges the kidney to excrete it in massive amounts will also cause a transient high blood urea level, since even a healthy kidney sometimes cannot cope with this situation. Such rapid, excessive breakdown of protein occurs in burns and destruction of tissue, hemorrhage within the intestinal tract with the consequent absorption of blood (which is rich in protein), and tissue breakdown due to tumors. So a *high urea level usually, but not always, means kidney failure.*

Certain drugs hurt the kidney and reduce its ability to excrete urea nitrogen. These include diuretics, some antibiotics (such as tetracycline, especially if expired, and gentamicin), sedatives, and blood-pressure-lowering agents. Their effect is not permanent.

When the offending agent is discontinued, the urea levels return to normal.

How We Test for Liver Function

The liver is a key and complex organ involved in many different life processes. As such, it is subject to a great many disorders. It can be infected by viruses, bacteria, and parasites; it may be the site of cancers originating within it or spreading to it from other organs. It can be damaged by toxic drugs and alcohol, and it may be swollen by virtue of blood backing into it from a failing heart.

A diseased liver can be detected grossly, as we've seen in the section on physical examination, if it is large, swollen, and tender. But when the derangement is early and subtle, only blood tests can indicate trouble. For example, in hepatitis from blood transfusions or infected needles, or the viral hepatitis developing under crowded living conditions (jails, boarding schools, and other institutions), or that which is sexually transmitted, early in the disease there may be no abnormalities on the physical examination. The patient may even feel well, and the diagnosis is made in the laboratory.

We do more than just one blood test in evaluating the status of the liver because it has so many functions. These are performed by several different kinds of cells in the liver, not all of which are affected at the same time and to the same extent. So we routinely perform a *battery of liver function tests,* the most important of which are the following: levels of proteins (albumin and globulin), alkaline phosphatase (not to be confused with the acid phosphatase test for cancer of the prostate), two very important enzymes called SGOT and SGPT, and bilirubin. Let me tell you briefly about each.

Albumin, the All-Purpose Protein

Albumin is an important protein with many functions and is synthesized in the liver. By its physical presence in the blood, it draws fluid to it and keeps it within the blood vessels. (This is its osmotic effect, for those of you with a physics background.)

When the albumin level is too low, fluid passes out of the blood vessels into the surrounding tissue. The result is generalized swelling. A low albumin occurs in severe liver disease (wherein not enough albumin is made), in kidney disease (in which instead of reabsorbing the albumin coming to it in the blood, the damaged kidney allows it to escape into the urine), and in severe malnutrition (because enough protein is simply not being eaten from which the liver can make the albumin—remember the pictures of pitifully starved youngsters in famine areas whose big potbellies are full of fluid). The measurement of albumin levels in the blood reflects the status of one of the liver's major functions. Unlike many other tests in which there may be too much or too little of a given chemical in the blood, *there is never too much albumin, only too little.*

Globulin (a Defense and a Warning)

Globulin is another blood protein, physically larger than albumin. Like calcium and phosphorus, albumin and globulin are measured together, even though the liver makes only a small amount of the total body globulins. Their main function is related to our defense mechanisms—providing immunity against infections. Globulin is not as important in keeping fluid within the blood vessel wall as is albumin. But when albumin is low and fluid seeps out the blood vessel wall, the body often makes more globulin. So when the albumin level goes down, there is a compensatory increase in the amount of globulin.

A chronic infection (for example, a parasite lodged somewhere) or a festering cancer, each of which is constantly challenging the body to defend itself, stimulates the production of more globulin. *So too much globulin, whatever the cause, is a sign of trouble.*

Will You Need a Gamma Globulin Shot?

With newer biochemical techniques, we've been able to separate different types of globulin, the most important of which are alpha, beta, and gamma. I trouble you with these details because *gamma* globulin is the one that has to do with immunity and your resistance to infection. That's why when you are going to an area where there is a lot of disease like hepatitis, or when you have been intimately exposed to someone with hepatitis, your doctor may recommend a shot of gamma globulin. Some people are born without the ability to make enough gamma globulin, and have recurrent infections throughout life. They require injections from time to time to maintain their immunity.

Bilirubin and Jaundice

Although bilirubin is not made in the liver, it is nonetheless a very important test of liver function. It is the pigment that makes you jaundiced. Where does bilirubin come from? Why, if the liver has nothing to do with making it, does an excess often reflect liver disease?

Bilirubin is derived from the red blood corpuscles, which survive in the body for about 120 days. The spleen is their main mortuary. This organ picks out from the blood circulating within it those red cells that are at the end of their life-span, and breaks them down. New cells are formed at a corresponding rate in the bone marrow. Think of the marvelous balance that the healthy body affords, with an exactly equal rate of breakdown and manufacture of the red blood corpuscles.

The Body's Recycling Program

The constituents of the old, broken-down cells are recycled. Remember that the main function of the red blood cells is to circulate through the body delivering oxygen to every organ and tissue. Oxygen is carried inside the red cell by a protein called *hemoglobin*. When the old cell is destroyed in the spleen, the hemoglobin within it is degraded or converted into the yellow pigment bilirubin. Think of the last time you were injured or bruised, and bled a little under your skin. Remember how the bruise was first reddish, then purple, and with time, how it changed in color to a yellowish hue? That yellow color was due to the bilirubin.

Whither Bilirubin?

After the old red blood cells disintegrate in the spleen, their bilirubin pigment goes to the liver to be excreted. It's the liver's job to keep getting rid of the bilirubin which is constantly coming to it from the spleen. It does so by incorporating it into and excreting it with the bile into the intestines and then out through the bowel.

Jaundice Without Liver Disease

You can now understand two basic circumstances under which there will be an excess of bilirubin in the blood, giving you jaundice. The first is when, for some reason, there are many more red blood cells destroyed than should be. This occurs when any toxic agent—a medicine to which you become sensitive, or a poison, or some disease—breaks them up. This process is called *hemolysis* (*hemo* meaning blood, *lysis* breakdown). Excessive red-cell breakdown means a large load of bilirubin needs to be excreted, more than even a healthy liver can handle. As a result the concentration of bilirubin in the blood goes up, and the patient becomes jaundiced, an example of how you can become "yellow" in the absence of liver disease. In an attempt to get rid of the bilirubin, the body tries to pass it through the kidney. Consequently, the pigment-loaded urine is very dark. The liver is also passing as much bilirubin as it can out the bile ducts, which empty into the gut, so the stool is a deeper brown than usual.

And When the Liver Is Sick

Bilirubin levels are high and jaundice is present in another circumstance—when the amount of bilirubin produced is normal, but some disease or injury of the liver affects its ability to excrete it. This happens in viral hepatitis, for example.

Light Stool and Dark Urine

Obstruction to the flow of bile in the ducts that carry it to the intestine from the liver may also cause jaundice. The bile then backs up into the bloodstream, staining the tissues yellow.

When obstruction is present, the urine is dark because the bile gets into it from the kidney via the blood. The stool, however, is light because the bile is not passing down the ducts into the intestine. So if ever you notice that your urine is the color of strong tea or mahogany, and your stool is light or clay-colored, you may well have liver trouble. Remember that this may be due to scarring within the liver itself or obstruction outside it (gallstones or a tumor near the bile ducts pressing on them and closing them off). When the bilirubin is high, especially in the obstructive cases, the skin often becomes very itchy as well as yellow because the bile becomes deposited in the skin.

Alkaline Phosphatase—a Different Phosphatase

This is an enzyme found in many different organs of the body, but for the most part in the liver (almost 80 percent) and bone (nearly 20 percent). Unlike acid phosphatase, it's found in men and women. Its measurement affords a useful index of *liver and bone disease*. It reaches high levels when there is obstruction to the outflow of bile from the liver, and the values return to normal when the blockage clears. If you're passing a gallstone, you have pain, fever, jaundice, a high bilirubin, and an elevated alkaline phosphatase while the stone is still in the duct. After it passes, the pain and fever lessen, the jaundice begins to fade, and the bilirubin and alkaline phosphatase return to normal. But if the obstruction is due, not to a stone, but to the unrelenting and increasing pressure of a tumor nearby, the alkaline phosphatase remains high and the jaundice due to the elevated bilirubin persists.

The levels of alkaline phosphatase are also increased in any disorder of bone with breakdown of the skeletal structure and release of the enzyme, in fractures, and in growing youngsters.

It is quite possible that if you are in your fifties or older, your alkaline phosphatase will be high even though you feel well and are clearly not jaundiced. If that's the case, you probably have a mild form of *Paget's disease of bone*. This is a usually harmless condition in which small islands of bone, most often in the pelvis or in the skull, undergo some structural changes and liberate alkaline phosphatase into the bloodstream.

Other, more serious disorders of bone which will raise this enzyme level in the blood include overactivity or tumor of the parathyroid glands, too much vitamin D in the diet, and occasionally a number of commonly used medications including oral contraceptives, sedatives, oral antidiabetics, various hormones, antibiotics, pills to lower blood pressure, and the medicine used to prevent gout and lower uric acid level (Zyloprim).

SGPT and SGOT

(Don't try to pronounce them, they're initials, not words.)

SGPT, which stands for *serum glutamic pyruvic transaminase,* is an enzyme found in many organs and tissues. Its measurement is useful as an index of liver disease. When the liver is sick, the SGPT level in the blood increases. Another enzyme, *SGOT (serum glutamic oxalacetic transaminase),* is also present in the liver but is found in large quantities in heart muscle as well.

Both SGOT and SGPT appear in a higher than normal concentration in the blood when there is damage to the cells that contain them; the cell walls become permeable and allow them to escape into the bloodstream. When the liver is injured, both the SGOT and the SGPT are elevated. Soon after a heart attack, the SGOT from the heart is increased, but the SGPT remains normal. If you've had chest pain that is not typical of heart trouble, and the electrocardiogram is "iffy," we measure the levels of both enzymes. When the SGOT is elevated and the SGPT is normal, the trouble lies in the heart or other muscle and not the liver. In addition, newer, more sensitive enzyme determinations are now available and are used specifically for coronary patients.

BLOOD FATS—WHY ALL THE FUSS?

The role of the *blood fats (lipids)* in the causation of heart attacks, strokes, and arteriosclerosis constitutes a continuing controversy among doctors, government agencies, food producers, epidemiologists, and the "man in the street." The consensus seems to shift almost from day to day. I am rarely asked after a complete laboratory examination, "What is my alkaline phosphatase," or "Is my serum globulin level high?" even though these abnormalities have known and proven serious consequences. What seems to interest us most is "What is the cholesterol?"

There are several blood fats—triglycerides, phospholipids, free fatty acids, chylomicrons, and cholesterol—just to mention a few. The *triglycerides* are of two types: those you eat in your diet are "exogenous" (coming from outside the body), and those you make, "endogenous" (produced within the body). The *phospholipids* are blood fats with no known relation to arteriosclerosis. From the point of view of your health examination and what may have a bearing on your vulnerability to arteriosclerosis, *the important ones to remember are cholesterol and the endogenous triglycerides.*

Cholesterol, Almost a Dirty Word

How much cholesterol you have flowing within your arteries is measured very easily by means of a simple, inexpensive blood test. "Cholesterol" has become almost a dirty word these days. But despite its bad reputation, it happens to be vital for many body functions, including the manufacture of our sex hormones and all of the membranes that surround the cells in our bodies.

We get some of our cholesterol in the foods we eat (eggs, butter, other dairy products, fatty meats like marbled beef, and certain shellfish like lobster, crab, and shrimp). In addition to, or despite, what we eat, the liver continues to form its own cholesterol from some very simple chemical building blocks. In many of us, it makes too much. If you try to follow a diet with virtually no cholesterol in it—and that's not easy—we may still find too much in the blood when we measure for it.

A high cholesterol may also be due to specific malfunctions of the body, as, for example, kidney disease or low thyroid function. When these are treated, the cholesterol level returns to normal. A *low cholesterol* may reflect liver disease, since it is made in the liver, but may also be due to acute infections, starvation, and an overactive thyroid.

Why the Worry About Cholesterol?

Our concern about cholesterol stems from several important observations. When we measure it in thousands of people who have had heart attacks, we find higher values than in persons of the same age who are free of heart disease. The higher the average level of cholesterol in a country, the greater its incidence of heart disease. For example, in Japan where the mean cholesterol value is almost half what it is in the United States, the incidence of coronary artery disease is quite low. The same is true in Crete. Even in different parts of the same country, where geographic conditions are such that populations do not intermix very much—as, for example, in the mountainous and coastal areas of Norway—the incidence of arteriosclerosis varies with the cholesterol level.

Another important observation is that in arteriosclerosis the arteries are narrowed or completely obstructed by plaques of fatty material, which, when analyzed, are found to be rich in cholesterol.

Putting all these facts together, we seem to be left with the almost inescapable conclusion that high cholesterol is in some way responsible for the plaques in the arteries and the consequent heart attacks.

But Rabbits Aren't People

What's more, if we feed a rabbit, chicken, monkey, or other experimental animal a diet very rich in cholesterol, we can produce arteriosclerosis in its arteries within 12 to 18 months. The arteriosclerotic plaques can be made to disappear when a cholesterol-free diet is administered for the same length of time. You might think this experimental evidence wraps it all up. It does for many doctors—but not for all—because it's really not as simple as I made it appear. First of all, chickens, rabbits, dogs, and even monkeys are not people. The experimental diets required to cause arteriosclerosis cannot be compared with anything eaten by humans anywhere. Furthermore, many, many persons with "normal" or low cholesterol levels get heart attacks too. Why should they, if cholesterol is so important? Again, *only a very small percentage of those with high cholesterol suffer heart attacks*. If high cholesterol causes arteriosclerosis, why does it do so in only relatively few people?

Finally, lowering cholesterol levels by diet or drugs, at least in humans, has not been shown to protect against getting a heart attack. In any event, it is argued by some that maybe the high cholesterol level is only a signpost that something is wrong in the body, much like fever is the symptom of an infection rather than a disease. They believe that just as lowering the temperature in pneumonia doesn't cure the problem, so reducing elevated cholesterol levels may not cure or prevent arteriosclerosis.

Why Take a Chance?

The theory about high cholesterol predisposing to heart attacks is therefore still controversial. But active research and large-scale trials involving thousands of people with high cholesterol are now under way to settle the question. Half are being treated vigorously, the others (and the selection as to who gets what is a random one) are not. If these trials prove that lowering cholesterol is important in the prevention of heart disease—and I personally suspect they will—we would feel very sorry (and guilty) if we had not advised you about the suspicion that presently exists. So pending the final verdict, it is prudent to assume there is a connection, and act on that assumption. Why take a chance?

It seems logical to identify and correct an abnormally high cholesterol as early as one can. Waiting for adult life, or taking action after the first heart attack has occurred, is probably too late. A child with a high cholesterol level should eat a low cholesterol diet. If this substance ultimately is shown to cause arterial disease, that child will have a head start in life as far as his vascular tree is concerned.

What Is "Normal"?

Given these essentials of the cholesterol-arteriosclerosis debate, how do we go about measuring cholesterol and advising you in specific terms? I draw your blood for cholesterol—for which, incidentally, you need not be fasting—and report a number back to you. Is it "normal"? What is "normal"? There is no universal agreement about that either.

When we study thousands of healthy persons living in the

United States or Western Europe, we find that cholesterol levels vary and increase with age. The mean value for adults in the United States is about 250 milligrams percent. In children it is apt to be about 180 or 190, rising with every decade of life. In Japan and other Asian countries, a child will have a value of less than 150, an adult about 180.

Those who subscribe to the "cholesterol is bad for you" theory say that the 250 milligrams figure we use is *average but not normal.* According to them, it's wrong to consider this figure normal because there is so much arteriosclerosis in our society that what is average is still abnormal. Put another way, 250 milligrams percent is the average in a sick or vulnerable population. They would have us so modify our diet and methods of food production as to drop the mean level from 250 to the Japanese values of 180 or 190. If we were able to do this, they believe the incidence of arteriosclerosis and the death rate from heart attacks would drop significantly.

So What Should You Do?

My own feeling is that if your cholesterol level is somewhere in the middle range, say between 220 and 280, and you are middle-aged, try to reduce it by diet and weight reduction. I would not recommend any of the currently available drugs at these levels.

If you are below 220, you're entitled to feel happy; whichever theory is right, you're safe, statistically anyway. You're at greater risk driving your car or crossing the street than you are of getting a heart attack. If your cholesterol is above 300, you've got a problem, especially if there is a family history of premature (before age 60) heart disease. Follow a low cholesterol diet meticulously, avoid saturated fats (those that are hard at room temperature), keep your weight down, and consider, after consultation with your doctor, the use of a cholesterol-lowering agent (see later).

How Identical Cholesterol Levels Have Different Significance

Cholesterol does not just float around free in the bloodstream. It is attached to a variety of proteins. These have different physical structures and are grouped into the *high-density lipoproteins* or HDL (*lipo* because they carry the fat called cholesterol), *low-density lipoproteins* (LDL), and even *very-low-density lipoproteins* (VLDL). Interestingly, it has been noted that the more of your cholesterol bound to the high-density proteins, the lower the incidence of arteriosclerosis. In other words, if you have an elevated cholesterol, 300 for example, and also have a high HDL, you may be at less risk than if your HDL level is low. As a result of this observation, many doctors are now measuring the high-density lipoprotein values whenever they test for cholesterol.

Lowering Cholesterol by Pill

If we have tried without success to lower your cholesterol by diet alone, then medication should be added if your levels are above 300 and you have a bad family history. These include clofibrate (marketed in the United States as Atromid-S), cholestyramine (sold as Questran), Probucol, nicotinic acid (or niacin), neomycin (an antibiotic), Cytellin, thyroid hormone, and female hormone (estrogen).

Atromid-S will lower cholesterol level in certain cases as much as 25 percent. It is generally well tolerated, but can cause unpleasant side effects. (These are usually reversible, except for gallstones, and include anemia, impotence, liver damage, muscle cramps, and disturbances in heart rhythm.) When it works, it probably does so by reducing the amount of cholesterol made by the liver.

Cholestyramine and *Probucol* lower cholesterol too. Many patients have trouble taking cholestyramine because it gives constipation, cramping, and gas. But you should know that some investigators have found that in persons on a low cholesterol diet and also taking cholestyramine for long periods, there has been some reduction in the size of the arterial plaques. This drug reduces the cholesterol by a different mechanism than does clofibrate. It attaches to the cholesterol in the gut, preventing its absorption. Drug and cholesterol are then excreted together in the stool.

Nicotinic acid also lowers cholesterol. It causes a feeling of heat and flushing of the face, and if you've taken it for a while and then stop, you may get a rebound increase of the cholesterol level.

In addition to those agents specifically prescribed to reduce cholesterol, other substances may incidentally have a similar effect. For example, *thyroid hormone* and its derivatives will lower cholesterol, but should not be used for that purpose. It's one thing to take thyroid replacement because your body is low in that hormone, but quite another matter—and dangerous—to take it to lower your cholesterol. *More thyroid than you need constitutes a strain on the heart;* it may cause disturbances in cardiac rhythm and artificially speed up your metabolism.

Female hormone (estrogen) also reduces cholesterol. This was observed in men with cancer of the prostate who required this drug to prevent spread of the tumor. But unless you have such a prostatic cancer, it's better to have some cholesterol elevation than big breasts, small testicles, no sex drive, and a greater risk of heart attack—all of which high doses of estrogen may cause.

Persons who take a great deal of *aspirin* (more than 10 tablets a day) may have a low cholesterol, as do men who take male hormone (*testosterone*).

Did your grandmother ever tell you that garlic is good for you? Probably because it lowers cholesterol.

What Factors Raise Cholesterol?

In our preoccupation with lowering cholesterol, we forget about the nondietary factors that can increase it. Some of these are operative in our life-style. For example, heavy smokers have significantly higher levels than nonsmokers. Psychological stress, acute or chronic, will elevate the cholesterol. Students monitored before and after examinations have been found to have higher levels before the examination. Cholesterol, interestingly enough, is raised just before menstruation and falls after the period is over. Your cholesterol is apt to be higher by some 10 percent after you've been standing for a long time than if you have been recumbent. When a woman enters the menopause, her cholesterol level (together with her vulnerability to developing arteriosclerosis and heart disease) increases significantly. For some reason, the blind have higher levels. Patients with certain types of blood groups, for example, Type A, have a higher cholesterol than those with the other blood groups. In women who use oral contraceptives, if their cholesterol level was very low (like 180 or 190) before they started the pill, it is increased after they take it.

Cholesterol and Vitamin C

Some persons taking large amounts of vitamin C increase their cholesterol levels. Proponents of vitamin C say that this is a good thing, and results from the fact that the vitamin C sucks out the cholesterol from the blood vessel wall where we don't want it and into the bloodstream where it doesn't really matter.

Lowering Cholesterol by Diet

You can see from all the foregoing random, isolated facts how complicated the whole problem is. Should you decide that you want to follow a low-cholesterol diet, either because you are intellectually convinced that it is prudent to do so pending a final answer, or because your cholesterol level is frankly high and you are uncomfortable about it (and from a statistical point of view, you're justified in feeling that way), you should avoid or reduce the following foods in your diet: egg yolks, organ meats, beef, ham, pork, lamb, shrimp and excesses of other shellfish, whole milk, cream, butter, and cheese. Concentrate instead on fish, chicken, turkey, and veal. Drink skim milk. Eat baked goods prepared with egg whites and use plant fats (margarine) rather than butter.

Polyunsaturated fats (those of plant origin), like safflower oil, corn oil, and vegetable oil, may help lower cholesterol. These are preferred to the saturated fats of animal origin, like butter, and should be substituted for them.

Remember, too, that commercially prepared foods like cereals, bread, and cake contain cholesterol (largely due to egg yolk and saturated fats). I have long felt that government regulatory agencies should make the exact listing of all food ingredients mandatory.

What About Triglycerides?

The importance of triglycerides in the development of heart disease is also controversial. Some cardiologists feel that measuring cholesterol alone is enough and that the triglyceride level doesn't add anything really significant. Others feel that high triglycerides not only are important but may be causative, and should be reduced. They point to the fact that more people with coronary disease have elevated triglycerides than have high cholesterol. Besides which, a diet calculated to lower your triglycerides will also help you lose weight. So if your triglycerides are high, try to lower them even for this secondary benefit. When your blood is drawn for cholesterol, your stomach needn't be empty, but the same is not true for triglycerides. Unless you have been fasting for at least 14 hours before your blood is drawn, the triglyceride level will be falsely high. Some doctors and many patients do not appreciate this fact and as a result are unnecessarily concerned about a spuriously elevated triglyceride.

Are You Type 2 or Type 4?

All kinds of combinations of blood fat abnormalities have been worked out and numbered, but there are two important categories. If your triglycerides are high and the cholesterol is normal or elevated, you are Type 4. A normal triglyceride and a high cholesterol make you a Type 2. From a dietary point of view, the Type 4's must basically avoid alcohol and foods high in simple sugar like glucose. Patients in the Type 2 category should concentrate on low cholesterol foods, but may eat normal amounts of sugar and drink in moderation. Cholestyramine is most effective in the Type 2 group, whereas Atromid-S is most likely to lower your cholesterol if you are a Type 4.

THYROID FUNCTION STUDIES—CHECKING YOUR THERMOSTAT

Laboratory evaluation of thyroid function is not routinely included in the automated series of blood tests. However, I do it as part of the checkup in new patients or if I have the slightest suspicion that your thyroid gland is underactive or overactive.

Evaluating your thyroid function usually involves only analysis of blood, sometimes radioactive scanning, and occasionally a basal metabolism test (the old "breathing test").

Your blood tells us how much thyroid hormone is actually circulating in your body (T_3, T_4). The old PBI test is no longer used and has been superseded by newer types of analyses. One of these, the thyroid-stimulating hormone (TSH) test, indicates whether the brain is giving the appropriate signal to the thyroid gland. Remember, the thyroid is not its own boss.

Radioactive Techniques for Thyroid Testing

When the blood tests raise the suspicion that the function of the thyroid gland is awry, or if I have felt a lump in the gland during the physical, we proceed with radioactive techniques. These are done in a hospital clinic or other specialized facility. They are simple and painless, but expensive. You drink a small amount of absolutely tasteless "water," containing a tracer dose of radioactive iodine which goes to the thyroid gland. If the thyroid is underactive, very little of the tracer will end up in the gland. If it is overactive, the thyroid will extract a large amount of the radioactive substance from the blood.

The Geiger Counter Scan

The day after you have taken the iodine drink, you come back to the laboratory and we see just how much of the tracer has ended up in your thyroid. You lie down and a Geiger counter scans your neck, telling us exactly how much radioactivity is present in the gland. If your thyroid is enlarged and made up entirely of functioning tissue, the Geiger counter will reproduce an image of the whole gland.

Hot and Cold Nodules

If you have a "hot" nodule (a lump of thyroid made up of functioning tissue), the radioactive material will show up on the scan either in normal amounts or, if the nodule is overactive, in higher concentrations. In the case of a "cold" nodule (tissue within the gland not producing any hormone), there will be a "hole" in the representation of the thyroid scan, indicating the size and location of the nonfunctioning area. This is important information, since such "cold" nodules may be malignant and require surgical removal.

Treating the Sick Thyroid

Treatment of an *underactive thyroid gland* is very simple and consists of replacement therapy—usually 2 to 3 grams of thyroid per day. We work up to this level very gradually. Too much too fast causes palpitations and rapid heartbeat, loss of weight and nervousness, and may be dangerous if you have underlying heart disease.

If you are *hyperthyroid,* we have three treatment options. We may recommend surgery if the gland is diffusely enlarged or has lumps in it. If not, we give you radioactive iodine with treatment (not tracer) doses. One of the problems with this iodine therapy is gauging exactly how much radioactive material is needed to destroy the overfunctioning tissue, yet to leave enough of the gland intact so as to ensure enough thyroid activity. Realistically, most of the patients who are treated with radioactive iodine require additional thyroid years later, because the radioactivity destroys too much normal tissue. Some doctors prefer to control symptoms in yet a third way, using drugs for six to twelve months. In about half the cases, this does the job. The rest relapse when the treatment is stopped, and then require surgery or radioactive iodine.

OTHER BLOOD TESTS WE MAY WANT TO DO

This sums up the blood analyses that are normally done in the course of a routine examination. There are, of course, literally dozens of others that can be performed, when there is some special reason. For example, we can measure your iron and vitamin B_{12}, as well as various hormone levels. We can determine the amount of alcohol in your blood. Supposing an unconscious individual is brought to the hospital with alcohol on his breath. Is he drunk, or in a coma due to a stroke? Has he suffered a head injury, or does he have either advanced diabetes or too much insulin? One diagnostic step along the way is to measure the amount of alcohol in the blood.

We use blood tests to assess other poisons and drugs (including barbiturates) that may have been taken deliberately or accidentally.

Blood Donors, Hepatitis, and Australia Antigen

Blood transfusions are, of course, lifesaving, especially after blood loss from injury or during surgery. But they are not without risk. *Serum hepatitis* from infected blood is a serious illness most often contracted in cities where blood donors are paid for their contribution or where the blood is collected by less than reputable commercial laboratories. The financial incentive for such donations has prompted derelict drug users, many of whom are themselves infected with hepatitis to earn some extra cash by selling their blood. Fortunately, in recent years it has been found that blood which is infected with the hepatitis virus often contains a substance called *Australia antigen* which can be detected by special tests. Blood banks in many states now use this discovery to screen all blood donors, a procedure that, though not foolproof, is now saving thousands of lives each year.

Anticoagulant Precautions

If you are taking anticoagulants because of heart disease, recurrent blood clots, phlebitis, or artificial heart valves, your blood must be monitored regularly to ensure that the proper level of control is maintained. Too much anticoagulant may make you hemorrhage, too little permits you to clot. The test for this, called *prothrombin time*, should be done at least every three or four weeks, after a stable anticoagulant dosage has been determined and maintained.

What's Your Blood Type?

Patients often want to know their blood type "in case I need blood in a hurry." Remember that if you get a transfusion, knowing your type isn't going to make much difference. The blood given to you is always first tested against a mixture of your own anyway. If the two are incompatible, the blood cells can be seen to clump under the microscope. This procedure, which is called *blood typing and crossmatching, is an absolute must before you're given any blood—even if you know your blood type.* But routine blood typing is a good idea. You may want to donate blood in special circumstances—for example, to friends or relatives who need it.

In pregnant women, Rh typing is important for the following reason. *Rhesus factor* is present in the blood of about 85 percent of the normal white population and in 93 percent of blacks. The problem arises when an Rh-negative mother is carrying an Rh-positive baby. This can lead to destruction of the baby's red blood cells and even death. It happens this way. Someone who is Rh-negative cannot tolerate Rh-positive blood. Since the fetal and maternal bloods are mixed together during development, the embryo's Rh-positive blood stimulates "antibodies" (to the Rh factor) in the Rh-negative mother. These recirculate to the fetus, and cause clumping of its blood.

Drugs in Your Blood

Thanks to the development of radioimmune assay techniques (for which Dr. Rosalind Yalow, the American scientist who developed them, received the Nobel Prize in 1977), we can now measure tiny amounts of many drugs and hormones circulating in your bloodstream. This is very useful in many cases. Consider digitalis, for example. As you know, this drug is used to treat various forms of heart disease. When there is too little in the circulation, it is ineffective. Too much is toxic and potentially lethal. It is not always easy to know whether symptoms like nausea, vomiting, and visual disturbances are due to too much digitalis, since many who require this drug have other disorders as well—especially of the kidney and liver—which can give similar symptoms. So, to be able to measure the amount of digitalis in the circulation, using radioactive tracers, is a great advantage.

How Are Your Hormones Doing?

The concentration of various hormones in the blood can also be measured—for example, cortisone (vital to so many metabolic functions), adrenaline (which raises the blood pressure), and the pituitary hormones (which are produced in the brain and stimulate other target glands like the thyroid, sex glands, and adrenals). When I suspect some hormonal imbalance, a complete glandular workup can be performed by the precise measurement of these hormones.

Testing for "Kissing" Disease

Infectious mononucleosis (glandular fever, "kissing disease") is common among young people. It is suspected whenever we see sore throat, enlarged lymph glands, and generalized weakness in younger people. We confirm the suspicion by identifying the *heterophil antibody*. This can be done in the doctor's office.

You May Even Have Malaria

During your travels you may have been in an area where malaria is common. It is a very important disease of mankind. Should you come back with unexplained fever and chills, I will have a malaria smear done. A drop of your blood is put on a glass slide and looked at under the microscope. If the test is done shortly after a chill, the causative parasite is seen inside your red blood cells.

CHAPTER **16**

WE'RE IN THE LAST STRETCH

You've now provided the urine specimen; your blood has been drawn and is on its way for analysis. You won't have the result of those tests for one to five days depending on which specific analyses have been ordered and where they are being done. But you're not through yet. There are several other procedures to be completed or scheduled before you leave.

Regardless of the complaints that you volunteered or were elicited from you in the history-taking, and despite what the physical examination did or did not reveal, you will still need a chest x-ray and an electrocardiogram (ECG). What's more, if you're over 40 years of age and the ECG is normal, a tracing taken during and after exercise should be done as well. I will also arrange a barium enema if you haven't had one in the past two or three years and you are over 45 years of age.

THE CHEST X-RAY

It's a good idea to have a chest film every year, especially if you're a heavy smoker and at risk for developing lung cancer. The chest film tells me about your lungs, your heart, the major blood vessels in the chest, and the bony cage that houses the thoracic contents. It takes just a moment to do, involves very little radiation, and is inexpensive.

The lungs consist of two air sacs, one on each side of the chest. The x-ray cannot "photograph" air, so when you look at your chest film, the black portion represents the lungs. The white parts are denser structures like bone—that is the ribs and spinal column—and the heart. The white strands in the black air space of the lungs of healthy persons are the bronchial tubes and blood vessels, coursing through the lung tissue. When there is a tumor or an infection in the lung, a white "spot" appears in the otherwise black area, indicating that the air has been replaced by densities which shouldn't be there. Also, if there is fluid in the sac around the lung, that will also appear white on the x-ray picture. When the blood vessels in the lung are engorged because blood has backed into them from a weakened, failing heart, such congestion is apparent in the chest film.

"Is That Me?"

I'm not telling you all this in order for you to read your own chest x-ray. That requires a great deal of skill. It isn't always easy to distinguish normal "shadows" in the lung from those that represent disease. But so often a patient will look at his chest film and ask with incredulity, "Is that me?" Then a worried expression will often cross his face. "What's that big white thing? Should it be there?" That "big white thing" is your heart. I evaluate its shape (for if any chamber of the heart is enlarged, it will confer a distinctive configuration upon the shadow), its size (a rule of thumb is that the heart should not be greater than half the width of the chest), and its position within the chest cavity. (It can be pushed and pulled too much to the right or left by disease of the lungs themselves.) I also look for the aorta—the big vessel that comes up out of the heart and then courses downward toward the abdomen—to see if it is widened (as in an aneurysm) and if it contains any calcium or evidence of arteriosclerosis. Then I look at the rib cage itself. If you have emphysema, the spaces between the ribs will be wider than normal and your ribs will have lost their usual curvature. Also, your diaphragm will have been depressed by the overinflated lungs, making the chest longer and giving the diaphragm less opportunity to move up and down with respiration. I look for fluid in the pericardium (the sac around the heart), as well as in the pleural spaces (the envelope surrounding the lungs). I also search for enlarged lymph glands—evidence of chronic infection like TB or tumor.

Why Two Views of the Chest?

If you have viewed a chest x-ray taken head-on, you may remember seeing the big white heart, a little to the left of center, surrounded by the black lungs on either side. Nothing in the lung behind the heart can be seen in such a frontal view. That's the reason we turn you sideways and take another film. It enables us to see evidence of disease behind the heart and, in the presence of cardiac enlargement, to determine which chambers are too big.

Swallowing Barium for the Heart X-Ray

Sometimes, if I have heard a heart murmur I think may be significant, I will have you swallow some barium and then take the chest x-ray. Barium is an opaque substance that stands out on the x-ray film. When swallowed, it highlights the food pipe, which lies behind the heart, so that I can see whether any cardiac chambers are pushing it backward or otherwise distorting it.

Chest X-Rays and the Lungs

How useful is the chest x-ray? If you are being treated for an acute lung disease like pneumonia, it tells me whether or not treatment is effective, whether the antibiotic prescribed is working. If you have cardiac trouble, x-rays at regular intervals indicate whether the heart is getting bigger or smaller in response to treatment.

The chest x-ray is also useful in "normal" people who don't have any symptoms. For example, I may see a "shadow" in your lung. This could be a sign of old healed tuberculosis and of no consequence, or it may represent a burned-out fungal infection. It may also be due to a small patch of pneumonia masquerading as "the sniffles." It may reflect an old "silent" blood clot which made its way to the lung without your knowing about it and which resulted in some scarring. Finally, and most important, it may be a tumor.

The Shadow

The discovery of a *new* shadow in the chest film is a very disturbing finding which may require a whole series of further investigations and eventually culminate in an operation to find out precisely what it means and to make sure it isn't an early cancer.

You have probably heard people say that once evidence of a cancer appears on a chest film, it is too late to cure—so why take the x-ray in the first place? This simply isn't true. A significant percentage, perhaps 20 or 25 percent, of cancers of the lung can be detected early enough to cure—and that figure is constantly increasing. So when we see a shadow for the first time in someone who is totally without symptoms, we must determine what it is.

An "Unnecessary" Operation

Have you ever seen a large scar from an old operation on someone's chest—in a locker room, in a swimming pool, or at the beach? If they tell you it was from an "unnecessary" operation, this is probably how it happened:

Your friend went for a routine examination and was found to have a "shadow" on the chest x-ray. He had no complaints—no cough, fever, or chest pain. He was asked to bring in some old x-rays for comparison. He did. They showed nothing. This was a new finding. The possibilities considered were TB, a bacterial or fungal infection, a blood clot in the lung, and cancer (especially if the patient was a cigarette smoker). What did his doctor do?

First, he reexamined him very carefully, looking for glands in the spaces above the collarbones, in the neck, and throughout the body. If he detected an enlarged hard gland, he removed it and looked at it under the microscope to see whether it contained any cancer or infectious tissue. (Enlarged glands may be due to old inflammation or infection and may have nothing to do with the shadow on the lung.) If he had found evidence of cancer in the gland, the story would have ended there, and your friend probably would not now be around to tell it.

If no glands were present, a variety of skin tests were used. If these had been positive, some fungal infection, old or recent, was a possible but not definite cause of the shadow.

The Tomogram—a Chest Film In Depth

He was then sent for a *tomogram*. This is a series of chest x-rays in which the depth of the ray is varied so as to get slices of the shadow in question from front to back, the purpose being to evaluate its shape and density. We can often tell from this procedure whether we are dealing with a benign fungus, the cavity of tuberculosis, some other infection, or a tumor.

During this phase of the evaluation the doctor also tried to get your friend to cough. If he managed to bring up some sputum, it was sent to the lab, where it was cultured for bacteria, TB and fungus, and carefully looked at for cancer cells. If the sputum was negative or unrevealing, and if the location of the shadow in the lung was such that it could be reached with a bronchoscope, I suspect your friend was now subjected to the next step of the investigation.

Bronchoscopy—Not As Bad As It Used to Be

This procedure is not as bad as it used to be only a few years ago, when the instrument inserted through your mouth into the air passages was fairly large and rigid. Today, we use a thinner flexible fiberoptic tube. Under local anesthesia, this scope may be inserted through your nose and eased down the windpipe without too much discomfort. The tube has a fiberoptic cold light source which permits the operator to look at the lining of the air passages all the way down into the lung. If he sees a growth there, he can snip a piece off for study. He can also inject some solution into the bronchial tube to wash the lining, suction the liquid back out and look for evidence of cancer cells or infection. In many cases, especially when the area under suspicion is accessible to such bronchoscopy, the diagnosis can be established by this technique.

Scalene Node Biopsy

But sometimes, bronchoscopy doesn't clarify the picture either. That usually happens when the shadow is in some portion of the lung not accessible to it. That must have occurred with your friend. So the next step (although some physicians do it before bronchoscopy) was to nick the skin in the neck on the same side as the shadow, behind the collarbone, and remove some small glands which cannot be felt from the outside but which may become involved by spread of infection or cancer of the lung. This is called a *scalene node biopsy*.

Needling the Lung

If these glands did not show any evidence of disease and the doctor was still in the dark about the nature of the shadow, there were only two courses left. If the shadow was large enough and in a suitable place, that is, close to the chest wall, he introduced a needle through the chest wall. If such a *needle biopsy* can hit the shadow in question, it may yield a sliver of tissue for further study. Presumably, that was not feasible here.

The last recourse, and the one that gave your friend the scar you saw, was an operation to remove the section of the lung containing the abnormal-looking shadow. Since your friend is alive to tell the tale, they probably found a benign chronic infection (or conceivably a small tumor that was completely removed). But it took all that trouble to make the diagnosis. There are many people around who have had such an "unnecessary" lung operation. You now understand why it had to be done.

Other Lung Tests You May Need

If you have chronic lung disease or complain of shortness of breath which doesn't appear to be due to your heart, I will have you perform some *pulmonary function tests*. You breathe into a recording device which is capable of measuring the capacity of your lungs. The amount of air you can blow out rapidly is also measured. These tests indicate whether your ability to ventilate your lungs is reduced. For example, when disease of the chest wall limits its motion, the lungs cannot expand normally and their capacity is low. In conditions like asthma or chronic bronchitis, the narrowed bronchial tubes interfere with the passage of air in and out of the lungs so the amount of air forced out is reduced. Such abnormalities become apparent during the pulmonary function testing, which can be done in your doctor's office, if he has the equipment, or in a special pulmonary laboratory or hospital.

Prognosis For Cancer Patients

At this point I would like to make one or two points about the outlook for cancer of the lung and cancers in general. Malignant disease remains for the most part a fatal disorder, but there have been a few significant developments permitting earlier diagnosis and more effective management. These make a nihilistic approach to cancer totally untenable. For example, we have found that certain anticancer drugs when given alone have very little effect on tumors. But when combined, they cause significant slowing of growth, improvement of symptoms and prolongation of life. In addition to conventional surgery, radiation with new high-powered machines, and drug therapy, the field of cancer immunotherapy is also very promising. *Immunotherapy* refers to the way that the body's own defenses can be stimulated to fight cancer cells. It has been applied successfully to cancers of the skin, breast, bone, lung, and bowel; and the field is expanding every day with new agents being developed and produced. If you are told that you have a growth which may be malignant, your chances of cure or control today are better than ever and improving all the time.

Chest X-Rays and the Heart

What does the heart shadow reveal in a normal healthy person during a routine chest x-ray? First, its size. You may have had some elevation of blood pressure over the years, of which you were unaware. This often results in *cardiac enlargement*, indicating that even though the blood pressure elevation was mild, and you were without symptoms, it was nevertheless enough to affect the heart. As you will see in the next section, borderline or "non-specific" changes may appear in the electrocardiogram which are difficult to interpret or evaluate. When these are associated with even slight enlargement of the heart, they assume a greater significance.

Many *heart murmurs* are innocent, reflecting mild turbulence of blood flow across a valve. Others, however, are important and due to changes in the structure and function of the heart. Sooner or later, these will be reflected in the chest x-ray, as either cardiac enlargement or an alteration in the shape of the heart.

Shortness of Breath

This is a fairly common complaint in older, overweight and sedentary, but otherwise "well" persons. Their physical examination may be normal. But if a routine chest film shows the heart to be enlarged, early heart failure or disease of the heart muscle (as opposed to coronary artery disease) must be considered as a cause of the symptoms.

THE ELECTROCARDIOGRAM (ECG, EKG)

The ECG is an integral part of the routine examination not only of the adult but at any age, especially when a cardiac disorder is suspected. The tracing is an indirect reflection of the heart's electrical activity obtained from a machine called an *electrocardiograph*.

What Makes the Heart Beat?

The heartbeat is initiated by a "pacemaker," a tiny focus of special tissue within the right atrium which controls the cardiac rhythm. Under normal circumstances, the pacemaker "fires" 60 to 100 times a minute at regular intervals. The impulse originating here spreads like the ripples in a lake after a stone is thrown in, through a relay station, toward the powerful ventricles. It then passes into specialized conducting tissues which carry it to all parts of the heart. The path of this electrical impulse is identified in the electrocardiogram by a series of characteristic waves which are altered if there is any interference with the normal conduction of the impulse—through the conducting tissue or any other part of the heart through which it travels. Such interference may result from damage or strain of the heart or from drug effect.

When an ECG is taken, ten electrodes are placed on your hands, feet, and across your chest and are connected to the electrocardiograph machine. Every time I turn the knob on the ECG machine, I switch *leads,* thereby activating a particular set of electrodes and affording a different electrical viewpoint of the heart. The waves that appear on the ECG differ in shape, size, and direction, depending on which lead is being looked at—whether we are viewing the electrical activity of the heart from below, in front, or behind.

What Can the ECG Tell Us?

What abnormalities can we identify in the electrocardiogram? It is the best way to document disturbances in heart rhythm when the heartbeat is irregular. This may be the result of a toxic effect on the pacemaker (depressing or irritating it) or on various portions of the heart through which the electrical impulse travels. *Rhythm disorders* can also be produced by failure of the heart's "escape" or backup mechanism. When the main pacemaker is injured and so fails to generate electrical impulses, other areas of the heart farther along the pathway take over and initiate the impulse, usually at a slower rate than the original pacemaker. If, for any reason, this protective mechanism doesn't come into play, then no impulse is formed, the heart doesn't beat, and the patient suffers *cardiac arrest.* Although such an arrest or "standstill" may occur suddenly and without warning, routine electrocardiography often reveals clues that the patient is vulnerable to such a catastrophe.

Predicting Sudden Death

If you complain of palpitations, and I detect an "extra" or early beat when listening to your heart or taking your pulse, I will want to know where in the heart it originates and its frequency. This is usually possible only by means of an electrocardiogram. Those who die suddenly and without warning do so because their heart undergoes a series of rapid, consecutive, chaotic, and ineffective extra beats lasting only a minute or two. And that's enough to cause death. Such beats often occur first in isolated form, without your necessarily knowing about it. They can be detected in the ECG and, if necessary, treated with the medication now available to prevent sudden death.

Another cardiac abnormality that can be recognized in the electrocardiogram is enlargement of the heart. As a matter of fact, this is often more easily done on the electrocardiogram than in the chest x-ray. Here the electrical impulse takes longer to complete its cycle and gives bigger, wider waves (complexes) because it has to pass through thicker muscle. Depending on which ECG complexes and leads show these changes, we can tell which of the four heart chambers are enlarged.

Heart Attack (Myocardial Infarction, Coronary Thrombosis)

The electrocardiogram reflects heart damage caused by a heart attack. This may have occurred with or without your knowledge. Suppose one of your coronary arteries has been closed off (by thrombosis) and that portion of the heart muscle dependent on it has died because of blood deprivation. (We call this *myocardial infarction.*) The muscle is now biologically inert and can no longer conduct the electrical impulse going through it. The current has to make a detour around the dead area. This changes the shape of the normal wave in the electrocardiogram. *At least 25 percent of heart attacks are "silent,"* that is, they occur without being recognized as such. At the time, you may have thought you were suffering from a muscle spasm, "acute indigestion," "gas," or arthritis. Had you "pampered" yourself and gone to a doctor then and there, he would no doubt have recorded the diagnostic changes in the electrocardiogram and hospitalized you. But you didn't and fortunately survived all the same. Now, months or years later, on routine examination you are found to have this pattern of old infarction.

Before the Heart Attack

Before a heart attack actually takes place, there is often a pe- riod during which one or more of the coronary arteries are nar- rowed. They can deliver enough blood only for modest activity, but not for more strenuous effort. The electrocardiogram not only is able to detect the damage caused by an infarction, but may also indicate that the heart is getting an inadequate amount of blood or, in other words, that there is an *insufficiency*. This is not always accompanied by chest pressure or pain, and the only warning may be an abnormal ECG. (The converse is more often true—that is, you are apt to have chest pain or pressure without any changes in the ECG, except when the tracing is taken during an episode of symptoms.)

What's a Bundle Branch Block?

One day, in the course of a routine examination, your doctor (or insurance agent) may frighten the life out of you by telling you there is a "bundle branch block" in your ECG. It sounds ominous—but isn't necessarily.

The electrical impulse associated with cardiac contraction trav- els from its origin in the atria across a relay system into the thick- walled ventricles. The pathway it follows in each ventricle is called a "bundle." The "right bundle" is in the right ventricle, the "left bundle" in the left ventricle. The left bundle subdivides into progressively smaller "branches" as it penetrates deep into the ventricular muscle.

The Bundle Branch Block

When something interferes with the normal conduction of the electrical impulse through these specialized bundles, slowing it down or "blocking" it, the result is a "left bundle branch block"

(LBBB) or a "right bundle branch block" (RBBB), depending on which bundle is involved.

What causes bundle branch block? What does it mean when you have it? Can the heart still function if the impulse is blocked?

LBBB is usually more significant than RBBB. Injury to the "bundles" or their "branches" is almost always due to some reduction in their blood supply, such as occurs in coronary artery disease. After a heart attack, scar tissue may form around the bundles and their branches, interfering with the spread of the impulse through them. When that happens, an alternate pathway of conduction must be used. This takes a little longer (perhaps three or four hundredths of a second)—but in the end, the muscle contracts quite normally, although perhaps less synchronously.

Bundle branch block may be intermittent, so that sometimes you have it, then you don't. This may happen when the heart rate varies. In vulnerable persons, faster rates tend to result in bundle branch block because the conducting tissue fatigues more easily and can't cope with an impulse presenting itself before the bundle has recovered from transmitting the last one.

Suppose that in the course of a routine examination you are found to have a bundle branch block. What should you do? If you are young, without symptoms, and this, your very first ECG, shows an RBBB pattern, ignore it. Most insurance companies will offer you standard rates if you can show that you've had this finding all your life. If it is a new finding, you will have to undergo a complete cardiac evaluation to determine its significance.

It is much less likely that LBBB is a harmless variant, although it may be. If you are under 40, perfectly healthy without other evidence of heart disease, and your first ECG reveals an LBBB pattern, don't worry about it even if an insurance company does not want to do business with you. But if you have a bad family history for heart disease, are diabetic, or have high blood pressure, it should constitute an important warning sign. A change in your ECG from normal conduction to LBBB is significant, and must be evaluated by your doctor, even if you have no symptoms.

When You May Have Problems with Bundle Branch Block

Although bundle branch block itself in most cases requires no special treatment, there is one exception—when such a pattern appears in your ECG and is accompanied by evidence of additional interference with the transmission of the electrical impulse within the heart. For example, combined right and left bundle branch block is a threat. Such findings may not be accompanied by symptoms, but predispose you to *complete heart block,* with slowing or standstill of the heart. This leads to decreased blood flow to the brain, loss of consciousness, and possibly death. Happily, such electrical abnormalities are not necessarily accompanied by weakness or damage of the heart muscle itself—and can be very easily treated with a pacemaker. If you have any symptoms due to a slow heart rate, your doctor may recommend an artificial pacemaker.

So You Need a Pacemaker

This leads us into the subject of pacemakers. Hundreds of thousands of people need them, have them, and lead perfectly normal lives with them.

The pacemaker is not an artificial heart. It will not prevent a heart attack—that is, the closure of a coronary artery. *If your heart muscle is weak, the pacemaker will not strengthen it.* Its only function is to ensure that the electrical system in your heart will not go awry. A good analogy can be made with your automobile. The heart is the motor; the pacemaker is the battery. No matter how good the rest of the car is, you're in trouble if the battery won't start. If that happens, you get a new battery for your car—or an artificial pacemaker for your heart. You wouldn't think of getting a new car because the battery is dead, nor should you think your number is up because you need a pacemaker.

Many patients have perfectly good hearts, but the cardiac electrical system is sick. The heart may then beat erratically, too slowly, or run the risk of stopping. In such cases, the pacemaker is lifesaving. If you're advised to have one put in, don't panic or get depressed. First of all, it's very easily done and does not require opening the chest or the heart. An incision is made usually in the chest or abdominal wall. The battery that powers the pacemaker (smaller than a pack of cigarettes) is sewn in under the skin, usually only with local anesthesia. Current models are barely noticeable. A small wire is then threaded through a vein directly into the right ventricle. It all takes less than an hour and you need to be in the hospital only a few days, until the skin overlying the pacemaker heals.

You Won't Know You Have One

Once it's in, you are not aware of the pacemaker's action. You can lead a perfectly normal life with it—running, swimming, playing ball. You should, however, avoid microwave ovens. One hidden benefit is that you will be excused from going through electronic censors at airports. Most models are set to work on demand, that is, they trigger the heart to beat only if your own mechanisms fail. The unit is set to fire at a certain rate, for example 65 or 70 beats per minute. As long as your heart beats at that rate or faster, the pacemaker will just sit there and do nothing. But if, for any reason, your heart slows below that figure, the pacemaker takes over, ensuring the minimum heart rate.

Every so often you need to check with your doctor to make sure the pacemaker is working properly. This can easily be done by telephone. You buy a transmitter (under $200), again the size of a pack of cigarettes, place the phone mouthpiece over it and call the doctor. A unit at his end decodes the signal, indicating whether battery strength is normal and if the unit is functioning properly.

Modern pacemakers need a battery change every five to eight years or so (older models lasted only two to three years), depending on how often the pacemaker is called upon to fire. A nuclear-powered unit, with a battery duration of ten to twenty years, is also available, but is used mainly in children who need pacemakers because of a congenital heart problem or as the re-

sult of surgery which inadvertently injured their cardiac conducting system. As they become cheaper, older age groups will
also be using them.

In summary, then, the electrocardiogram identifies disturbances of cardiac rhythm, indicates enlargement of various portions of the heart, reflects damage due to any previous heart
attacks, and can reveal evidence of inadequate blood flow or coronary insufficiency. Having said that, let me offer two important
warnings. The ECG is only a gross indicator of what is actually
going on in the heart. It is, after all, an indirect recording device
that reflects electrical activity recorded from the surface of the
chest. Also, there is a great variation or range of normality in an
ECG. Too much significance can be attached to minor changes,
but there is also the danger that they will be erroneously dismissed as insignificant.

Put another way, the electrocardiogram is vulnerable to yield-
ing "falsely positive" interpretations or "falsely negative" ones.
The ECG of female patients often shows spurious changes which
may be overinterpreted. Nervous individuals too may have "abnormalities" in the ECG, while blacks often have changes that
mimic but do not reflect disease.

Whenever I read an electrocardiogram, I always ask if there is
an old one with which I can compare it. In this way, even minor
or subtle changes that have suddenly appeared can be interpreted more accurately.

Finally, and most important, *a completely "normal" electrocardiogram does not exclude the presence of coronary heart disease.* In my
experience, at least 60 percent of persons with symptoms of angina have a normal electrocardiogram. This probably accounts
for the popularity of the story so commonly heard at cocktail
parties: "My friend went for a complete examination the other
day, was told by his doctor that his ECG was normal, and
dropped dead later that day from a heart attack."

If the majority of people with symptoms of heart disease have
normal ECG's, how do we ever establish the diagnosis? That
leads us to a discussion of stress testing.

ECG Taken During and After Exercise

When an ECG taken at rest is normal, that does not exclude the presence of coronary heart disease, coronary insufficiency, or angina pectoris, all synonyms for a compromised blood flow within the heart which renders you vulnerable to a heart attack. Almost fifty years ago astute observers conceived the idea of recording a tracing after some kind of physical stress, like running, jumping, bending, or hopping.

The Master Two-Step Test

The most persistent of these cardiologists was Dr. Arthur Master. He designed the "Master two-step test," in which he calculated, on the basis of observations in normal men and women of different ages, how many times a healthy individual should be able to ascend and descend two steps each 9 inches high in a period of three minutes without causing ECG abnormalities. This procedure has been modified over the years, and the interpretation of the ECG changes noted after exercise has been continuously updated. It is still probably the most widely used stress test to elicit diagnostic ECG abnormalities, as it can be performed in the doctor's office without any additional equipment, is safe (the level of exercise demanded is not excessive), and is reliable. In our office, as in many others, we still use it as the initial screening exercise test for the clarification of chest pain. It is particularly useful if you complain of symptoms that suggest angina pectoris and your electrocardiogram at rest is normal. But even if you have no symptoms, I will still ask you to do it because so much coronary heart disease is "silent" or its symptoms misinterpreted.

Bicycles and Treadmills

More vigorous stress tests are also widely used in cardiologists' offices, hospital laboratories, or special clinics. They involve either a *bicycle ergometer* (a stationary bicycle on which you pedal against a progressive increase in resistance at a specific rate) or a *treadmill,* whose speed is increased and its incline raised. These procedures differ from the Master Test in that the level of exercise they require as the test progresses is much more strenuous. (Some cardiologists believe that the workload in the Master test does not raise the heart rate enough to constitute an adequate challenge to it.)

Another feature of the more vigorous testing procedures is that they permit us to record the electrocardiogram not only after you have finished the exercise but while you are actually performing it. This adds another dimension to the kind of information obtained. Certain disturbances of rhythm and other changes may be present only during exercise, and not after the test is completed. More sophisticated measurements based on blood pressure changes, heart rate variations, and the amount of exercise performed can be computed. We then determine what workload will produce a "strain" on the heart. Based on these measurements and on the electrocardiographic response noted at different heart rates, we can prescribe exercise programs for healthy persons as well as for those with heart disease.

In addition to unmasking coronary insufficiency, the stress tests may induce disturbances of heart rhythm that were not present on the resting ECG. Although some of these are perfectly harmless, others may warn us that certain levels of exertion are dangerous for you because they may trigger the kind of rhythm disorder that can result in sudden death.

Even though accidents during the various forms of stress testing are extremely rare, you will still be asked to sign a release stating that the risks were carefully explained to you and that you consented to undergo the test. Laboratories where these procedures are performed have the appropriate equipment and trained personnel to deal with any such emergency situation. If a certain amount of exercise is potentially dangerous to you, it's better to learn about it during a stress test with a doctor nearby than jogging in the park alone or in the company of your tailor.

I will have you perform the bicycle ergometer or treadmill test if the Master two-step test is borderline, questionable, or abnormal. In my experience the more strenuous exercise tests are (a) a little more reliable, (b) a little more dangerous, and (c) a lot more costly than the original Master test.

The abnormalities that may be observed during and after exercise consist of evidence of "strain" or "insufficiency," suggesting that at certain workloads and heart rates, the blood supply to various portions of the heart muscle may be inadequate. These abnormalities may be seen in persons who are not aware of any unusual symptoms as well as in those who do experience shortness of breath, chest pain or pressure with physical or emotional stress.

Ambulatory Monitoring: Taking Your ECG on the Tennis Court

Dynamic or ambulatory ECG monitoring has already become virtually routine in the cardiac evaluation performed by many cardiologists. It permits an ECG to be recorded over a period of up to 24 hours—during which time you perform your usual everyday functions. You come to the ECG laboratory in the morning and the apparatus is attached to you. This involves placing three small plastic electrodes very much like the ones used in a regular ECG on your chest. These are connected by thin wires which are slipped through your shirt to a small recording device weighing about a pound and a half. It either fits around your belt or can be carried like a pocketbook. Inside this device is a miniature tape recorder with a cassette that revolves very slowly for 24 hours, constantly recording your electrocardiogram. If you should lose your temper, have an emotional crisis, indulge in sexual intercourse, eat, play tennis or move your bowels, any change in the ECG associated with or precipitated by these events will be documented. More important, if you have some rhythm disturbance of which you are not aware or which was not picked up in the resting or stress ECG, it too will be documented. The next day you return the machine, and the tape is processed on a rapid playback device which permits the 24-hour record to be analyzed in a few minutes. This machine, which was devised by Holter several years ago, represents a major advance in diagnostic cardiology. We use it in patients with definite angina, persons with puzzling cardiac symptoms, or those who have been discharged from the hospital after a heart attack. It provides a great deal of additional information not otherwise available. The widespread use of this technique will surely identify more and more persons who have silent heart disease or who may be vulnerable to sudden cardiac death and in whom preventive measures may be instituted.

ECG by Telephone

Another new diagnostic capability is the telephone-transmitted ECG. Suppose that every few days or so, unpredictably, you experience a certain symptom which we think may be due to heart trouble. It may take the form of an uncomfortable pounding of the heart, an irregular pulse or one that is briefly too fast or too slow, chest pressure, light-headedness or dizziness. Like the toothache that disappears when you go to the dentist, the symptom is usually not there when you happen to be in the doctor's office. Even a stress test may not uncover the disorder. If it occurs episodically, the 24-hour tape may not show anything either on the day you happen to be hooked up. You can then borrow a small battery-operated ECG transmitter which weighs a few ounces. When the symptom in question appears, you simply place one electrode in each armpit, put the transmitter over the telephone mouthpiece (as with pacemaker transmission), and dial your cardiologist, the cardiac clinic, or coronary care unit. A small apparatus hooked up at the other end to a regular electrocardiograph will receive the ECG. Elusive disturbances in heart rhythm can often be picked up by this technique.

Two Questions Often Asked About the ECG and Heart Disease:
1. What to Do About Silent Coronary Disease?

Suppose that in the course of a routine examination I find your ECG shows evidence that you actually had a heart attack in the past without knowing it. To the best of your knowledge you are now and always have been perfectly well. Is this finding of value to you? Would you not have been better off psychologically if you hadn't been told about it?

Opinions differ concerning the management of such a situation. It poses no problem for the insurance companies. They simply jack up your premium—if you can get any insurance at all. Some doctors choose to conceal the finding from you, their philosophy being "why worry a perfectly well patient simply because you find evidence of an old small scar in his electrocardiogram which probably isn't going to cause any harm anyway?" This position is basically a nihilistic one and reflects lack of candor between doctor and patient. My view is that you go to the doctor to determine the state of your health and what you can do to preserve it. ECG evidence of a previous myocardial infarction indicates that you were vulnerable in the past and may be again in the future. Given this surprise finding, it behooves me to evaluate you very carefully concerning how best you can avoid a future attack. The next one may not be so mild as to go unrecognized and may not be without complications.

While the causes of heart attacks and arteriosclerosis are not completely understood, we have nevertheless made several observations which may have a bearing on your vulnerability. We think that intervening in some areas can make a significant difference to you. For example, if you're overweight, a silent heart attack may really motivate you to reduce. If your cholesterol and triglycerides are very high, you will want to normalize them by diet and perhaps by drugs. If your blood pressure is elevated or even borderline, you will now surely adhere to a dietary and medication regimen to normalize it. If you are a smoker, you will finally be convinced to stop, because cigarette smoking contributes directly to coronary artery disease. And if you are physically inactive—don't exercise nor even walk—you will decide to spend some time each day taking some exercise, which may open up new arteries within the heart (collateral circulation) and improve your outlook.

If nothing else, all these alterations in your life-style will make you feel a lot better and convince you that you are in fact doing something useful. So if you've had a silent heart attack sometime in the past, I'll tell you. It's better to hear it from me than from your insurance agent.

2. What to Do with an Abnormal Stress Test?

Suppose that your resting electrocardiogram is normal, you have absolutely no symptoms of coronary insufficiency, and your

ECG response to stress is abnormal. What do we do about that? First, let me emphasize that a small number of people, mostly women, have a normal coronary circulation but for some reason, as yet poorly understood, manifest abnormal stress tests. These are the so-called *false-positive* reactors. If you are taking various drugs like digitalis or certain blood-pressure medication, you may also have an abnormal ECG response to exercise. However, if such noncardiac causes are ruled out and your postexercise tracing is abnormal, I think you should take the same measures I listed for people found to have had a silent heart attack. Statistically, no matter how you feel, an abnormal ECG response to exercise places you at greater risk for suffering a heart attack sometime in the future. I have seen improvements in these abnormalities in many patients who subsequently engaged in a supervised exercise program. *Cardiac rehabilitation* centers are located in some eighty cities throughout the United States and various parts of Europe. Ask your doctor, local Heart Association, or YMCA if there is one in your community.

CORONARY ARTERIOGRAPHY (ANGIOGRAPHY)— WHEN AND WHY

While on the subject of evaluating your cardiac status, let's discuss *coronary arteriography,* what it is and when it should be done. The procedure involves the insertion of a long thin rubber tube (catheter) into an artery in the groin or the forearm. This is then threaded slowly forward until its tip enters the heart. An opaque dye is injected into the tube and goes out through a hole at the tip, into the aorta and the coronary arteries. X-rays are then taken in rapid sequence and a video film is also recorded, enabling us to see what the coronary arteries actually look like, whether there are any significant obstructions in them, and where they are located. This test also tells us how well the heart contracts and whether there are any areas of muscle that are not moving at all or are contracting poorly. In short, it provides fairly definitive information about the coronary circulation and heart function.

Is It Dangerous?

Coronary arteriography used to be riskier than it is today. Most medical centers with good equipment and experienced personnel who are doing the procedure frequently now report about one to three complications in every thousand cases. This is not very much, considering that those tested have significant heart and vascular disease.

Although you remain awake during the procedure, you are given a sedative to reduce anxiety. The test itself is not really painful or uncomfortable, although you may be apprehensive about it. The site of insertion of the catheter is frozen, so you don't feel any pain there. Passage of the catheter into the heart itself is not uncomfortable, though the injection of dye sometimes causes temporary nausea, chest pain, headache, or a burning sensation in the face.

When to Have It Done

Some physicians, in my opinion, send patients for coronary arteriography too casually. They're apt to do so if they themselves are experienced technicians in this field, or if they are working in a sophisticated university hospital where active research is being carried on and new information being sought. Most cardiologists will recommend arteriography only when you have chest pain for which there is no satisfactory explanation— when the clinical history is not typical of one cause or another, or the ECG and stress tests are not diagnostic, and where both doctor and patient feel an answer is absolutely necessary. Everyone agrees that arteriography should be done if you need surgery (aortocoronary bypass) because of severe angina pectoris not responding to medical treatment, and symptoms so debilitating that your life-style is drastically compromised. In this situation, the surgeon needs to know whether he can help you, and which of the coronary arteries are diseased, where, and to what extent.

Angina with Normal Coronary Arteries

Before leaving the subject of coronary arteriography, let me give you one additional piece of information which will baffle you as much as it does me. From time to time a patient, usually female, has symptoms typical of angina pectoris. The pain is relieved by the usual medication—nitroglycerine under the tongue—and is documented by electrocardiographic abnormalities at rest and/or after exercise. But when we do an arteriogram, we find the coronary arteries wide open without any evidence of disease. We are not sure what this means. The pain may be due to transient spasm of the arteries without permanent obstruction or perhaps to some disturbance of oxygen transport within the heart itself. Whatever the mechanism, these patients, who have no abnormality that the surgeon can correct, do well over the long term when treated with the conventional drugs for angina (nitroglycerine, coronary artery dilators, and propranolol).

AORTOCORONARY BYPASS SURGERY

As Common as the Appendectomy

Since 1970, an ever-increasing number of patients have undergone bypass surgery because of heart attacks or angina pectoris. In 1977 more than 80,000 such operations were performed in the United States alone, and the procedure is also now being done virtually everywhere.

What is the bypass operation? Who should have it? Who shouldn't? What will it do for you?

When one or more of your coronary arteries (there are three major ones within the heart, plus their branches) is severely narrowed or blocked, you may have chest symptoms on exertion—or ultimately, a heart attack. In the aortocoronary bypass operation, one end of a piece of vein removed from your leg, or a small artery from your chest wall, is sewn into the aorta. The other end is swung around the diseased, narrowed part of the coronary artery and inserted into the unaffected area beyond it. The block has thus been "bypassed." Three, four, and even five such grafts can be put in.

What are the technical requirements to make the operation possible? *There must be good portions of artery below the block.* What's the point of attaching a vein graft to a vessel riddled with disease throughout its entire course? Another requisite for a successful operation is that the heart muscle must still be good enough to benefit from the new blood brought to it by the bypass graft. A scarred, enlarged, weakened heart—one that is in failure—may not tolerate the stress of the operation and, even if it does, may not benefit from it.

Does It Work?

Despite what seems like a logical way to correct impaired blood flow within the heart, there is still controversy about the bypass operation. There are enthusiasts (mostly among heart surgeons) who believe that anyone with a demonstrable, significant blockage of one or more coronary arteries should have a bypass even if there are minimal symptoms. Such "silent" obstructions are usually found as the result of coronary arteriography done when an ECG or exercise stress test turns out, unexpectedly, to be abnormal. Other physicians feel the operation is indicated only if you have severe symptoms of coronary disease. Finally the majority of us believe a bypass should be recommended only if (a) you have heart pain not responding to the modern drugs now available or (b) the site of the blockage is very high up in the coronary arterial system, so that if complete occlusion should occur, a large portion of the heart would suddenly be deprived of blood (this is referred to as a "left main stem lesion").

Why the Controversy?

When we follow patients with coronary artery disease—those who have had corrective surgery and those who have not—we have thus far found surprisingly little difference in survival or in the incidence of subsequent heart attacks. The operation does control angina pectoris in some 85 percent of cases, making life more comfortable, but does not necessarily prolong it. So if your pain is severe and unmanageable, an operation will almost certainly help. Statistical studies have shown that if only one artery is involved, you're just as well off leaving it alone. If two or more vessels are diseased, you are a good candidate for it, provided that (a) it can be done and (b) you have symptoms despite optimal medical treatment.

Long-Term Follow-Up

What happens to you after a bypass operation? Chances are you'll lose the pain, but for how long? If you're lucky, for years. If you're not (about 20–25 percent of cases), the new graft itself may clot, at which point you may be back where you were before the operation, since the diseased, bypassed artery is still there. But if in the meantime the latter went on to close, your angina may recur or be worse than it was prior to surgery. Often, the graft itself remains open, and you may still have a heart attack or a return of the angina. That happens because the arteriosclerosis, which gave you the trouble in the first instance, continues unabated, and now involves an artery or portions of arteries previously free of disease and therefore not bypassed. *Bypass is not a cure.* It is at best palliation. It buys time. How much time depends on you and the rate of progress of your particular disease. So even after a successful bypass operation, it's still important to follow the principles of cardiovascular preventive medicine.

BARIUM ENEMA

We now come to the last routine procedure that you will have to endure in the course of your checkup—the barium enema. It is generally not done on the day of your complete examination, because you have to be prepared for it with an empty bowel. You will be asked to remain on a diet of clear liquids the day before the test. That evening, you take a mild laxative and then nothing further by mouth until just before the procedure in the morning, when you may have some tea and toast. After your bowel is cleaned out with an enema, barium is inserted through a tube into the rectum, and x-rays are taken. Occasionally, air is also introduced to improve the visualization.

Although healthy subjects tolerate the procedure without any problem, the barium enema x-ray is tiring and uncomfortable especially for the chronically ill. It should be done gently and with care in older patients, those who have heart disease or who are otherwise sick. I rarely allow it to be done within eight weeks of a heart attack.

Why It's Done

The purpose of the barium enema is to detect various growths (polyps, tumors) of the large bowel, colitis, and any structural abnormalities like diverticula (small fingerlike outpouchings of the bowel often seen in healthy people).

How Often?

A barium enema should be done approximately every three to five years after the age of 50, if there is a family history of colon cancer, or if you have had a polyp removed sometime earlier, even if you have no symptoms. It is *essential* whenever blood and pus are seen in the stool, when a lump is felt on examination of the abdomen, when there is unexplained weight loss or anemia, or when any disease of the large bowel is suspected. There is also some evidence in humans, supported by experimental animal studies, which suggests that the higher the fat intake, the greater the risk of colon cancer.

If for some reason the upper gastrointestinal tract is to be studied too, the barium enema is done first.

17

NONROUTINE TESTS THAT ARE FREQUENTLY PERFORMED

AT THIS POINT in the checkup we will sit down and discuss what we have found out so far. I will not ask you to undergo any other testing unless something in your history or physical examination suggests it is necessary. Let me describe a few other nonroutine procedures and tell you why, and under what circumstances, I will recommend that they too be performed.

X-Rays of the Spine

Spinal films are not done routinely. I will send you for them if you have pain in your back or have been injured. If you complain of pain in your arms or your chest, or if you have numbness and tingling of your hands made worse by movement of the neck, x-rays of the cervical spine may explain them. If you have sciatica and low back pain, x-rays of the lower spine may reveal a disc problem.

In older persons, x-rays may show demineralization of the spine and fractured vertebrae of which the patient is unaware. But remember that even when you have considerable arthritis and pain, the spinal x-ray may be normal. It takes fairly advanced disease to be visible in the films. *A negative x-ray does not exclude the possibility of arthritis.*

X-Rays of the Stomach and Upper Intestinal Tract

X-rays of the esophagus, the stomach, and the duodenum are not routine because, unlike the lower bowel, cancer or other disease in these areas is less common and usually produces symptoms. So I will arrange to study this portion of your intestinal tract only if you complain of pain. If you're passing black stools, or have a lot of "gas," if you have chest pain not explained by the electrocardiogram or spinal films, we will have a "gastrointestinal series" done. In addition, if I suspect some disorder of absorption or inflammation farther down in the small bowel beyond the duodenum, we will get a "small bowel series," in which we follow the course of the swallowed barium beyond the duodenum well into the small bowel. Whereas the upper gastrointestinal series takes about half an hour, it takes the barium as long as five or six hours to pass through the small bowel.

You are required to fast between midnight and the time of your upper GI series the next day so that your stomach is empty. You will then be given barium to drink, which is often flavored and not unpleasant. The barium renders the gut opaque to x-rays and then passes unchanged through your gastrointestinal tract. Your stools will remain white for a couple of days after the procedure, and you may need a laxative to eliminate the barium.

Endoscopy (Direct Visualization) of the Upper Intestinal Tract

Occasionally the x-ray suggests the presence of a tumor or polyp somewhere in the upper intestinal tract. In order to know whether or not it is malignant, we may want to pass a thin, flexible tube down your food pipe to look at it directly or even get a piece of it to view under the microscope. This instrument, called a fiberoptic *endoscope,* has a light at the end of it and a tiny camera which can photograph the interior of the organ under investigation.

The availability of these thin, flexible instruments has made endoscopy much less unpleasant than it used to be. Your throat is first "frozen" with a local anesthetic; you are given a tranquilizer, and the tube is passed. The whole procedure takes up to an hour, depending on which part of the upper intestinal tract we're looking at. If it's only the top portion of the esophagus, we'll be through in fifteen or twenty minutes. But if the scope has to be manipulated through the stomach into the duodenum, it takes longer. Aside from perhaps a sore throat due to irritation of the tube, endoscopy is well tolerated. Make sure you remove your dentures before you have it done if your doctor doesn't remind you to do so. You don't have to be hospitalized for this test, but it is usually done in an outpatient department clinic so that you can be observed for several hours afterward.

If in the course of your barium enema a polyp is seen in the large bowel, the same type of procedure is performed, but from the other end. It is then called *colonoscopy.* A flexible fiberoptic scope is inserted into the rectum and pushed gently up the large bowel to the site of the area under study. It permits biopsies to be taken and polyps to be removed. The big advantage of this innovation is that it eliminates the need for exploratory surgery in some cases.

X-Rays of the Gallbladder (Oral Cholecystography)

The gallbladder is not routinely studied but maybe it should be in patients over 50, so common are the symptoms of gallbladder disease. If you have a lot of "gas," particularly a couple of hours after eating fatty or fried foods, if you suffer from recurrent pain in the right upper portion of your abdomen, and if you have intermittent jaundice which suggests the passing of stones, then a gallbladder x-ray will be done. A high cholesterol level and a strong family history of gallbladder disease are additional reasons for doing the x-ray. Years ago, patients with typhoid bacillus in their stools used to get gallbladder disease. It has also been observed that those with rheumatic heart disease, particularly involving the mitral valve, are prone to gallstones and should be x-rayed for them. Finally, if you have palpitations and chest discomfort, the fault may lie in your gallbladder, not your heart.

It's such an easy test to do and so relatively inexpensive that I don't hesitate to order it if I have the least suspicion that the gallbladder is diseased. You take six tablets of dye at the rate of one every five minutes about nine o'clock the night before the test. You should have had a fat-free supper, and after that you should not take anything by mouth until the next morning, when you may have water, tea, or black coffee. The x-ray is taken with you lying in various positions on a table. No needles, no enemas, no tubes. The dye tablets have laxative properties, so don't be alarmed by the sudden onset of diarrhea.

If your gallbladder has accepted the dye and is visible on the x-ray, any stones present will usually be seen. You will then be given a fatty drink to see whether the organ contracts. Remember that the job of the gallbladder is to squeeze out the bile (which it stores) into the small bowel to help digest any fat there. If the gallbladder is working, when you drink the fat it should contract, forcing bile out. If it isn't functioning well, the contraction will be poor or absent.

Sometimes six tablets of dye will not cause the gallbladder to be visualized. In that event, we repeat the test the next day using six additional tablets. If the gallbladder still does not take up the dye, we assume it's diseased. We can then do an intravenous cholangiogram, especially if we suspect the presence of stones in the gallbladder ducts.

Intravenous Cholangiogram (When the Oral Dye Doesn't Show Up)

In this procedure the gallbladder dye is not taken by mouth but is injected into a vein. X-rays are then done every twenty minutes for about two hours. This technique shows up the bile ducts as well as the gallbladder, and is therefore especially useful if we want to see whether they contain any stones. Sometimes, years after the gallbladder has been removed, stones or sludge form in the remaining ducts. Since we cannot do an oral gall-bladder x-ray because there's no gallbladder, the intravenous procedure has to be used if you have symptoms suggesting obstruction to the flow of bile.

Special Ways to Examine the Nervous System

A thorough clinical examination by an experienced neurologist is sometimes not enough to clarify neurological symptoms. When we look for the cause of headaches, strokes, muscle weakness, backache, paralysis, behavioral changes, or want to rule out infections or tumors of the nervous system, we rely on a battery of diagnostic procedures. Let me briefly describe some of them so that you will know what's involved in the event that you ever have to have one.

Remember how we went step by step trying to clarify a shadow on the chest x-ray? We do much the same with a neurological problem. Whenever we investigate symptoms in any part of the body, we start with those tests or procedures that are least dangerous, uncomfortable, and expensive.

When there is reason to suspect some disease within the brain or the skull, we order x-rays after the usual clinical and blood tests. Skull films may reveal the presence of tumors in the brain. They also give some indication of bone disease, ranging from fractures to various malignant processes that spread there.

Electroencephalography (EEG, the Brain-Wave Test)

Whenever disease of the brain is suspected—for example, if you have fits (seizures), or unusual headaches, or bizarre behavior—an EEG is obtained. This test is to the brain what the ECG is to the heart. Just as we put electrodes on your chest to record your ECG, they are put on your scalp in order to study the brain. To get a complete electrical picture, electrodes are placed over representative areas of the brain. You just lie back while lights are flashed at you and you breathe in and out deeply. Sometimes you will be asked to try to sleep. Your head does not have to be shaved. Areas of abnormal electrical activity may indicate epilepsy, tumor, infection, or hemorrhage.

Computerized Transverse Axial Tomography (CTT or CAT Scan)

This fairly new technique has revolutionized the field of diagnostic radiology. First developed for evaluating the brain, it is now being used for the entire body. In effect, it enables us, for the first time, to "see" tissues without the use of contrast dyes. This is done by taking x-rays in several different planes and expressing the various absorption qualities of different tissues in numbers, which are then analyzed by a computer. The final print-out of the scanner is in the shape of the organ studied.

Radiation exposure with CAT scanning is considerable, as is the cost, so it should not be done for trivial reasons.

In many cases, the brain scanner, as it is called, has eliminated the need for invasive procedures of the brain such as arteriography, where dye is injected into the arteries of the neck or elsewhere to see the blood vessels going to the brain. The brain scanner can detect tumors, hemorrhages, areas of damage due to blood vessel blockage (infarcts), and injuries to the brain where pools of blood have formed. In the abdomen similar scanning can be performed. It makes possible the detection of tumors deep within the abdominal cavity that cannot be seen by conventional x-rays. Cancer of the pancreas is a good example of the great use of the body scanner. When suspected, pancreatic cancer previously required an arteriogram of the abdominal vessels, looking for their distortion, or an exploratory operation. Today, the diagnosis can be made painlessly and quickly. The CAT scanner should not be confused with radioactive tracer "Scanning" techniques described elsewhere.

Lumbar Puncture (Tapping Your Spine)

Where there has been a "vascular accident" within the brain, and it is not clear whether we are dealing with a clot that needs to be anticoagulated or a hemorrhage where anticoagulation is dangerous, we frequently do a lumbar puncture or spinal tap. If there is some infection of the nervous system (meningitis) and we need to identify the organism, or if we want to know about the pressure of the fluid surrounding the brain or spinal cord, there is no substitute for a lumbar tap.

Usually done in the hospital, it simply involves the insertion of a small needle between two vertebrae in the lower back and into the space where the spinal fluid circulates. The skin in the area is "frozen" first. (Spinal anesthesia is also administered in this way.) The pressure of the fluid is recorded, and a small amount is then withdrawn. We immediately look at a few drops under the microscope, and send the rest to the laboratory for chemical and bacteriological study.

When a brain tumor is present, the spinal fluid pressure is frequently elevated, it contains more protein than normal, and tumor cells may be visible under the microscope. If there is an infection in the brain, the sugar content of the spinal fluid is diminished, pus cells are seen under the microscope, and the fluid is cloudy. Bacteriological investigation will determine which bug is causing the infection. If there is a hemorrhage in the brain, the spinal fluid may be bloody. If the bleeding occurred days or weeks ago, the spinal fluid is yellow because of the release of bilirubin from the red blood cells that have broken down.

After a spinal tap, it's best for you to remain flat for several hours in order to minimize the occurrence of a postspinal headache.

Myelogram—Lowest Test on the Popularity List

If you have severe back pain believed due to a slipped disc, and if conservative measures such as heat, rest, and appropriate exercises have failed, surgery is considered. You will then need a myelogram to identify for the surgeon exactly where the problem lies within the spinal cord. This involves the injection of dye by the lumbar puncture route into the spinal canal followed by x-ray pictures. It can be a painful procedure and is very unpopular among patients, but at the moment there is no alternative technique that will provide the same information.

Testing for Glaucoma

Glaucoma, or increased pressure within the eye, is an important cause of blindness. You should suspect it if you have chronic headaches, deteriorating vision, or see a halo around lighted objects. Glaucoma can be detected early by measuring the tension within the eyeball. This is done by pressing a tonometer (which measures the resistance or pressure beneath it) against the eyeball. Tonometry is painless, and though done by some internists, it is more frequently performed by the eye specialist. It should be done every year in persons over 40, and whenever you have your glasses checked or changed.

Sonography or Ultrasound Techniques

Scientists are always trying to develop diagnostic procedures that are painless and do not involve breaking the skin or introducing catheters and dyes into the body (*noninvasive techniques*). Sonography is the classic example of such a noninvasive procedure. The procedure itself is based on *sonar*. High-frequency sound waves are directed at the organ under study and partially reflected by it. The time of travel of the sound wave to the target and back is measured. The returning echo is processed by sophisticated machines which give a multidimensional, detailed view of the internal organs. Such ultrasound techniques are available for use in many different parts of the body—for example, in the heart, kidney, brain, pregnant uterus, liver, spleen, eye, and pancreas. If we see a mass on the x-ray and can't tell whether it is a solid tumor or a cyst (a sac filled with semisolid material, which is usually benign), a sonogram easily makes the distinction.

Echocardiography—Looking at the Heart with Sonar

Whereas sonography gives a picture of internal structures, echocardiography, which also utilizes ultrasound, is able to evaluate heart motion, so that the status of the valves and movements and thickness of the walls can be assessed. Echocardiography is one of the most important diagnostic techniques in cardiology.

It analyzes valve function, detects heart tumors, and indicates the presence of fluid in the sac around the heart. Many structural disorders of the heart that formerly required cardiac catheterization are now detected by echocardiography, a painless, convenient, and fairly inexpensive procedure.

Cardiac Catheterization

Once a diagnosis of valvular disease has been made, and an operation deemed necessary, cardiac catheterization is almost always done to confirm the precise anatomy of the disorder so that the surgeon knows exactly what to expect when he enters the heart. This technique also measures pressure in the various heart chambers, to determine how well the heart is functioning and to predict whether the patient will, in fact, benefit from surgical correction.

Cardiac catheterization, as in the case of coronary arteriography, involves introducing a catheter into a blood vessel in the arm or leg and advancing it into the heart. If the right side of the heart is to be studied, the catheter is inserted into a vein, usually at the groin or in the forearm, since these vessels lead directly to the right side of the heart. If the left side of the heart is to be studied, then the catheter is inserted into an artery, which leads directly back to the aorta and the heart. Once the catheter is in place, pressure is measured in the various chambers, the concentration of oxygen is assessed in different parts of the heart, and dye is injected so that x-rays can be taken of the cardiac interior.

Angiography—Looking at the Major Arteries Outside the Heart

In addition to studying the interior of the heart, it is sometimes necessary to take a look at various arteries in the body, for example, in the legs, abdomen, or neck. We've already seen how pain in the legs on walking may reflect severe arterial narrowing, or how we can find an aneurysm of the aorta in the abdomen. There are operations to correct these disorders, but before the surgeon knows whether he can help, he must look at the arteries to see where they are blocked, to what extent, and whether and where a graft can be accepted. This involves introducing dyes into the arteries through a needle or catheter, and then taking x-rays.

Venography—Studying Your Veins

When pain and swelling of the leg are due to phlebitis, anticoagulants must be given. Sometimes, however, a muscle tear or an injury may mimic phlebitis, and then anticoagulation is unnecessary and undesirable. In order to be absolutely sure about the phlebitis, a venogram is done. Dye is injected into the vein at the top of the foot, and photographs are then taken to see whether and where a clot is present. When there are recurrent emboli, this procedure indicates where they originate, and whether any of the large veins leading to the heart should be tied off.

Additional Tests of the Respiratory System: Laryngoscopy

We've already discussed bronchoscopy and the circumstances under which it is necessary—namely, to clarify the appearance of a shadow in the lung or to obtain a piece of tissue for biopsy. A much less involved procedure for studying the *vocal cords* in cases of chronic hoarseness and suspected tumor is called *laryngoscopy,* in which an instrument with a light attached to it is passed through the mouth. Also if a foreign object has been swallowed and is stuck in the area, laryngoscopy permits it to be seen and removed.

Bronchography—Putting Dye in Your Lungs

If you have chronic bronchitis, resulting in severe and recurrent episodes of pneumonia, and we want to know whether an area of the bronchial tree is diseased and to what extent, the procedure called *bronchography* is performed. Here, we anesthetize your throat, and then insert into your windpipe (trachea) a thin tube into which a dye or contrast material is injected. The bronchial tubes can be outlined on the x-ray pictures subsequently taken.

Thoracentesis—Draining the Chest of Fluid

If you complain of shortness of breath, chest pain, or fever, and a chest x-ray shows fluid in the lining around your lungs, I will want to remove some of it to analyze it and also improve your breathing. Heart failure is most commonly at the root of the problem, but various infections and malignant tumors of the lung can also give such fluid.

The procedure is very simple. The surface of the skin is frozen, a small needle is inserted into the area where the fluid is known to be, and some of it is drawn off. The only precaution we have to take is to make sure that the needle doesn't penetrate the lung, causing it to collapse. After thoracentesis, a chest x-ray is taken to see that the lung is completely inflated.

Hysterosalpingography

(Now there's a mouthful.)

When a woman complains of infertility, one of the procedures that may be recommended is hysterosalpingography. An opaque solution is introduced through the vagina into the fallopian tubes, which lead from the ovaries to the uterus. If the tubes are obstructed, usually due to chronic infection, which is an important cause of sterility, the dye will not fill the entire tube.

Intravenous Pyelography—Important Kidney X-Rays

A very important series of x-rays called *intravenous pyelography* involves looking at the kidneys, ureters, and urinary bladder. It is done whenever kidney disease is suspected—tumors, high blood pressure in persons under 40, stones somewhere in the genitourinary tract, or a large prostate is causing obstruction.

Dye is injected into an arm vein and is taken up and then excreted by the kidneys; then the x-rays are taken. In some allergic persons the dye may cause an acute reaction. So if you are generally sensitive, especially to shellfish, tell the doctor about it.

An Alternative

The urologist may also want to look directly into the bladder, the openings of the ureters, and the urethra to obtain additional information. He introduces into the urethra a cystoscope—a thin tube with a light at the end of it through which he can look into the bladder and, if necessary, remove any polyps from that organ. He can also shoot dye through the cystoscope into the ureters, viewing the kidneys from below. This procedure sometimes has to be used when a patient is sensitive to dye and cannot have intravenous pyelography. Because dye introduced through the cystoscope does not enter the bloodstream, sensitivity reactions do not occur.

Nuclear Medicine

There is a new and rapidly growing field of diagnostic procedures that are usually done in a hospital clinic or other specialized facility. The principle is to use tiny (tracer) doses of radioactive isotopes which combine with chemical compounds that are normally picked up by specific organs—for example, iodine to the thyroid, thallium to the heart, and so on. These substances are either taken by mouth or injected into a vein. After the radioactive material makes its way to the organ under study, the amount of radioactivity it contains and the pattern of distribution are determined by instruments which scan the involved area.

These procedures are just beginning to be used clinically in heart disease. However, bone scans are done frequently—to find evidence of cancer or infection when patients complain of bone pain and the usual x-rays are normal. Thyroid scans, described earlier, are also very useful.

Liver scans too are common, as are lung scans, used to identify the presence of clots in the lung. The lung scan not only confirms the diagnosis but also indicates what part of the lung is involved and how much has been damaged by the clot. Virtually any organ—the pancreas, the kidney, the spleen, and even the placenta of the pregnant woman can now be assessed by radioactive scanning, thereby reducing the need for more hazardous invasive techniques and even exploratory surgery.

CHAPTER **18**

AFTER ALL THAT, YOU FOUND
NOTHING WRONG?

Now you know (or should) what it's all about. If you have an appointment to see the doctor because you have specific symptoms, refer back to the appropriate section in this book. You will then have a pretty good idea of what your complaints mean, what questions you're likely to be asked, what important information you should volunteer, how you will be examined, and what tests will be performed.

If you've already had the examination, you now understand the nuances of your dialogue with the doctor, each step of his physical exam and how it related to your symptoms, why he ordered the tests he did, and why he emphasized certain aspects of the physical.

On the other hand, if like millions of others you have no specific complaints, but are going for a "health maintenance examination" or "checkup," you now appreciate what's involved and why, as well as the kinds of early warning signs that will be looked for and the silent diseases that can be detected.

We are living in a very exciting medical era. Modern technology, popular interest, and government support are speeding the pace of discoveries that will prolong life and improve its quality. Though still stumped by the mysteries of cancer, arteriosclerosis, arthritis, and many of the lesser diseases that afflict mankind, medical science can control or cure the major killers of yesteryear—tuberculosis, bacterial infections, polio. Others like smallpox have been virtually wiped out. Many of nature's faults— from harelip to holes in the heart—can now be corrected surgically. Since 1972, there has been a continued decrease in deaths from high blood pressure, strokes, and heart attacks.

And there is much more on the way. The artificial heart is being developed cooperatively by the United States and the Soviet Union. Pacemakers are now smaller and last for eight or more years before needing replacement. Nuclear-powered models are already available for selected patients. Rejection phenomena which prevent organ transplants are gradually being overcome. There is experimental work on an artificial pancreas for severe juvenile diabetes, which now tragically shortens the life-span. Lung and liver transplants are already being tried, though still without much success. Mechanisms of heredity are now so well understood that we may one day be able to "program out" birth defects and the susceptibility to terrible diseases.

New diagnostic techniques will, in the future, eliminate many of the tests I have described in this book. For example, we are anticipating the imminent availability of a simple test using a drop of blood which will tell "healthy" persons whether they have a cancer anywhere in the body, where it is, and its stage of development.

The list is endless. Suffering and death from whatever cause is the stimulus for the research to overcome it. Your doctor's office is where that research is translated into action. What you have read in the preceding chapters tells you where it's at now. Keep an open mind and a healthy interest in future developments.

There should be no mystery in medicine for you—its ultimate recipient.

Do not, as a result of reading this book, make the mistake of diagnosing your own or anyone else's symptoms. Remember, although I have tried to highlight the most likely causes of these complaints and findings, they may in fact be due to something else. Only your doctor can tell for sure. That's why he's a doctor and you're not. By the same token, do not treat yourself on the basis of a diagnosis you have made. You are not now a diagnostician, but an informed patient. That means you know how to work more effectively with your doctor.

INDEX

abdomen, 217–30
abortion, 244
abscess, 223–24, 229, 232
acid phosphatase, 299–307
acne rosacea, 163
acupuncture, 183
Addison's disease, 151, 298
adenoma, 173
adrenal glands, 69, 76, 139
adrenaline, 321
advertising, 83, 84, 169
age and aging, 45–46, 109, 152, 153
  and retirement, 48
  and sex, 68–69
albumin, 303–4
  in urine, 272–73, 274
alcohol, 39, 160, 220, 316, 318–19
  and diabetics, 295
  and insomnia, 64–65
  myths about, 59–60
alcoholism, 58, 59, 60, 160, 224
  symptoms, 39, 40, 41, 162, 164
Aldactazide, 299
Aldactone, 68, 75, 199, 203, 299
Aldomet, 68, 75, 146, 237

alkaline phosphatase, 303, 307, 308
Alka-Seltzer, 145
allergy, 47, 94–97, 162
  in families, 52, 55
  and pets, 95
  treatment of, 96–97
allopurinol, 296
American Society of Internal Medicine, 67
aminophylline, 96
amphetamines, 71, 77, 85–86
Ampicillin, 95
Amplivix, 296
anemia, 69, 71, 214, 313
  and aspirin use, 75, 280, 286
  causes, 285–86
  and iron deficiency, 83, 113
  pernicious, 39, 150, 164
  sickle-cell, 289
  and skin color, 41, 150
anesthesia
  spinal, 354
aneurysm, 228
  aortic, 113, 176–77, 226, 324
angina, abdominal, 230

363

HB5H